Due Back. Class H

D1587664

This book is to ...
the last da...

23 OCT...

THE STORY OF
THE GROWTH OF NURSING
As an Art, a Vocation, and a Profession

THE STORY OF
THE GROWTH OF
NURSING

as an Art, a Vocation, and a Profession

by

AGNES E. PAVEY, S.R.N.

Diploma in Nursing, University of London. Sister Tutor's Diploma, Battersea Polytechnic. Formerly Sister Tutor at the Central Middlesex County Hospital, London. Also formerly Tutor at the East Suffolk Hospital, Ipswich; Queen Mary's Hospital for the East End; and Government Hospital, Southern Rhodesia.

With a Foreword by
Sir John Weir, K.C.V.O.

LONDON
FABER AND FABER LIMITED
24 Russell Square, W.C. 1

First published in January 1938
by Faber and Faber Limited
24 *Russell Square London W.C.* 1
Printed in Great Britain by
R. MacLehose and Company Limited
The University Press Glasgow
Second edition 1944, *reprinted* 1947
All rights reserved

" History is the tale of the spirit of man unfolding itself."

DR. CHARLES SINGER

DEDICATION

To the Memory of my Father, without whose influence and early teaching this book could not have been written.

FOREWORD

To those interested in the care of the sick the reactions of past ages to sickness and suffering make fascinating reading. And here we have, briefly recorded, the heroism and devotion of those ancient kings, queens, and commoners alike, whose efforts have become historical.

Miss Pavey's book really needs no Foreword. Anyone who dips into its pages is bound to read on. They are full of interest; a mass of facts, plainly and tersely set forth, and pre-eminently readable.

We heartily congratulate the Author, marvelling at the amount of wide study the writing of such a book has entailed. One envies her. It must have given her immense happiness in the midst of a busy and exacting life.

JOHN WEIR

47 WELBECK STREET,
CAVENDISH SQUARE,
LONDON, W. 1

November 15th, 1937

ix

AUTHOR'S PREFACE

IN this book I have tried to tell the story of the birth and development of each phase of nursing from its earliest beginnings to its present form, and I have endeavoured to make the information given therein as accurate and reliable as possible. I am, however, acutely conscious of shortcomings and omissions, and I ask the indulgence of readers who may feel that their particular branch of the work has not been given the prominence that they could have wished for it.

Many widely diverse external factors have influenced or determined the lines upon which nursing grew. I have tried to give perspective to the more important of these factors by showing them against a briefly sketched-in background of contemporary social conditions and historical events. In this, I have written for the general reader and for the senior schoolgirl who hopes to become a nurse, as well as for those already engaged in nursing or medical work.

Each branch of nursing is described in the country of its origin, and I have tried to give some account of the characters and personalities of the instigators and pioneers of each movement, but not of their successors except where further development followed along new channels. I have shown how the various branches which originated in other lands eventually spread into England, and I have given some account of their progress in this island; but space would not permit of descriptions of relative development in other countries.

The present standards of nursing education require a sound knowledge, not only of nursing technique, but of many related subjects—hygiene, anatomy, physiology, chemistry, physics, pharmacy, and psychotherapy—if a nurse is to be really proficient and bring an intelligent understanding to bear upon every phase of her work. Therefore, it seemed to me that some account of the origin and development of all the sciences that have an essential place in the curriculum of a nurse's training fell within the scope of a book that endeavoured to tell the story of the growth of nursing. That is my justification for including some subject matter which might have appeared irrelevant in a formal History of Nursing.

My very grateful thanks are due to all who have helped me to obtain the information I needed, especially to the Staff of the College of Nursing, whose courtesy and interest have enabled me to overcome several difficulties, to my brother-in-law, Mr. A. Allen, for his constructive criticism of the manuscript, and to Dr. C. E. Wheeler, Consultant Physician to the London Homœopathic Hospital for his great kindness and patience in reading the proofs, and for his encouragement.

May I also express my deep appreciation of the honour that Sir John Weir has accorded me by writing the foreword?

AGNES E. PAVEY

January, 1938

CONTENTS

PART I. An Art

PERIOD. The Dawn of History to the Fourth Century A.D.

PART II. A Vocation

PERIOD. The Beginning of Christianity to about 1850 A.D.

PART III. A Profession

PERIOD. About 1850 A.D. to the Present Time

Part I : An Art

CHAPTER I

INTRODUCTION

Primitive psychology—Influence of primitive religion—Primitive pathology—Curative procedures—Superstitions and folklore—Primitive medicine—Influence of wars—Influence of science

WHEN we reflect that birth, sickness, accidental injuries and death have played an inevitable part in the life of every human being who has ever sojourned on this earth, we cannot but realise that nursing must also have had its origin with the beginning of life itself, although we search in vain among the records of ancient peoples for any definite account of such work, or even allusions to the part that women must have played in the care of the helpless and sick of their time. So that it would appear that in any attempt to uncover the origins and early progress of nursing we must trace out the beginnings of curative work in general, and assume that in every age and in every race women have taken their place in the fight that humanity wages against 'the ills that flesh is heir to'. Other branches of that work—medicine, surgery, hygiene, chemistry, massage, light treatment—have their undoubted origins and early development among a definite race and in a known locality or country, determined, probably, by the conditions under which that people lived and the beliefs they held.

Primitive Psychology.

Man has always reacted to his environment, not only in his physical, but also in his mental development—he entered into his life on this planet with no heritage of knowledge, but en-

3

dowed with a faculty for remembering, reasoning and imagining. He took cognisance of the world around him, and bent his faculties to the understanding and utilising of the forces of nature in the furtherance of his own well-being. He was not always right in his conjectures, he blundered badly at times, and yet, even in his wildest theories with regard to mankind and his place in the eternal scheme of things, there is to be found *some* kernel of true and sound reasoning—some stumbling across a great truth of natural law.

But we must look to his idea of himself in relation to the world around him, to his idea of his origin and ultimate destiny, in order to understand his attitude to his physical body and its needs. How will he arrive at any conclusion in regard to these matters? Only by observing and reasoning, and storing his impressions in his mind for future reference.

Life is exemplified by the power of movement; and, in his attempt to interpret the ways of nature, primitive man confuses life with motion and thinks that every moving thing must be alive—the rustling of leaves in a forest, the roaring of wind and rain, the crash of thunder and lightning, the flickering of shadows in sunlight or firelight, the fire itself, the echo of a sound —all have life, and all have power to help him or to harm him; so that he must learn something of the nature of these forces and of ways in which he can gain control over them, in order that they may contribute to his comfort and not to his undoing.

He observes the phenomena of sleep. He seeks his rest in a sheltered spot, in a few moments, or so it seems to him, his environment changes, he goes on journeys, meets and overcomes dangers, fights his enemies, and is endued with greater strength and endurance than in his waking hours. He sees and talks with a friend whom he afterwards learns was far away at the time. He observes the sleep of his fellow man, and notes the powerlessness of the sleeper's body and his oblivion to the sights and sounds around him. Then the sleeper awakes and relates his dream. The observer knows that his friend's body has not moved, nor have those with whom he held 'dream converse' visited the spot. What then? Man must have two selves, a visible and an invisible entity —the latter being by far the more powerful, and yet needing the former for its effective operation, the body being inert and defenceless when the spirit, or invisible self, is not present. And sometimes the spirit goes on a long journey and does not return. Then many unpleasant things happen to the body. Degenerative and decomposing changes take place, the flesh is eaten by jackals or wild beasts—and if after many wanderings the spirit returns, where will it find a home? It will lurk in all sorts of places—in trees, in rocks, in rivers, in an animal, or it will seek to enter another human body. But it is still powerful, and may be a valuable ally if it is the spirit of a friend. How difficult to cope with, however, if it is the spirit of an enemy no longer having a visible body to be attacked or avoided! So, to the primitive man, every stick and stone, every mountain and torrent, every cloud or star in the sky is animated by an invisible, yet powerful spirit. In a later stage of man's development these spirits become grouped under the sway of a few more powerful spirits—beings like himself, and guided by feelings and emotions similar to his own. Some of these spirits are ready to help him when occasion arises, others are seeking his destruction. In order to cope with these powers he must, in all times of stress, invoke the aid of the friendly spirits and propitiate the unfriendly—and therein lies the germ from which his religion will develop.

Influence of Primitive Religion.

What do we understand by 'religion'? That is a word capable of so many interpretations that it may be well to define it in order to avoid any confusion of thought; and of all the available definitions, that given by Max Müller, perhaps, best meets the present requirements. He defines religion as 'the worship of a higher power from a sense of need'. Now that involves several ideas—first, the belief in the existence of a power outside, and above, that possessed by human beings; secondly, the belief in the ability and the willingness of that power to be affected by the worship, and to grant the requests, of the devotees, and thirdly, a realisation of a human need.

Now, primitive man's needs are all on the physical plane, he needs protection from his enemies, from wild beasts and from the elements, he needs warmth, food, shelter, relief from pain, and recovery from illnesses. He believes in a whole hierarchy of benign and malevolent spirits, demons or gods; and he thinks that these are the agencies responsible for the abundant growth or the destruction of his crops, for the welfare or sickness of his cattle, for birth and healthy development, or for the sickness and death of his family. Thus, not only is his religion determined by the realisation of his bodily needs, but his attitude to his body will be, to a very great extent, dependent upon his religious beliefs.

In this way we arrive at the conclusion that of all the factors which profoundly influenced the development of medicine, and therefore of nursing, in the ancient world, none were so deep or so far reaching as religion, and we can understand medical customs only in so far as we attempt to understand the mentality of the people, and the religious beliefs they held. One cannot separate primitive medicine from primitive religion, and the common point of convergence in the medical 'folklore' of all nations is the belief that spirits, or other supernatural agencies, are responsible for disease and death. Therefore, much of the medicine of ancient times was an attempt to direct or to control these agencies. Whether the attempt was made by the priest, the physician, the witch or the 'medicine-man' did not really affect the issue.

As civilisation advanced and man's horizon widened, ideals of conduct were formulated; and his needs, and therefore his religion, became infinitely more complicated, but the essential underlying principles still remained very much the same.

6

Primitive Pathology.

It is not assumed that the thought processes of primitive man were logical, or even coherent, but in a somewhat vague and unformulated way he worked out a pathology rather on these lines: disease resulted from one of the following causes:

(1) An evil spirit had been projected into the body—it might have been breathed in, it might have been swallowed with food or drink, or have gained entrance through the skin.

(2) A good controlling spirit had been taken from the body, or had left it of its own accord.

(3) Sorcery had been effected upon some part of the body, or upon an object belonging to, or given to, the victim.

If we examine these beliefs we cannot fail to be astounded by their very close analogy to modern teaching. An invisible living agent entered the body to distress it by its living activities. Whether the term 'evil spirit' or 'bacterial infection' is applied to that invasion it does not materially affect the result, or the need of the patient. Neither does it matter, essentially, whether the 'good controlling spirits' are now understood as ductless gland secretions, or the third cause as 'infection by fomites'.

In practically all uncivilised races we find a belief that power to control the forces of nature is given to a few chosen individuals, and that the man who could influence the sunshine, the rain and the winds, who could direct the mysterious forces that granted success in war, abundance of crops and fertility amongst cattle, could also aid his fellow man when stricken with disease or incapacitated by wounds. *He* was the mediator between the unseen powers and the visible people dwelling upon the earth; and he had the ability to cure his friends and to cause disease among his enemies. Often this power was believed to be hereditary and definitely restricted to a particular family or caste, usually that of the chief of the tribe; and women as well as men might be endowed with this indefinable but natural gift. It could not be communicated to those of different families, but, being present, it could be developed and strengthened by the training and instruction given by the father to the son, or by the mother to the daughter.

Curative Procedures.

How did this primitive medicine-man strive to cope with disease? We find that he instituted ritual sacrifices in order to divert the attentions of the evil spirits. He tried by rites of propitiation, purification and atonement to arrest the progress of the malady, and to drive out the tormenting spirit. His medicine was often an affair of charms, incantations, spells, plant-lore and psychotherapy, designed to stave off the effects of the supernatural agencies. Naturally, the personality of the healer played a great part in curative work then, as now: but his powers were often sadly misapplied. As a means of driving out the evil spirits he used purgatives, emetics, hot and cold applications, cauterisation, blistering, cupping, sweating, massage—which was a pummelling of the body—hypnotism, nauseating drugs and deodorants. He aimed at making the body such an uncomfortable abode for the evil spirit that it was forced to leave it. Surgical practices also made their appearance amongst ancient peoples, for example, trephining for epilepsy—which was making a hole in the skull so that the evil spirit could get out—the bits of the cranium afterwards being used as charms or amulets.

Superstitions and Folklore.

It will be seen that the genealogy of many of our present-day treatments leads us back to the very remote past, but these procedures were thickly overlaid with superstitions, many traces of which still remain, even among people with a long history of civilisation. Everyone knows the rural superstitions relating to the causation and cure of warts, and nearly every county in England has its pet superstition with regard to the avoidance and cure of whooping cough. To give a few examples, Norfolk

8

countryfolk tie a spider in a piece of muslin and pin it to the kitchen mantelpiece, in Suffolk a child is held head downwards in a hole dug in a meadow, in Yorkshire owl-broth is considered a certain cure, and in yet another county a beetle in a bottle is thought to be efficacious—the idea probably being derived from the potency of the ancient Egyptian scarab. Gilbert White, in his *Natural History of Selborne*, tells of the belief that passing a child through a cleft in an ash-tree is a certain cure for hernia. There is such a tree in Richmond Park, and another in Suffolk, and the practice is described as having been followed less than forty years ago, but with what result is not recorded. In many English counties we meet with a belief that a cleft or hole in a tree or a rock is endowed with magical properties. There is a holed-stone in Cornwall, near Lanyon, through which children with spinal deformities or skin diseases were passed naked—and were said to be cured. The persisting superstitions with regard to herbs, numbers and colours, the meeting with a piebald horse, a load of hay, a person with a squint, are all too well known to need more than a passing mention; but they all, undoubtedly, had their origin in antiquity. These beliefs are interesting and comparatively harmless, but there was another type of a very different quality, perhaps the most terrible superstition that has ever tormented mankind—the almost universal belief in witchcraft. The appalling results of this amongst uncivilised races forms one of the saddest revelations of historical research. It is, of course, an extension of the demonic theory of disease, but its reappearance in Christian Europe during the Middle Ages brought torture and death to many thousands of innocent human beings. The physical and mental agony caused by this terrible delusion has no parallel in the history of the world.

Primitive Medicine.

Herb-doctoring is a feature of all primitive medicine. Man soon perceived that some poisons were remedies under certain conditions, and he came to know which was the most fatal arrow

9

poison, and which herbs and grasses to seek as antidotes. He knows the virtues of vegetable drugs, and how to prepare them for administration. He dresses wounds and ulcerated surfaces with moss and fresh leaves, and sucks poison from wounds, or cauterises them.

All these methods of treatment can be seen even at the present time in primitive people, for example, among the natives of Africa—and the writer speaks of this from personal experience. With the use of something in the nature of a herb pack the native can often heal an extensive ulcer which has defied all the treatments of the white man. The patient has, perhaps, begged to be allowed to go back to his native kraal, and then in a few weeks he has reappeared with the wound completely healed by the ministrations of the black medicine-man. But the secret of the remedies used are jealously guarded, and the white doctor will seek in vain to discover exactly what line of treatment was adopted. Undoubtedly, it was accompanied by more or less elaborate therapeutic ritual, which may have exercised some control over the patient's movements, and so favoured the healing. To this day some African tribes believe that fever or ague can be transferred to a tree, or its owner, by cutting off a hank of the patient's hair and pegging it into a groove in the tree trunk; but one finds that, in addition to this, some native concoction had been administered.

Influence of Wars.

Although, as we have seen, the continuous development and progress of medicine and surgery is, to so large an extent, coloured by the religious outlook of the people, that is not the only powerful factor which has had, and still has, a great influence on advance. Every war, whether it is merely a tribal affair, or involving such a large area of the world as did the Great War of 1914–1918, so stupendously increases the toll of human injuries and suffering that man turns his mind and his energies to the task of finding new remedies and new methods of treatment.

Then again, war always attracts so much limelight, it involves the greatest in the land quite as much as those of lesser account to the country as a whole; infinitely more nursing is required than in times of peace, for not only are there the wounded to be tended, but in the wake of war comes famine and pestilence. In these times of national crisis the women of all ranks have undoubtedly responded to the call for their services, although in the writing of an Iliad or an Odyssey we find but scant mention of the part they must have played. Even when women have not been allowed to accompany armies they have tended their sick and wounded men-folk on their return to their homes. And it is not only the war itself, but the awful aftermath of suffering and disease, of maimed bodies and tortured souls, that has been the spur upon the heel of progress. Every age and every race has known war, therefore any survey of nursing history must include some history of wars; and yet, when one considers how many weary centuries of bloodshed were endured before the necessary organisation was effected that would link up the wounded man on the battlefield with those who were eager to help him, one is conscious of a shock of consternation and surprise. Such organisation must, of course, include first aid, transport, and efficiently equipped hospitals with sufficient medical and nursing staffs.

Influence of Science.

There is also a third great factor. Gradually the human race has learned to perceive, and to assign, the right causes for phenomena in the human body and in the world around. With the increase of knowledge new treatments have arisen and old methods have needed to be analysed and revised. In every home and in every hospital the nursing treatments of thousands of years ago are still being carried out—not in an indiscriminate and haphazard attempt to cope with sorcery and evil spirits, but in the clear light of scientific knowledge, with understanding of the structure and functions of the human body, of the origin and course of the disease, and of the aims and objects of the treatments given.

All this has by no means been a continuous upward and forward progression—the true pathway has often been broken and even at times obliterated, and has needed to be entirely rediscovered, sometimes after a lapse of many centuries, whilst false tracts have been made which led nowhere except to the establishment of useless and often cruel practices, or to barren deserts of speculation.

In the following chapters we shall endeavour to trace these pathways, to see how the ill-defined tracts made in the remote past all tend to converge towards the broad, illumined road which we of the twentieth century are treading; and in all humility to give the meed of sincere, appreciative honour—the due of all honest human endeavour—to those races and individuals who have blazed the trail, even though that trail often led through intricacies which, for a time, almost hid its direction, and its goal.

12

CHAPTER II

CRETE

Geographical and historical note—Hygienic building construction—Literature and pictorial art—Position of women—Legendary references to Crete—Cretan religion—Sanitation

A Lost Civilisation of the Ancient World.

THERE is a long, narrow island lying to the south of the Ægean Sea which sixty centuries ago was the centre of a civilisation that was remarkable for its commerce, its architecture, its sculpture, its gem and ivory and inlaid metal work, its textile manufactures, its dress fashions and its sanitation. This is the island of Crete, undoubtedly the cradle of the civilisation which enabled the Greeks to create their own with such artistry. Its wonders were undreamed of by any recorders of history until, in the first years of this century, the excavations of Sir Arthur Evans and Jacques de Morgan uncovered the buried palaces of Knossos and Phaistos.

Knossos, which was obviously the capital, and the home of the monarch, was unearthed by Sir Arthur Evans; and it consists of three cities built on the top of each other. It is thought that each may, in turn, have been buried by some great earthquake calamity—the second arising over the ruins of the first, and the third over the remains of the second. Historians now refer to three periods in this civilisation, the early, the middle, and the late Minoan periods, each of which is again subdivided into three. This civilisation was completely forgotten, and no mention of it appears in any history written previous to those excavations, although broadly speaking, the era extends from 3400 B.C. to

13

1200 B.C. The King was called Minos, in the same way as the Egyptian monarch was called Pharaoh, hence the adjective 'Minoan', which is always applied to the things pertaining to ancient Crete.

Hygienic Building Construction.

The chief source of our information regarding this people is the unearthed palace of Knossos—a stately, many-storied building having monumental stairways, labyrinthine corridors and colonnades of cypress wood, and showing elaborate domestic and sanitary arrangements complete with ventilating devices, waterways for drainage, and bathrooms and lavatories with running water which excel in their construction anything of the kind used in Europe before the nineteenth century.

Literature and Pictorial Art.

The Minoans had a system of writing, utilising about 70 characters which show that they had passed from picture writing to sounds. A great number of manuscripts on clay tablets have been found. Unfortunately, the key to their deciphering has not yet been discovered, so the history of the race can only be reconstructed from the unearthed remains. As yet, nothing is known of their medical work—there are no pictures or sculpturings showing attendance upon the sick or injured, although there are many depicting games, sport, warfare, religious ceremonies, court scenes, and incidents in the life of the common people. It may fairly be assumed, however, that a people who had such a developed sanitation must have known something of means to maintain and to restore health.

Position of Women.

Then undoubtedly, women held a high place in the social and intellectual life of the community. Why else should the textile industries have reached such a stage of perfection, or the fashions in women's dress have become so sophisticated? The frescoes and

14

reliefs show ladies at receptions and feasts in very décolleté bodices, with small corseted waists and flounced skirts almost identical with Victorian styles, and they were adorned with very elaborate jewellery. Some of the statuettes of fashionable ladies are exquisite in their detail and colouring. They dressed their hair in dainty curls, with long ringlets hanging over their shoulders, and down their backs, but they left their breasts completely uncovered. Some very beautiful examples of these statuettes can be seen at the British Museum.

That women were in no way subservient to men is shown in all the art of the period, and in the beauty and elaboration of the Queen's apartments at the palace. The Cretan artists show highborn women standing up in chariots and holding the reins—they are seen hunting; and Crete obviously had its female pugilists and toreadors. In other scenes women are depicted in loggias and gardens, mingling with men in court and social functions, and in betrothal ceremonies, where each is standing erect and fearlessly facing the other, with no hint of anything but a gracious equality in their bearing; but until the Cretan alphabet gives up its key we cannot know what part they took in conserving the health of the race. At present we have only material evidence, and that is of an hygienic nature.

Legendary References to Crete.

We have said that, although the culture lasted over twelve hundred years, there is no record of it in history. There are, however, many references to such a people in the great epics of the Greek mythology. It is obvious that such a brilliant civilisation and artistic development could not have come about on a small island without constant intercourse with countries overseas, for many of the materials used had to be imported. It is assumed that Cretan sovereignty of the seas probably lasted through 1,000 years of the Bronze Age, and we read, in the *Odyssey*, that 'the dark-prowed ships were borne to Egypt by the force of wind and rain'. Were they from Crete? Then, the

15

story—which was thought to be entirely mythical—of a great king who lived in a labyrinthine palace, and there kept a horrible monster known as the Minotaur, to feed which he levied a tribute of youths and maidens from the Athenians, might easily have had an historical basis. For that epic tells of the journey of Theseus across the seas in the quest of the monster, and of how Ariadne, the daughter of Minos, showed him the way through the labyrinth, and of how he slew the Minotaur. The description of the palace given by Homer tallies with that of the palace of Knossos.

Cretan Religion.

The principal divinity of the Cretans is a Goddess Mother, and priestesses bring humanity into touch with divine power. The goddess appears to be the patroness of childbirth, and in many frescoes and statuettes she is shown as a serpent goddess. When we reflect that in every known religion a serpent divinity is associated with wisdom and knowledge—especially with regard to the physical functions of mankind—that a serpent is often the symbol of rejuvenescence and immortality, and that it is, in fact, the symbol *par excellence* of the medical art, it seems reasonable to suppose that it had some such significance for the Cretans.

Maybe, if it were possible to interpret Minoan writings, we should find much of medical interest which would throw light, not only on their own ideas and practices, but also on the later Greek development. At present we can but observe Cretan sanitation, and draw our own conclusions with regard to its medicine.

Sanitation.

Crete is an island subject to torrential rainfall, so naturally the builders had to give special attention to the problem of carrying away storm water. Below the Palace of Knossos there are great water channels. The rain water from the terraces and the waste water from the different floors descended by large shafts into

16

underground conduits, which were strongly cemented and covered with flat stones. The drains were large enough to allow a man to walk about in them without difficulty. Two branches met and discharged into the main drain which descended into the river, receiving other affluents on the way. Two large stone basins form the heads of drains. The water from the neighbouring roofs was carried into these by cemented shafts built against the walls, which led by a zigzag course from terrace to terrace. The same system was employed for the houses and streets in the towns, and the rain water was used to carry off waste from baths and lavatories. As an example, there is to be seen in the Queen's apartments at the Palace of Knossos an installation on the ground floor which is repeated on the first floor. Immediately above the drain is a recess which communicates with it by two holes. A groove in the wall about 20 inches above the floor shows where a wooden seat was fixed. Certain details have suggested that there was a balance flap; but however that was arranged, the opening above the drain secured adequate flushing and ventilation.

There is equal evidence with regard to the fresh water supply, and its arrangement shows very competent engineering work. Professor Gustave Glotz[1] describes the water-supply system thus: 'In the Palace of Knossos a very monument of hydraulic science has been preserved. Alongside a stairway which descends towards a stream there is a runnel, so that the water, instead of falling down a series of vertical steps in violent cascades, flowed in a succession of parabolas; at every bulge the current was broken, and by the time it had reached the bottom of the stair and turned a sharp double corner it had lost its force. At this point the runnel was deepened to form a kind of basin in which the current was slowed down still more, so that the water left any impurities behind before turning a right angle and finishing its course. Not one of the laws which should be observed in order to

[1] *The Ægean Civilisation*, by Gustave Glotz (London and New York, 1925), p. 117.

check and clarify a flow of water seems to have escaped the builder of these waterworks.' In his further description he tells of the distributing pipes of terra-cotta.[1] 'These pipes are manufactured and set in place with incomparable mastery. They are of a fine well-baked clay, and were joined with a cement of such good quality that it still sticks to the joints. One end being wider than the other they were fitted into one another, and they were furnished with stop-collars; the diameter is 17 centimetres at the wide end and half as much at the other. This difference no doubt increased the pressure.'

Can we doubt that a people who had such an advanced system of sanitation also had a developed medical and nursing service? How was it that such a civilisation could be so completely wiped off the face of the earth, and its advances and attainments forgotten? Probably some great physical calamity befell the island—for example, an earthquake followed by fire. Shall we ever know, and shall we ever read the manuscripts that escaped destruction? If so, there will be, doubtless, valuable additions, not only to the knowledge of the world in general, but also to the history of our own profession.

[1]*Ibid*, p. 116.

18

CHAPTER III

CHALDEA, BABYLONIA AND ASSYRIA

Geographical note—General history—Social conditions—Intellectual development—Medical customs and literature—The Legal Code of Hammurabi

THE stretch of land between the Eastern Mediterranean and the Persian Gulf was, in ancient times, one of the most fertile tracts known. Through it flowed two great rivers—the Tigris and the Euphrates. Their tributaries, with abundant springs and probably wells, provided a trustworthy supply of water at every season of the year. There was fodder for animals, food for human beings and building materials for their houses, in a climate of enduring sunshine.

Herodotus, the great historian of the fifth century B.C., tells us that in Mesopotamia wheat yielded a hundredfold to the sower, that there were two crops a year and that the leaves and stalks provided fodder for sheep. Date palms were abundant and grew untended, and many other plants grew in profusion. The clay became hard brick in the sunshine. The only other region in the Near East having such favourable conditions for human habitation *en masse* was Egypt, and therefore these two countries became great settlements very early in the known history of the world. The richest soils, however, were always the most subject to a change of masters—and no stretch of territory underwent that change so frequently in ancient times as did Mesopotamia. This resulted in an intermingling of races having different temperamental characteristics and different ideas and customs. Each developed on its own lines in medical work as in all else; but also

19

borrowed and assimilated much from its neighbours, most of whom were Semitic races.

General History.

It may be well, perhaps, to give a brief résumé of the history of this country in order that one may understand its comparative poverty of logical medical customs. It was originally known as Sumer to the south, and Accad to the north, and as such is mentioned in the Book of Genesis. The first great leader in its history is Sargon I. who, about 2750 B.C., united the Semitic tribes under one rule and extended his sovereignty from the Persian Gulf to the Mediterranean, forming the first Sumero-Accadian Empire, which lasted for over 200 years; but Semitic races were in the ascendant in this country for a period of over 2,000 years —that was, until the fourth or third century before Christ.

After about a hundred years of warfare the empire of Sargon was conquered by the Amorites, who became masters of all Mesopotamia under a great King—Hammurabi, who founded the first Babylonian Empire—about 2100 B.C. Further north on the banks of the Tigris another Semitic people, the Assyrians, were building cities, of which Nineveh and Assur were the chief. They developed their military forces, intrigued with Egypt against Babylon, became very clever raiders and exactors of tribute, and introduced war chariots and horses. They were conquered by Babylon and later became free again. Eventually under Tiglath Pileser I. they subdued Babylon; and then for many centuries power swayed between Nineveh and Babylon, sometimes the monarch, who claimed to be 'King of the World', was an Assyrian, and sometimes a Babylonian.

From the north they were frequently hampered and harassed in the extension of their Empire by another race—the forerunners of the Syrians. In 745 B.C. Tiglath Pileser III.—mentioned in the second Book of Kings, xv and xvi—conquered and ruled the whole of Mesopotamia, founding the New Assyrian Empire. His son Shalmaneser died during the siege of Samaria—2nd

Kings, xvii—and was succeeded by a usurper who took the ancient Sumero-Accadian name of Sargon II. He armed his forces with *iron* weapons. It was his son, Sennacherib, who led the Assyrian hosts against the Israelites, where they were smitten by a pestilence. There is an interesting Biblical account of this. Isaiah had prophesied, 'Thus saith the Lord God of Israel, "that which thou hast prayed to me against Sennacherib, King of Assyria, I have heard, . . . He shall not come into the city, nor shoot an arrow there, nor come before it with shield, nor cast a bank against it".' The prophecy was fulfilled thus—'And it came to pass that night, that the angel of the Lord went out and smote in the camp of the Assyrians an hundred, fourscore and five thousand: and when they arose early in the morning, behold, they were all dead corpses. So Sennacherib, King of Assyria, departed, and went and returned, and dwelt at Nineveh.' His grandson Ashurbanipal did succeed in conquering Egypt, and ruled over it for a time. He is known to the Greeks as Sardanapalus, and he became a great collector of the clay documents of the past, in the cuneiform script of the country. His great library of ancient writings at Nineveh, which has now been unearthed, is one of the most precious sources of historical knowledge in the world. He was almost the last of the Assyrian Emperors—the Chaldeans came from the south-east, and, assisted by the Medes and Persians from the north, they took Nineveh in 606 B.C., establishing the Chaldean—or Second Babylonian—Empire, which three centuries later was conquered by Alexander the Great of Macedonia.

Social Conditions.

With all this interaction of nations, involving an interchange of ideas in building, in writing, in agriculture, in trade, in art and in invention, it is difficult to say what each brought to the sum of the whole. There were wars and massacres and pestilences, there was great intellectual development, there was an advanced sanitation, and there was a legalised medical service. There must also have been nurses, but whether these were men or women, or what status they held, is not known. It is certain that there was not the equality of the sexes in Babylonia that we have reason to believe existed in Minoan Crete—all the evidence is against it. A girl's life was completely controlled by her father, who gave her in marriage as he thought fit. Men were held responsible for the chastity of their women and for the moral laws—which were very strict, and also for enforcing the penalties for breaking them; but we hear nothing of women's achievements, so it is fairly obvious that they were allowed very little scope for development.

Intellectual Development.

The Babylonians were skilled in mathematics and astronomy. They originated the decimal system of notation and a system of weights and measures, and they gave us our calendar—that is, they made division of time into years each having twelve months, they divided months into weeks, and weeks into days each having twenty-four hours of sixty minutes, and each minute having sixty seconds. They divided the circle into 360 degrees, as we do; and they invented a cuneiform system of writing, reading from left to right.

They studied all the affairs of public and private life in relation to the changes of the moon, the courses of the stars, the appearances of comets and eclipses, and so on; and concluded that human life was controlled and governed, to a great extent, by these agencies. They believed that some numbers were lucky and some were unlucky. Seven was a lucky number, except for days—the seventh, fourteenth, twenty-first and twenty-eighth were sacred days, but they were days of misfortune for the activities of mankind—the Babylonians neither baked nor roasted, permitted medical treatment nor performed public acts on these days; and this may have been the prototype of the Jewish sabbath. Twelve was always propitious, it was easy to divide in all sorts of ways, into triangular threes and square fours. It was a noble, generous and familiar number, and were there not twelve months in the year and twelve signs of the zodiac? Thirteen was awkward and impossible to divide, and was looked upon most unfavourably.

Medical Customs and Literature.

Of their earliest medicine Herodotus[1] tells us that 'they bring their sick to the market place, then those that pass by the sick person confer with him about his disease, to discover whether they themselves have been so afflicted or have seen others in like condition, and advise him to have recourse to the same treatment as they have previously known to be effectual. And they are not allowed to pass by a sick person in silence without inquiring into the nature of his distemper.' A very simple way of providing for a medical service, but it undoubtedly had its drawbacks.

Our knowledge of Babylonian medicine is mainly derived from some 700 medical tablets which formed part of the great library of Sardanapalus, found during excavations on the site of Nineveh in 1849 by Sir Henry Layard. There were some 12,000 of the tablets discovered, and they are now in the British Museum. The original collection probably numbered 100,000. These medical tablets show that the Babylonians eventually reached a stage when they had a doctor for every disease, and the patient had a choice as to whether he would use charms or medicine. The prescriptions used included a great number of drugs, both vegetable and mineral, although their nature cannot always be determined. They warded off disease by the wearing of charms and amulets, and by incantations. They were strong in their conviction that illness and death were due to the agency of demons, and they instituted many cruel practices in order to free the patient from the molestations of these evil spirits. But in spite of their demon theory, these writings show that the Babylonian and Assyrian physicians had at least reached the border of

[1]Book i, 197.

23

scientific medicine, for they describe such treatments as poulticing, bandaging, massaging, sponging and the dressing of wounds. They prescribed diet and rest, enemata and suppositories. Their personal hygiene was of quite a good order and so was their sanitation; from that, too, we can deduce a common-sense knowledge of medicine and disease. A letter written by a physician named Arad Nanaï to the Assyrian King Esarhaddon in the seventh century B.C.—obviously in answer to an enquiry by the king with regard to a man in whom he was interested, is translated thus—'It is well with the poor man who has eye trouble. I have applied a dressing to his whole face. Last night I undid the bandage which fastened the dressing and took it off. There was pus on the dressing, a spot as big as the tip of my little finger. If one of thy gods has taken the matter in hand he has put everything right. Let the heart of the king, my master, rejoice; in seven or eight days he will be cured.'[1]

The Legal Code of Hammurabi.

One of the most astounding discoveries of recent times was the unearthing, at Susa in 1902, of the now famous legal code of Hammurabi (2100 B.C.). This is engraved on a large stone with a bas relief showing Hammurabi worshipping the sun-god Shamash, from whom he is receiving the laws. The Code is most comprehensive in its scope, but only the clauses 215 to 223 are relating to the legal control of medicine. They have to do with the fees to be charged. No. 215 reads—'If a physician operates on a man for a severe wound (or makes a severe wound upon a man) with a bronze lancet and save the man's life, or if he open an abscess (in the eye) and save that man's eye, he shall receive ten shekels of silver.'

No. 221—'If a physician set a broken bone for a man, or cure his diseased bowels, the patient shall give five shekels of silver to the physician.'

[1] *Mesopotamia*, by L. Delaporte (London and New York, 1925), p. 351.

24

217 and 223 both read—in connection with each of the above clauses, 'If it be a man's slave, the owner of the slave shall give two shekels of silver to the physician.'

If the doctor caused the patient to lose his life or his eye, he had his hands cut off if the patient was a nobleman, and had to render value for value in the case of a slave.

But these fragments of knowledge do not amount to anything very instructive in an account of *nursing* through the ages. They are given here because of their value in linking up with the developments in other empires, and in order that the perspective of the whole shall be as true as it is possible to show it. It is thought, too, that this culture filtered through to India— whether by land or sea is not definitely known—probably by sea. With regard to the belief in the potency of charms and amulets, surely something of that has come down to us. Few of us are so logical and strong-minded that we have entirely broken away from these beliefs. How many nurses go to their hospital or State examinations without *some* lucky charm or mascot? These things do not supply the requisite knowledge, nor do they influence or control the questions asked; but that does not appear to affect the faith of the examinee. Doubtless, they have a 'psychological effect'. Why? Must we not look to man's remote past for the answer?

25

CHAPTER IV

THE JEWS

Early history—Effect of Babylonian captivity on Jewish development—Jewish religion—Medical and hygienic customs—Preventive medicine—Anatomy and physiology—Jewish hospitality

FOR a history of the Jews in ancient times our standard authority is, of course, the Old Testament. We know of their captivity in Egypt, which was probably about 1400 B.C., of their forty years of wandering in the desert, and of the establishment of their small kingdom of Judea. This strip of country, by its very position on the eastern shores of the Mediterranean, between Egypt and the lands of the Hittites, Syrians, Assyrians, and Babylonians, was predestined for a stormy history. It was such an important trade route, and whichever of those eastern Powers was in the ascendent at the moment harried it from that side, whilst Egypt attacked it from the west. Judea could not have been of consequence to the great Empires of the time for any other reason than as a trade route—it was too small, and it had neither mineral wealth nor agricultural possibilities.

As we have already mentioned, in the eighth and seventh centuries B.C. the Assyrians were heading for Egypt and their way lay through Judea—hence all the attacks mentioned in the second 'Book of the Kings'. The Jews were engaged in warfare successively by the Moabites, the Canaanites, the Midianites and the Philistines. They were in captivity to the Assyrians in the eighth century B.C., but they became free again. Eventually, Judea fell, and then came the Babylonian captivity of the Jews: 'and them that had escaped from the sword carried he (Ne-

26

buchadnezzar) away to Babylon; where they were servants to him and his sons until the *reign of the kingdom of Persia*' (2 Chron., xxxv. 20).

Effect of Babylonian Captivity on Jewish Development.

This captivity lasted for two generations, and when, having regained their liberty, they returned to Jerusalem the Jews were a changed people. It has been said by H. G. Wells that 'The Jews went to Babylon barbarians and returned civilised'. That may be rather an over-statement, but they certainly returned with most of the material for writing the Old Testament. Sardanapalus had already collected his great library, and it was an age of great learning and historical enquiry in Babylonia. Many of the stories of the Old Testament, for example, of the Creation, the Flood, and of the birth of Moses and his concealment in a basket made of bulrushes and bitumen, have their counterpart in *antecedent* Babylonian literature.

Jewish Religion.

The Jews, however, were the first monotheistic people. From the dawn of their history they worshipped a sun-god Jehovah— a God above all other gods. They developed an ideal of righteousness; and Jehovah became the Righteous God of all the earth, and they were the chosen people of the Most High. They believed that misfortunes and illnesses were the expressions of the wrath of God, and they relied on divine more than on human help; but they retained the 'serpent myth' with regard to knowledge and wisdom in all things pertaining to the body and its functions.

Medical and Hygienic Customs, and Surgical Advances.

The Jews instituted ritual circumcision by the use of chipped flint We read in Exodus iv, 25, that Zipporah the wife of Moses, 'took a *sharp flint* and cut off the foreskin of her son'. They had professional pharmacists and professional midwives. They

27

dressed wounds with oil, wine and balsam—the usual methods of the time—they used sutures and bandages, and freshened the edges of old wounds in order to promote healing.

Moses instituted strict supervision of foods, including inspection of meat, and laid down dietetic restrictions and commands. There were ritual fasts, and the use of hyssop as a purgative agent. They were familiar with such procedures as cupping, venesection and the application of leeches. Among their 'major surgery' is mentioned Caesarean section, amputations and trephining, preceded by the giving of a sleeping draught. They also made crutches and artificial limbs. It is thought, however, that their hygiene was, to a great extent, borrowed from Babylonia and Assyria. In former days it was considered to be essentially a Jewish phenomenon, but it is no longer correct to regard it so, for in the tides of racial intercourse flowing between the Nile and the Euphrates, the Jewish people were exposed to cultural currents from which they undoubtedly absorbed much. The Jewish sabbath, giving a seventh day of rest, had a definite health value both for body and mind, but it has already been pointed out that this may have accrued to them from Babylon.

Preventive Medicine.

The Hebrews, nevertheless, come into their own in this history as the founders of preventive medicine and public health measures. They enforced a ritual cleanliness in the touching of unclean, or infected, objects, the purification of women after childbirth, and in the hygiene and nutrition of the newly born. They gave very clear and detailed instructions for the prevention of the spread of contagious diseases, for the segregation of all those suffering from communicable diseases, and for the subsequent disinfection—even to the burning of a patient's garments and the scraping of the walls of a house. Leviticus, xiii–xv gives an account of the diagnosis and prevention of leprosy and gonorrhœa. The Jews were the first people to attempt to deal with infection in a rational manner.

28

Anatomy and Physiology.

The Talmud gives some account of the current ideas of anatomy and physiology, the former was probably learned in the slaughter-houses by inspection of carcases. It is stated that the skeleton has 248 bones. The respiration is likened to burning, the liver is believed to elaborate the blood—which is the vital principle—and the heart is the organ which is the most essential to life. Other physiological ideas, however, are certainly rather fantastic and wide of the mark; but that was so with those of all other races for many centuries after this time.

Jewish Hospitality.

A characteristic of the Jewish religion which must have had an effect upon the care of the sick, was the duty of hospitality, not only to their own people but also to 'the stranger within the gates'. This developed into a systematised charity which organised 'houses for strangers' and arranged for the visiting of the sick. Their religion demanded that they should give a tenth of their possessions towards charitable work; and the knowledge of the laws of health was disseminated amongst the people from the time of Moses onward. Before that, it had been the treasured possession of the priestly caste, as it was amongst most other nations.

CHAPTER V

INDIA AND CEYLON

General history—Invasion from the north-west—Legendary origins of Hindu medicine—Medical progress—Surgery—Royal hospital foundations and medical education—Ethical standards—End of scientific medicine in ancient India—Indian influences in Ceylon—Royal founders of Cingalese hospitals

General History.

SOMEWHERE about 2000 B.C. a nomadic, Aryan-speaking people who were in occupation of Northern Persia and Afghanistan had come down through the north-west passes into India. They fought their way, eventually, through the whole peninsula, but they never attained to any definite unity. There were numbers of rival princes and kings, and small republics. The various rulers fought amongst themselves occasionally, but with these exceptions there was peace, and the conditions under which the ancient Indians lived were less fierce and probably happier than those of the more western races. They had a warm climate, a prolific soil and trustworthy seasons, their wants were few and there was no trading with other countries, indeed, they were probably unaware of the existence of any other of the great empires of the time.

India's natural barriers rendered her comparatively secure from invasion, no great ambitious chieftains had arisen within her, and there was no sea life. Some of the rajahs tamed elephants, killed tigers, and built cities and palaces wherein they lived in great splendour, being the possessors of almost fabulous wealth.

Epic stories were composed and handed down by word of

30

mouth, and there was a great deal of thoughtful speculation with regard to life and its mysteries. The people recorded, in songs, their feasts and social customs, the happenings of ordinary life and events of agricultural importance. They worshipped many gods, the chief of which was Brahma—the sun-god—until the coming of Buddhism in the sixth century before Christ.

Invasion from the North-west.

After their conquest of Babylonia the Persians had invaded India, but without much success; and then, about 376 B.C., Alexander of Macedonia came down through the Khyber Pass in his search for more worlds to conquer. He fought a great battle against the very tall and chivalrous King Porus—who had included 200 enormous elephants in his entourage. The Macedonian *infantry* fought and defeated these huge opponents; but Alexander's troops were weary and refused to follow him farther, otherwise he might have travelled eastwards over the desert to the valley of the Ganges. However, he built a fleet and returned to the mouth of the Indus; but he did not invade the country again. And so it happened that, through all these centuries, Indian civilisation was developing on lines of its own, uninfluenced by any of the cultures we have been considering in the foregoing chapters.

Legendary Origins of Hindu Medicine.

The ancient Indians had a 'serpent god of a thousand heads' who possessed all the wisdom of the earth. One of their legends tells that Brahma, in pity for the sufferings and sorrows of humanity, gave his twin sons, Ayur and Veda, to the world, and endued them with all the wisdom and knowledge of this serpent god, that they might teach mankind 'the way'. A less picturesque version of the origin of Hindu medicine is that, of the four sacred books of the Vedas—the oldest Sanscrit documents—one is known as the 'Ayur-Veda', or 'Science of Life'. This was in four parts, and dealt with medicine and surgery, ophthalmic work and children's diseases; and it was compiled by a great physician named Susruta. But then, the works of Susruta were believed to have been dictated to him by the divine physician Dhanwantari; and the story of the birth of this medicine god is quaintly told in the ancient Hindu writings.

Drought and pestilence had fallen upon the land, and the gods had declared that only by obtaining the 'Amrita', or drink of immortality, might the ills of mortals be assuaged. The only way to secure this marvellous drink was to churn the 'ocean of milk' from which rose the mountain Mandara; and for this purpose gods and demons forgot their hostility and united their powers. The great serpent, Vasuki, twined himself around the base of the mountain, and then the immortals grasped the monster by the head and the tail and twirled the mountain in its ocean bed. The labour was long and arduous, and the story of it is told with much fantastic detail; but at length the herculean task was accomplished, and there arose from the churned ocean, first, the moon, then a very wonderful tree, the sacred cow, the goddesses of Love, of Wine, and of Beauty, and last of all, the white-robed physician Dhanwantari holding the cup containing the Amrita in his hands. After this, out of infinite compassion for the sufferings of humanity, he caused himself to be born on earth as a prince of Benares, becoming incarnate for the purpose of dictating his Ayur-Veda to Susruta, a son of the famous warrior-sage, Visvamitra.

Susruta is undoubtedly an historical personage, but there is a great difference of opinion regarding the age in which he lived. Some writers, relying upon the fact that both he and Charaka—the second of the famous physicians of ancient India—are mentioned in the great epic, Mahabharata, consider that the works attributed to them are at least as old as the Homeric poems; but recent Sanscrit scholars assert that they were written not long before the Macedonian invasion, and possibly even a century or two later than that.

By far the oldest of the sacred books of India is the 'Rig-Veda',

or 'Knowledge of Praise', which is believed to date from about
1500 B.C. It is a collection of songs or hymns telling of agriculture,
social customs, illnesses and their conquest; and containing sup-
plications to Ayur and Veda—for sickness was considered to be
a manifestation of anger on the part of the gods. It mentions a
special class of physicians, and it contains passages which praise
the healing powers of herbs and water, and acknowledge at least
two diseases—leprosy and phthisis. A third book is the 'Atharva-
Veda', or 'Knowledge of Spells', and this is also pertaining to
medicine, although it is really a 'science' of charms and invoca-
tions. The 'Ayur-Veda' is considered to be the second of the
books.

Medical Progress.

From 800 B.C. to 1000 A.D. was the most brilliant and opulent
period of Indian civilisation; but although medicine was entirely
in the hands of priests and scholars there was definitely a centre
of medical education at Benares. The two outstanding physicians
of the early part of this period—Susruta and Charaka—both collected medical literature into a compendium, or samhita. Charaka's knowledge and skill was said to have been revealed to him
by the great god Indra through the medium of a sage. Of the two
samhitas, that ascribed to Susruta is the more remarkable; it en-
umerates over eleven hundred diseases arranged in two great
classes, natural and supernatural; and mentions 760 medicinal
plants. Among the medical and nursing treatments described are
baths, enemata, emetics, vaginal and urethral injections, venesection, gargles, and inhalations. Susruta emphasises the fact that
practical and theoretical knowledge must be combined—'He
who is versed only in books will be alarmed and confused, like a
coward on a battlefield, when in face of active disease, he who
rashly engages in practice without previous study of written
science is entitled to no respect from mankind, and merits
punishment from the king; but he who combines reading with
experience proceeds safely and surely, like a chariot on two

D   33

wheels.' He warns his pupils against unintelligent repetition from books, the student who thus obtains his knowledge 'is like an ass with a burden of sandal-wood, for he knoweth the weight but not the value thereof'.

Surgery.

Nowhere else in the ancient world did surgery develop to such a high level as it did in ancient India. The Hindus used cannabis indica and hyoscyamus as narcotics—anæsthetics were not known then—and their methods of cataract extraction, excision of tumours and skin-grafting did not differ greatly from those of the present day; except that they do not appear to have used ligatures. They checked hæmorrhage by pressure, cauterisation and boiling oil. From the books of Susruta we learn that they divided the supra-orbital nerve for neuralgia, and performed laparotomy and suture of the bowel for intestinal obstruction, and for injury. He describes more than one hundred instruments, the first and best of which is the 'hand'. Plastic surgery —especially rhinoplasty—is described in detail. Such operations were practised on dead animals. A favourite form of punishment seems to have been to mutilate or cut off the nose; perhaps this accounts for the Indian proficiency in this particular branch of plastic surgery. New noses were made by taking flaps from the cheek or forehead.

The Indians of this period also realised the importance of pre-natal influences, and the care needed both before and after childbirth.

Their knowledge of anatomy and physiology was surprisingly full and accurate, and was based upon actual dissection. The bodies of children under two years of age were used for this purpose, but the bodies of all persons over that age had to be cremated.

Royal Hospital Foundations and Medical Education.

The greatest of all the monarchs of ancient India was King Asoka, who reigned from 264 to 227 B.C., and his dominion extended from Afghanistan to the province which is now Madras. In an inscription on a rock he records the building of hospitals. He had gardens laid out especially for the growing of medicinal herbs, which were gathered with ritual ceremony similar to that employed by our own mediæval doctors and of which magic was an important feature. Asoka also organised the digging of wells, the founding of public gardens and the planting of trees for shade throughout his territory. He made provision for the education of women, and gave vast wealth to the Buddhist teaching orders. All this must inevitably have had a profound effect upon the medical work of the country, but, of course, there was still much magic and superstition.

One form of treatment that appears to have originated with the Indians is hypnotism. It apparently developed in the early days of Buddhism, and, with it, migrated to China. The only survival of these practices among the Indians of the present day seems to be the strange cult of the Swamis and the Mahatmas.

In both India and Ceylon there was a fairly widespread acceptance of the doctrine of metempsychosis, or transmigration of souls. Men and women were believed to pass through successive stages in a series of reincarnations ere they eventually attained to the perfect life of the hereafter. This doctrine made people very careful in their treatment of the sick and the destitute, and also of injured or ailing animals, because they were never sure that some dear departed friend might not be incarnated in the body of a wandering beggar suffering from some loathsome disease, or even in that of a starved or maimed dog or other animal—and that might also be their own fate at some future time. Hence it behoved them at all times to show compassion to suffering humanity and to make proper provision for the destitute. This was extended to include animals, who shared in the organised care that was given to the sick and needy, special hospitals being built and equipped for their accommodation.

35

Ethical Standards.

The standards of conduct demanded from those who attended upon the sick were of an exceptionally high order. The nursing of patients seemed to have devolved, primarily, upon men, although in the very nature of things women must have carried on a great deal of unrecorded work. Speaking of these attendants upon the sick, we are told[1] that they must be 'of good behaviour, distinguished for purity, possessed of cleverness and skill, endued with kindness, skilled in every service a patient may require, competent to cook food, skilled in bathing and washing the patient, rubbing and massaging the limbs, lifting and assisting him to walk about, well skilled in the making and cleansing of beds, ready, patient, and skilful in waiting upon one that is ailing, and never unwilling to do anything that may be ordered'. Susruta says, 'The physician, the patient, the drug and the nurse are the four feet of medicine upon which the cure depends.' He then explains how each may be a true foot (pada). The nurse is a 'pada' when he is kind-hearted, without false shame, strong, trustworthy, and mindful of the physician's orders.

The End of Scientific Indian Medicine.

In the eighth century A.D. the Arabs translated portions of the works of both the great Hindu physicians, but after the Mohammedan conquest all the systematic care of the sick in India seems to have been completely lost. Why it should have vanished so mysteriously is not clearly understood. The reintroduction of Brahmanism with its strict caste prejudices and its endless formalities and inhibitions was probably a great factor; but it could hardly have been the whole story.

[1]*Charaka-Samhita*, vol. i, section xv.

36

CEYLON

During the period of ancient India's greatest brilliance Ceylon also had a developed and intellectual civilisation. It had well-planned cities, good roads, and beautiful public gardens. Its chief city is said to have been twenty square miles in extent; it had lovely architecture, and its palaces, temples and other buildings were entirely of white marble.

Indian Influences in Ceylon.

King Asoka sent missionaries into Ceylon—as well as to many other countries—to spread the doctrines of Gautama (Buddha), and they taught the faith of the great leader himself, without any of the preposterous accretions it has gathered through the centuries since that time. We find a history of philanthropy, with records of the building of many hospitals, and of the nursing work that was carried on in them, in the Sacred Books of Ceylon; particularly in the first book, Mahavansa, or the Cingalese Chronicle. Hospitals for animals, as well as for human beings, were founded in both India and Ceylon; and the great love of animals which existed in these two countries may possibly account for an extraordinary passage in the Samhita-Susruta, which forbids medical aid to hunters and to all who trap animals.

Royal Founders of Hospitals.

The most noted king of that age was King Dutha Gamani (sometimes called Dootoogameny), who died in 161 B.C. He is credited with the building of eighteen hospitals, to each of which he appointed physicians to attend the sick. The records show that he also supplied the patients with proper food and medicines from his own stores.

Other stories are told of King Buddhadasa (A.D. 341), who ordered hospitals to be erected and physicians appointed for all the villages in his domain, and he built asylums on the principal

37

highways for the blind and maimed. He collected the medical knowledge of his country into one manual, and caused a copy to be given to each physician as a guide in his practice. He was himself a skilled surgeon, and it is recorded that he always carried a case of surgical instruments when on journeys, so that he might minister to any of his subjects who needed his help.

King Parakrama (Parackramabahoo), who reigned from A.D. 1164-1189, built the most famous of the Cingalese hospitals. It contained a large hall which could accommodate several hundred patients; and he supplied it with all the equipment available at that time, for the proper carrying out of the treatments ordered. 'To each patient he assigned a male and a female servant, that he might be cared for night and day, and he prescribed the necessary diets as well as the various kinds of foods. He also built many granaries, which he filled, taking care to place therein everything requisite for the physicians . . . and since he had a heart filled with kindness he looked upon the patients with eyes full of pity, and being eminently wise and skilful in the healing art, he would call before him the physicians who were employed there and would minutely question them as to their methods of treatment, and if he found that these were not good, the king, who was the best of masters, showed them where they were mistaken, and clearly pointed out the road they should have followed according to the principles of science, whilst to some patients he offered medicaments with his own hands.' (From Tournour's translation of Mahavansa, revised and completed for the Ceylon Government by C. J. Wigesintha in 1889.)

CHAPTER VI

CHINA

General history—Legendary origins of medicine—Chinese anatomy and physiology—Medical and nursing treatments—Pharmacy and hygiene —Women workers

General History.

THE Chinese are not only one of the oldest races, but also one of the largest nations in the world—and China still belongs to the Chinese, whilst so many other of the ancient civilisations have long since passed away. The Chinese were probably not the first inhabitants of that country. Some authorities suppose that they originally lived in the valley of the Tigris and Euphrates— which seems to have been the earliest settling place of humanity —and that somewhere about fifty centuries ago they migrated eastward into what is now the valley of the Yellow River.

Chinese historians consider four periods in their civilisation:

(1) Ancient or Legendary Period—from 2967 to 1122 B.C.

(2) Historical or Golden Period—from 1122 B.C. to A.D. 960.

(3) Mediæval or Controversial Period—from A.D. 960 to 1800.

(4) Modern or Transitional Period—from A.D. 1800 to the present day.

Only in the last of these periods have we any definite records of nursing work; but as with all other races, the present cannot be understood except against a background of the past, and therefore it is worth our while to consider the medical ideas and curative work of the ancient Chinese.

Their earliest period is characterised, as with all other races, by plant-lore, demonic belief and faith healing. Shen Nung is

39

venerated as the Father of Medicine. He was also a great ruler who was supposed to have reigned from 2838–2698 B.C.—a period of 140 years. To him is ascribed the writing of the Pen P'sao, or 'The Great Herbal'—the earliest Chinese treatise on medicine; and in most cities in China to this day a temple of medicine is dedicated to him, and incense and offerings are placed before his shrine on the first and fifteenth days of each month. Most drug stores give a ten per cent discount on purchases made on these days.

Modern authorities consider that the literary work ascribed to him bears evidence of being a product of a much later time—about the second century B.C.

Legendary Origins of Medicine.

Shen Nung was followed by Huang Ti, the Yellow Emperor, who is said to have visited the immortals and to have obtained his knowledge of healing from them. He went to the two goddesses, Scarlet and White, in the Golden Valley, and learned about the pulse and about the diagnosis of disease; and he made nine needles for acupuncture. There were 365 puncture points in the body, each having its own name and supposed relationship with internal organs.

Chinese Anatomy and Physiology.

The Chinese fantastic elaboration, and attention to numberless details, is very much exemplified in their attitude and beliefs regarding the human body. They have worked out a system of relationships and very complex associations between the various organs and structures of the body which is hardly comprehensible to the European mind; and their writings have a pedantic character, attaching undue importance to accessory details, and dazzling the reader by a display of learning.

As an example of their anatomy one might quote the following: 'The small intestine is attached to the spine behind and to the navel in front. It has sixteen convolutions. The large intes-

40

tine lies on the left side of the navel and has also sixteen convolutions. The total length of the alimentary tract is sixty-four feet and *four-tenth inches*.' This reads to us like a particularly glaring 'examination howler'. The physiology is not much better; the functions of the different organs are described thus: 'The heart is the prince of the body, the seat of the vital spirit. The lungs are the ministers who regulate one's actions. The liver is the general, the abode of stratagem. The gall-bladder is the central office, courage dwells in it. The pericardium is the ambassador who brings joy and happiness. The spleen and stomach are the granaries, the five tastes emanate from them. The large intestine is the organ of communication where matters are undergoing changes. The small intestine is the receiving organ, the place of digestion. Skill proceeds from the kidney, the seat of vigour and strength. The *san chiao* constitutes the sewage system which drains off fluids. The bladder is the reservoir storing up secretions, which pass out after having been interacted upon by vapour.' These are translations from the 'Nei Ching' or 'Canon of Medicine' published about 300 B.C., but thought to be much older. In the ninth century A.D. there were works on the diseases of women and children in circulation.

Medical and Nursing Treatments.

The treatments which the Chinese claim to have originated are acupuncture—which they brought to a fine art; the moxa—a very painful method of blistering by the application of cones of 'mug-wort' to the skin, which were then set alight—and massage. The massage movements practised in China from the beginning of its history were tapping, kneading, pinching, chaffing, and pummelling the body all over, producing delightful sensations and relief from tiredness. This treatment filtered across to Japan very early—and the Japanese became wonderfully clever masseurs. It has always been a profession followed specially by the blind in Japan; and their treatments have proved to be of value in muscular fatigue, lumbago, rheumatism, nervousness, headache and paralysis. It was first brought to European notice about A.D. 1800.

In dealing with any illness the Chinese physician took into consideration the physical temperament, the general condition, the state of mind, the influence of the atmosphere, the time of year or day, the positions of the stars and constellations, the colour of the patient's skin and other clinical features. Most important of all was the pulse, the art of feeling this being most complicated and mysterious; and the nature, the location, and the course and treatment of the disease often depended upon this alone.

The Chinese believed in a particular devil to cause each disease, in fact some diseases have a separate devil to cause each symptom. For example, malaria has three—one with a bucket of cold water to produce the shivering, one with a stove to set up the fever, and one with a hammer with which to belabour the victim's head, thus producing the headaches.

The introduction of Buddhism—a century or so before the birth of Christ—brought with it Indian ideas and therapeutics. Taoism, at the same time, invented a system of charms for the cure of disease; but the two systems flourished side by side, stress being laid upon the observation of the patient.

Pharmacy and Hygiene.

With regard to pharmacy, the Chinese knew of 365 drugs, of which 240 were of vegetable origin. The methods of compounding them were very elaborate and saturated with superstition. About A.D. 800 the Chinese herbalist was in a position to choose his remedies from no fewer than 11,886 recipes. The search for the Philosopher's Stone and the Elixir of Life started in China in the third century B.C., and continued through many ages. Its quest reached its zenith about 900 years later. The Chinese claim to have discovered general anæsthetics about A.D. 240, and to have performed major operations. The thyroid gland was used in the treatment of goitre in A.D. 627. Vaccination against small-

42

pox was started in the eleventh century, using the pus from a smallpox pustule. (*History of Chinese Medicine*, by Wong and Wu, published 1932.)

The personal hygiene of the Chinese was quite good—for example, their habit of drinking tea instead of unboiled water protected them from developing parasitic and infectious intestinal diseases. All the better class Chinese attached great importance to baths and the wearing of spotlessly clean linen.

Women Workers.

The first mention of women in connection with attendance on the sick was in the Hans dynasty (260 B.C. to A.D. 220). This dynasty was considered the most glorious in Chinese medical history, and during it lived three of the greatest physicians China has ever known.

A woman named Ch'un Yu'yen was called to the palace to treat the Queen, to whom she administered a pill composed of aconite. Another reference states that she was a midwife, and attended the Queen and other royal ladies at their confinements. The strict moral code handed down from very ancient times forbade the attendance of a male upon labouring women, so that this work was left to women. Probably they were uninstructed, for the mortality was high.

There is the mention of a daughter of a minister—the lady's name was Candida Hyu (1607–1680)—who became a convert to Roman Catholicism. She married at sixteen and was left a widow at thirty. Among her charities she established a foundling hospital and orphanage. As Du Halde says, 'Being sensible that numbers of poor people, for want of necessaries to support life, exposed and abandoned their children as soon as they were born, she . . . obtained permission to purchase a large house where she lodged the infants thus exposed, and *provided them with nurses*. The number of these children was so great that, notwithstanding all the care taken, upwards of two hundred died every year.'

With this exception, no mention of women nurses is found

until the latter part of the nineteenth century. The Chinese had seemed, until about the ninth century, to have been feeling their way towards a real science of curative work; and then, about that time, an 'intellectual blight' appears to have fallen upon them and all advance was arrested. During the last half-century China has made rapid progress in medicine and in all other sciences. Modern nursing training was introduced from America, by missionaries, about 1900. China has now many training schools both for general nursing and for midwifery, and their standard is equal to that of many European hospitals.

44

CHAPTER VII

EGYPT

General history—Religion and intellectual development—Medical literature and education—Practice of medicine—Egyptian anatomy and chemistry—Pharmacy—Hygienic customs—Bone diseases and injuries —Nursing—Later history

THROUGH all the fluctuations of the Empires and cultures we have been considering *one* realm and *one* people seem to have maintained a degree of stability unachieved by any other nation. Great Powers rose, developed their civilisations, fell, and passed away, and yet Egypt remained—a long narrow strip of rich black soil, flanked on either side by seemingly endless stretches of sandy wastes. Running through its midst was a broad grey river that opened at its mouth into a wide delta, not as we know it now, but cut across by many narrow streams that led into morasses fringed with reeds and grasses; and this country was inhabited by a people who seemed to have been there since the beginning of history. Through all these centuries the people of other races considered that 'to be learned in the wisdom of the Egyptians' constituted the acme of intellectual achievement. For over 4,000 years this people had a crowded and eventful history, and at times their conquests extended far and wide, so that no other people could compare with them in wealth, in power, and in dominions.

Egyptian chronology is a problem still far from solution; but even though the calculations of the most modern and scholarly Egyptologists differ widely from each other, especially with regard to the more ancient periods, all agree that the history of

45

Egypt should be considered in five outstanding divisions or phases:

(1) *The Pre-dynastic Period.*—Before 4000 B.C., during which time we conclude that the primitive Egyptians were not unlike other primitive people in many parts of the world.

(2) *The Old Kingdom.*—Begins about 4000 B.C. with the first dynasty, includes the Great Pyramid age, and ends in anarchy 2430 B.C.

(3) *The Middle Kingdom.*—From 2160–1788 B.C. It includes two great dynasties, the eleventh and twelfth, and also ends in anarchy.

(4) *The New Kingdom or First Empire.*—From 1580 to 1095 B.C. —a century after the fall of Troy. The Empire is now tottering; and the last of the Rameses, who was weak and lacking in personality, was its Pharaoh.

(5) *Brief Periods of Power.*—In which dynasties rise and fall, alternating with conquests by Assyria, Babylonia and Persia, until finally she is conquered by Alexander of Macedonia in 332 B.C. and he adopts the rôle of Pharaoh, or God-king. For the next three hundred years Egypt is ruled by the Ptolemies, the last of whom was the famous Cleopatra, and in 30 B.C., Egypt became the vassal of Imperial Rome.

There were originally 20 small states in Upper Egypt and 20 in Lower Egypt, each with its own ruler and special deity. They were united by the first Pharaoh, Mene, when he adopted the double crown of Egypt (upper and lower) and formed the first dynasty.

Religion and Intellectual Development.

The Pharaoh of Egypt was always considered to be divine— a God-king—and received worship as such. But the great God was Ra, a Sun-god, who later became worshipped as Amen-Ra, by his fusion with another great deity. There were also 39 lesser deities, probably one for each of the original states, although

46

this distinction was not maintained. The god of the underworld, or of life after death, was Osiris, and his consort was Isis. One myth tells that they taught the medical arts to their son Horus. Another version is that all knowledge was given, from the heavens, to Thoth, or Hermes, an ibis-headed god, to be communicated to man. He is accredited with the invention of language and writing, of geometry, arithmetic, astronomy, medicine, music, and rhythm—the latter including gymnastics and dancing. He was also believed to have introduced sculpture, painting and architecture—in fact, he was a sort of titular genius.

Medical Literature and Education.

The immense knowledge of the Egyptians is gathered into the forty-two volumes of the Hermetic Collection—the last six of which are concerned especially with medicine; the first deals with anatomy, the second with diseases in general, the third describes instruments, the fourth, drugs and medicine, the fifth, diseases of the eyes and their treatment, and the sixth, diseases of women.

Amen-Ra (the sun) was regarded as being responsible for generation and corruption, and therefore was the source of life, health, disease and death; but the true god of healing was I-em-hoteb—'he who comes in peace'. He is known also as 'the master of secrets' and 'the consoler of the afflicted'. He is the prototype of the Greek Æsculapius, the Indian Dhanwantari, and the Persian Thrita. All these are believed to have been historical personages who, because of their excellence as physicians, were deified by later generations. I-em-hoteb is thought to have lived about 2980 B.C. in the reign of Zozer, a king of the third dynasty,[1] and to have designed a terraced pyramid 190 feet high. An inscription on a tomb near the Pyramids shows it to have been his last resting place. He was the earliest known

[1]Sir Flinders Petrie puts this date much earlier, about 4900 B.C.

47

physician. In later years there was a temple with a medical library dedicated to him at Memphis.

Medical schools existed in Egypt as early as the first and second dynasties. There was a college at Sais where women were taught midwifery, and they in turn, gave instruction in gynæcology to the physicians.

A great deal of our knowledge is derived from unearthed manuscripts—papyri—which have been found during excavations, and from works of art. Papyrus was prepared from a long, broad reed, now extinct in Egypt, that grew abundantly among the marshes of the delta. Strips of fibre were laid side by side, and others placed at right angles across them, then the whole made into a compact sheet by running a kind of liquid gum between the fibres. These sheets were about fourteen inches wide, and of varying lengths, and when one sheet was filled, another was fastened to the end, and the story continued until often the papyrus had grown to many yards in length. It was then rolled up and stored away.

There are four principal medical papyri in existence:

(1) *The Ebers Papyrus.*—The best preserved of all. It was found between the legs of a mummy in a tomb near Luxor. It is a huge roll on which the writing stands out as clear and vivid as if it had been written only a day or two ago. It was advertised for sale, and was acquired by Professor Ebers in 1872; and he translated it into German. A second German translation was made by H. Joachim in 1890, and it was translated into English by Dr. Cyril Bryan in 1930.

(2) *The Berlin Papyrus.*—Found in an earthern vase at Memphis—the capital of Egypt during the first dynasty. This is now in the Museum at Berlin.

(3) *The Hearst Papyrus.*—This dates from the tenth dynasty— about 1700 B.C. It came from a ruined house in a small provincial town, and it is now in the British Museum.

(4) *The Edwin Smith Papyrus.*—Found at Thebes in 1862 by Edwin Smith, an American Egyptologist, and bequeathed by

him to the New York Historical Society. This is a sort of case-history and records 48 cases classified according to the organs affected, and includes all kinds of injuries affecting males. A very beautiful translation of this by J. H. Breasted, in facsimile, with the text and plates, was published in 1930.

These papyri, however, are by no means the only literature of ancient Egypt still in existence—there are many books in the museums of Cairo and Europe which undoubtedly belonged to the I-em-hoteb Library at Memphis, from which the Greeks derived so much of their medical knowledge.

Practice of Medicine.

Herodotus (fifth century B.C.) tells us that the practice of medicine was very widely carried out in ancient Egypt. Every physician was a specialist in that he applied himself to one disease only, and did not treat several classes of disease. There were oculists, dentists, specialists for diseases of the head, for diseases of the internal organs, and for abdominal conditions; and Egyptian physicians were esteemed for their skill and learning in other countries besides their own. Cyrus, the Persian king who conquered Babylonia in the sixth century B.C. sent for an Egyptian ophthalmologist, and Darius is also said to have employed a physician from Egypt.

But these 'specialists' were not working in the light of clear scientific knowledge—as are the specialists of to-day. There was a good deal of magic and superstition embodied in their beliefs and practices. There were three distinct classes of healers: (1) Those who carried out their work according to the books. (2) Practitioners who were known as 'exorcists', which, literally translated means 'a priest of Sekhet'. Sekhet was the lion-headed goddess of war, whose wrath produced a great number of diseases and the greatest mortality. The work of her priests consisted mainly in appeasing her, and thus exorcising the disease. (3) The charmer, who had neither the learning of the physician or the inspiration of the priest, but who recited formulæ, accom-

E

panied by gesticulations and ceremonies—the latter often including the administration of herbal remedies. He was quite ignorant of the meaning of his 'charms', but had acquired the routine from other practitioners. No doubt the treatment kept the patient amused whilst nature effected the cure—for everyone realises how greatly a patient's progress is facilitated when he or she is convinced that recovery is certain.

Egyptian Anatomy and Chemistry.

In anatomy, the knowledge of the Egyptians was evidently acquired before it was deemed an impious act to use a knife upon a corpse in order to discover any of the mysteries of the human body and its formation. There is a treatise in existence which is attributed to Athothis—the son of Mene, and the second Pharaoh—which deals with anatomy and the dissection of the human body. The facts given are rather fantastic, however, and the Berlin Papyrus tells us that 'the head has twenty-two vessels with which to draw the breath out of the heart, and from there to carry it to all parts of the body—there are two vessels in the breasts which conduct to the kidneys. There are two vessels in the legs, two in the arms, two in the forehead, two in the throat, two in the eyelids, two in the nostrils, two in the right ear through which the breath of life enters, and two in the left ear through which the breath of death enters'. Such knowledge would hardly be acceptable to a twentieth-century examiner, but it was a fairly good level of advance for nearly six thousand years ago. The science remained stationary, however, because of the great horror that developed during the following period in the minds of the ancient Egyptians towards any mutilation of the body after death—and here their religion shows its controlling influence.

They worshipped a sun-god—Ra—and every morning he appeared on the eastern horizon and began his daily journey across the sky in his chariot called 'Millions of Years'. On his way he looked down upon his people and saw their deeds of good and evil; and he gave them light and heat, the sources of all life and power. In the evening he paused in the west before dropping over the horizon in order to gather up the spirits of those who had died during the day. These he took to the underworld presided over by Osiris—hence the probable origin of the term 'going west' to signify an end, or death. The soul was then judged, the god Thoth standing beside the balance in which the good deeds are to be weighed against the evil; but one good deed might often overbalance a heap of evil ones. Then the soul was sent on a journey, during which it would encounter hardships and dangers, but would become purified in the process. It was then considered fit to enter the 'gardens of perpetual peace'. But the soul was homeless without the body, so that the whole hope of immortality seemed—to the ancient Egyptians—to depend upon the preservation of the body; for the soul might die if deprived of its body, or become a restless ghost, having no happiness and being a source of danger to mankind. So they bent their intellects and their energies to discover means of preventing the natural processes of decay—they studied the reactions of one compound upon another, and originated and developed the science now known as chemistry. The very word 'chemistry' is derived from 'chemi', the ancient name of Egypt. The word means the 'black land' and chemistry was known as the 'black art'.

Holding such religious beliefs, how could they have developed otherwise? After being embalmed, the body of a king or great noble was laid in a beautiful granite sarcophagus, the sides of which were carved with pictures of the journey through the underworld, and in it was placed the 'Book of the Dead', giving all instructions about the journey, although every Egyptian had learned this by heart during his life-time. Everything else that might conceivably help the soul was placed in the tomb; and there the body waited, in a calm and tranquil peace, for the return of the soul.

Professional embalmers, however, were always drawn from the

lowest stratum of society, and were held in hatred and abhorrence by all others. Embalming had to be done with the least possible delay, allowing no time for an extensive examination of the various body cavities and their contents. Even had this not been so, there was no social contact between the embalmers and the physicians and priests, so that any knowledge the former may have gained could not have been passed on to those who could have profited by it.

Pharmacy.

The Egyptians had an extensive and elaborate pharmacopœia, and they were skilled in the preparation of drugs for administration. The Ebers Papyrus tells of plasters, pills, pastilles, gargles, inhalations, fumigations, snuffs, salves, ointments, and emollients of many kinds. It also mentions suppositories and enemata, poultices and bandages. The marvellous skill of the Egyptians in the application of bandages is shown on the mummies—as much as a thousand yards being used in many cases, and remaining in position for thousands of years.

In the Berlin Museum there is to be seen a domestic medicine chest which belonged to the wife of the Pharaoh Mentu-hoteb, a ruler of the eleventh dynasty. This is a basket of straw work which was found standing in a wooden chest in the Queen's tomb. It contains six vases—one of alabaster and five of serpentine—with dried remnants of drugs, two spoons, a piece of linen cloth and some roots. Of course, this may have been a cosmetic chest, for there are many prescriptions for cosmetics given in the Ebers Papyrus.

Hygienic Customs.

Herodotus tells us of the hygienic customs of the Egyptians, their simple dress and frequent baths—'they purge themselves every month, three days in succession, seeking to preserve health by emetics and clysters, for they suppose that all diseases to which men are subject proceed from the food they eat'.

52

Divine ordinances regulated the cleanliness both of the person and of the dwelling place. Many temple inscriptions promised health and long life to the clean and temperate. The priests set the standard—taking a bath every six hours, shaving their bodies every three days, and always wearing spotlessly white garments. But there was probably no attempt to attain such standards on the part of the poorer people.

The teeth of many mummies appear to show that dentistry had reached a fine art—many have gold fillings, but these may have been put in after death. Dental caries, although extremely rare before the Pyramid age, became common as soon as the people learned luxury; after which tartar-formation, dental caries and alveolar abscesses were at least as common as they are in modern Europe to-day. But although every form of dental disease was prevalent among the wealthy, there was a relative immunity from such ailments among the poorer people who lived mainly upon a coarse uncooked vegetable diet.

Bone Diseases and Injuries.

The bones of numbers of mummies give evidence that they suffered from rheumatoid arthritis; the moisture of the climate during the part of the year that the Nile was in flood would probably have predisposed to such affections. As a result of a very extensive examination of mummies, Professor Eliot Smith reports that 'it can be quite confidently stated that no trace whatever even suggesting syphilitic injuries to bones or teeth was revealed before modern times, nor was any case of true rickets found in a human skeleton; although in some domestic animals—in particular some of the sacred monkeys kept at the temple at Thebes—distortions suggestive of rickets were found. Evidence of tubercular and malignant disease was also extremely rare.'

Many of the degenerative changes in the joints, and especially in the spine, may have been due to excessive strain. The glory of Egypt lay in its mighty monuments, erected by the mercilessly forced labour of countless thousands of workers. The hauling of an obelisk from a quarry is said to have taken 5,000 men, working under the lash of an overseer. Two of these great pillars stood behind the Hall of Columns at Karnac. One has now fallen, shaken by an earthquake, but the other stands tapering skyward as proudly as when it was first erected. It is a monolith of solid granite almost a hundred feet in length, polished smooth and having no join or division. Its top was once covered with pure gold, but that was stolen long ago. In the building of one of the Pyramids 360,000 men were employed for twenty years. This was mostly slave labour, and the strain of hauling must have been terrific.

In the treatment of fractures Egyptian methods must have been effective, for out of 100 ancient bodies showing united fractures, examined by Professor Eliot Smith, only one was observed to show any signs of suppuration. Splints for fractures were made of layers of linen impregnated with glue and plaster, and moulded whilst soft to conform to the shape of the limb.

Nursing.

That actual nursing was done, and was recognised to be necessary, is evident from the descriptions of nursing procedures given in the various papyri and other literature. The Edwin Smith papyrus give details of the method of feeding in tetanus—liquid food is administered by holding the mouth open with a 'brace of wood padded with linen'. A favourite dressing for wounds was fresh meat applied on the first day, followed by linen saturated in an ointment of honey and grease, which was bound on to the wounded area, and renewed daily.

But who administered all their medicines and treatments? Who made the beds and prepared the invalids' food, and attended to the daily toilet of the sick? Surely not the physicians or the priests, and surely not men for women patients! There is no mention of any special class of women for these duties. Some authorities consider that it was the work of handmaidens and personal slaves of the patient—and surely of wives, and of mothers!

Later History.

As time went on, Egyptian medicine became excessively formal. It was controlled by the priests, and physicians were bound to give those treatments that were established by written law and none other. It is known, from allusions to these writings by classical Greek and Roman authors, that because they were believed to be of divine origin they were not subject to improvement by man, subsequent transcribers being permitted to make marginal comments only. As the historian Diodorus Siculus—who lived in the first century A.D.—relates: 'If the doctors follow the recognised laws from the sacred books and are yet unable to heal the sick person they are guiltless and absolved from all blame. But if they do anything contrary to the written law they endure the death penalty, as the law givers would think that few persons would be more clever than the treatment observed for so long a time, and recorded by the best masters of the art.'

With such penalties there could be very little scope for further development. Brave indeed would be the physician who would risk his life by giving an original prescription. Only after the third day of treatment, if there was no improvement in the patient's condition, might an alteration be made.

55

CHAPTER VIII

GREECE

General history—Divine origin of medicine—Homeric accounts of wound dressings—Temple-hospitals dedicated to Æsculapius—Women's part in curative work, historical and legendary—Anatomy and physiology—Greek physical culture—Beginnings of scientific medicine—Hippocrates instruction in nursing duties—Hippocratic literature—The Hippocratic Oath

General History.

The Greeks make their first appearance in history as a wandering Aryan people, skin-clad and armed with bronze axes, coming over the Illyrian mountain crests into the Balkan peninsula. They consisted of many tribes, known collectively as the Hellenes, and in the south of the peninsula they came into contact with the civilised Ægean people whom they afterwards fought. Eventually, it is assumed, they conquered and destroyed the Ægean civilisation, on the ashes of which they built up their own. They spread eastwards and northwards into Asia Minor and the shores of the Black Sea, and westwards to Italy, and thence along the northern shores of the Mediterranean, where they founded the town of Marseilles on the site of an earlier Phœnician city.

They came as barbarian herdsmen-raiders into a world of old civilisations where there was already agriculture, shipping and trading, walled cities and temples, a developed system of writing and some literature. They did not slowly build up a civilisation according to their own ideas and their developing beliefs and customs; but they assimilated the cultures of the races with whom they mixed. That may account for their later freedom of thought

56

—they were untrammelled by old established beliefs in priest-kings, temple-states and powerful gods. They were nimble-witted and their minds were comparatively free to follow the flights of their reasoning without having first to break through the bonds forged by centuries of accumulated primitive beliefs in demons and magic and what not.

They wrecked existing civilisations and put various pieces together on the ruins, as it were, to form their own. They came into a heritage of knowledge from the past such as none of the people of the older Empires had done, and as they became more comprehending of underlying factors they became more religious and superstitious as a result of that heritage.

Divine Origin of Medicine.

For much of our knowledge of their earlier medicine we are indebted to the *Iliad* and the *Odyssey* of Homer. The gods of the heroic Greeks were glorified human beings, and they were not held in such overwhelming fear and awe as were the gods of the older civilisations, nor were they expected to perform miracles or to save men's lives. The god of Medicine was Æsculapius, held to have been the son of Apollo, and to have been instructed in the healing art by Chiron, one of the centaurs. The traditional story of his birth is that a maiden named Koronis, being with child by Apollo, fled to the mountains above Epidauros—the infant Æsculapius was born and his mother left him on the mountain, where he was tended by a goat and watched over by a dog. Homer does not speak of him as a god, but as the mortal king of Thessaly. His two famous sons—Machaon and Podalirius—accompanied Agamemnon and the Greek hosts on their expedition to Troy; the siege of that city representing an attack on one of the last of the Minoan strongholds. We are told that Machaon was 'a doctor worth many men at cutting out arrows and laying on gentle drugs'; and that Podalirius had 'cunning to find out things impossible and to cure that which healed not'. Of the six daughters of Æsculapius the most famous was Hygieia, the goddess of health. There was also Panacea, the restorer, and Meditrina, the preserver of health. Epigone, the wife of Æsculapius, is regarded as 'the soothing one'.

Homeric Accounts of Wound-dressings.

There are at least a hundred references in the *Iliad* to wounds inflicted by javelin, spear or arrow, or to the hurling of great fragments of rock; and there are accounts of the remedies applied. All these show a familiarity with anatomy, and with the essentials of surgical dressings. The following, from the fourth book of the *Iliad*, lines 230 *et seq.*, gives an example of Machaon's skill in attending the wounded Menelaus, King of Sparta:

'From the close-fitting belt the shaft he drew
With sharp return of pain . . .
And when the wound appeared in sight, where struck
The stinging arrow, from the clotted blood
He cleansed it, and applied with skilful hand
The healing ointments, which in friendly guise
The learned Chiron to his father gave.'

In the eleventh book, lines 755 *et seq.*, we read:

. . . 'then as he (Eurypylus) lay reclined,
Patroclus, with his dagger, from the thigh
Cut out the biting shaft; and from the wound
With tepid water cleansed the clotted blood,
Then, pounded in his hands, a root applied,
Astringent, anodyne, which all his pain
Allayed; the wound was dressed, and staunch'd the blood.'

In another passage we are told that Helen infused a drug, nepenthe, into the wine as an 'antidote to the pains of grief and anger—a most potent charm for ills of every name'.

Since Professor Schliemann's recent excavations on the site of ancient Troy it has been realised that Homer's *Iliad* is not merely a creation of his own romantic and poetic fancy, but is probably an actual narrative of events that occurred about 1200 B.C.

58

Temple-hospitals Dedicated to Æsculapius.

Æsculapius was publicly deified at Athens in 420 B.C. after having been held in reverence for many centuries. Numbers of temples, known as Æsculapieia, had been built in his honour; the more famous being at Trikka in Thessaly, at Cnidus on the coast of Caria in Asia Minor, at Cyrene on the Libyan coast opposite to the island of Crete, at Epidauros in Argolis, at Athens, and on the island of Cos in the Ægean Sea.

The priest-physicians were supposed to be descendants of Æsculapius, and no doubt many of them were. One can reconstruct the arrangement of these temple-hospitals from Professor Meyer-Steineg's account[1] of the excavations and surveys made on the island of Cos in recent years. This temple occupied an extremely healthy site on the northern slopes of a range of mountains which extended throughout the entire length of the island, and which have a maximum height of 3,000 feet. The temple and associated buildings were about two miles from the city, and about 300 feet above sea level. The heights behind were covered with pine forests which gave ample protection against the much dreaded and debilitating south wind. A large brook of very pure water passed through the temple grounds—the spring from which it had its origin was located 300 feet higher up the side of the mountain. In the same neighbourhood is a mineral spring containing both iron and sulphur. The temple itself was on three artificially prepared terraces, communicating with each other by a series of broad and massive steps, and facing northward towards the sea.

The curative agents utilised were sunlight, pure air and drinking water, dietetic measures, massage and physical exercises, and also the rational employment of drugs and surgical operations. The procedures were somewhat as follows: the patient underwent preliminary bathing and dieting, after which he was taken

[1]Th. Meyer-Steineg's *Kranken-Anstalten in griech.-röm. Altertum*, Jenaer med.-hist. Bietr. H.3, 1912.

into the temple enclosure and encouraged to pray and to make offerings to the god Æsculapius. He then settled down to sleep and it was thought that the lines of treatment and the remedies to be employed would be revealed in dreams by the god himself. Upon awaking, he told his dream to the priest-physician. Sometimes it was the physician who underwent the temple-sleep and dreamed the line of treatment to be adopted; but, in addition, it is presumed that he used his own powers of observation and his acquired knowledge. Often he watched whilst the patient slept, and every nurse knows how much valuable clinical evidence can be thus obtained.

The sacred emblems of the cult were the serpent—the symbol of physical knowledge, rejuvenescence and immortality; and the dog—probably symbolising faithfulness; but by the fifth century the dog was replaced by the staff, an emblem of the journeys to be made—mostly on foot. The staff and the serpent are the emblems of our own Royal Society of Medicine to this day.

It is thought that the cult of Æsculapius was assimilated, along with other cultural ideas, from the Phœnicians. The whole system was undoubtedly conducive to quackery and superstition, but the natural beauty of the surroundings, the rest and sunshine, and the healing waters all played their part in effecting cures.

The best known Æsculapian temple, both from literature and from excavations, is that of Epidauros. It is about 30 miles from Athens, and lies between two ranges of mountains. Its remains can still be seen by travellers, and it is said to have accommodated about 500 patients, to have had wards and corridors, baths, gymnasia, libraries, rooms for visitors and patients, and houses for priests and physicians. It was presided over by a head administrator.

Women's Part in Curative Work, Historical and Legendary.

The Grecian women of the fourth and fifth centuries B.C. did not participate in the scientific and intellectual development of their day. They lived, for the most part, in seclusion. There is no record of women nurses or attendants in the temple hospitals, although priestesses are mentioned. There were two grades of priestesses, one of which assisted in the temple rites and ceremonies, and the other in the more practical duties—they were known as 'basket-bearers', and the bath attendants, and those who waited upon the sick and carried the helpless, worked under their direction. Women doubtless did much noble, if unnoticed, work among the sick, and they evidently found a sphere of usefulness in midwifery. We are told that the mother of Socrates was 'a midwife brave and burly', so also was the sister of Pyrrho. Plato tells us that the practice of midwifery was confined to elderly and experienced matrons. It is quite obvious that there were women who attended upon the sick, either as doctors or nurses, for in *Hyppolytus* Euripides makes a handmaiden say to her mistress Phædra, 'If thou hast some ailment which thou dost not care to reveal to men, here are women who are competent to treat the condition properly.' And Plato in his *Republic* says,[1] 'There is not then, my friend, any office among the whole inhabitants of the city peculiar to the woman, considered as a woman, nor to the man, considered as a man, but the geniuses are indiscriminately diffused through both. The woman is naturally fitted for the sharing of all offices, and so is the man, but in all the woman is weaker than the man. Shall we then commit everything to the care of the man, and nothing to the care of the woman? How shall we do so? It is therefore, I imagine, that one woman is fitted by natural genius for being a physician, and another is not; one is naturally a musician and another is not.' (Translation by Spens.)

There were legendary women, also, who are revered as having helped to assuage human suffering. There is Hera, the divine midwife who aided women in labour. She is depicted in art with

[1] *The Republic of Plato*, Book 5, Chapter V (Henry Davis, London, 1854, Bohn's Classical Library).

61

scissors in her hand for the severance of the umbilical cord. Her daughter, Ilithyia was the goddess of maternity.

Then there are the divine witches—Cybele, the daughter of Minos, King of Phrygia, who is known as the 'Great Mother' and who invented liniments to assuage gripes in little children; Hecate who discovered aconite, which she obtained from the froth of Cerberus, and also belladonna. Circe and Medea were her daughters. Circe's draught was composed, probably, of the deadly nightshade, and Medea discovered colchicum, but these ladies made potions and love philtres which could turn men into swine and dignified persons into absurd sentimentalists. Rendel Harris, in *The Ascent of Olympus*, gives reasons for believing that herb gardens were cultivated in very early Greek times.

Anatomy and Pathology.

Dissection was being practised at this time, and therefore the knowledge of anatomy was becoming wider and more correct than formerly; but this science reached its great development at Alexandria about two centuries later. Descriptions of bones are quite accurate, even as regards the finer detail. Many pathological conditions were correctly understood, and one may see in the British Museum several very carefully modelled statuettes, which were recovered from the ruined Æsculapian temples, showing patients with facial paralysis, with ascites, and with cancer of the breast.

Greek Physical Culture.

By the sixth century B.C. most of the Greek city states had become aristocratic republics, but slavery was considered a natural condition and, on the whole, women were regarded as being unfit for freedom and political rights. Physical culture and sports of all kinds were most popular. Olympian games had been instituted in 776 B.C. and were held every four years afterwards. They consisted of foot races, boxing, wrestling, jumping, javelin and quoit throwing, and chariot and horse races. Greek intellect and the power of abstract reasoning were developing to an extent hitherto unknown in the history of the human race. The Greeks had conceived ideals of physical grace and perfection such as are consistent only with perfect health, and they immortalised those ideals in their sculpture and their art.

Beginnings of Scientific Medicine.

The Greeks had absorbed demonic ideas from Babylon and Assyria, but probably much valuable knowledge also, for Sardanapalus was then collecting all the medical lore of his country into his great library at Nineveh. They had probably absorbed hygienic ideas from the Minoans, and a knowledge of mathematics and drugs from the Egyptians, as well as the basis of their medical ethics. Many Æsculapian temples had developed into medical schools; but there was still a great deal of 'temple-jugglery'. It was about this time that Greek medicine began to be definitely scientific, to break away from quackery, superstition and magic, and to establish some of the traditions that govern it to this day. The Greeks were collecting and recording their observations regarding the facts of disease. There was an organised public medical service in the latter half of the sixth century B.C., which was regarded as being of importance to the state as a whole;[1] and the two hundred years that followed were the most brilliant in Greek intellectual and artistic accomplishment. Schools of philosophy were springing up in many centres. It was an age that produced Plato, Socrates, Aristotle, Sophocles, Euripides, Pindar, Aristophanes, and others whose names have been revered for their learning through the ages since that time.

During the middle part of the fifth century B.C. Athens was ruled by Pericles, a great statesman who combined extraordinary political ability with the most passionate striving for the deep and beautiful things of life; and it was during this age that Hip-

[1]Sir Clifford Allbutt gives a full account of these in his *Greek Medicine in Rome*, pp. 443–474 (Macmillan, London, 1921).

63

pocrates—considered to be the Father of modern medicine—
was born into the Æsculapian priesthood at Cos, in the year 460
B.C. Very little is definitely known about him, as historical fact—
he is mentioned by Plato, and about a hundred works have been
associated with him since antiquity, and are known as the Hippocratic Collection. These are certainly not all his writings, the
views expressed are often contradictory, and the authors obviously lived in different parts of the Greek world during periods
varying from each other by several centuries. The best of them,
however, contain an ideal ethical standpoint that is in accordance with all that is known of the man Hippocrates. Dr. Charles
Singer, in speaking of Hippocrates says:

'In beauty and dignity that figure is beyond praise. Perhaps gaining in stateliness what he loses in clearness, Hippocrates will ever remain the type of the perfect physician. Learned, observant, humane,
with a profound reverence for the claims of his patients, but an over-
mastering desire that his experience shall benefit others. Orderly and
calm, disturbed only by anxiety to record his knowledge for the use of
his brother physicians and for the relief of suffering. Grave, thoughtful and reticent, pure of mind and master of his passions, this is no
overdrawn picture of the Father of Medicine as he appeared to his
contemporaries and successors. It is a figure of character and virtue
which has had an ethical value to medical men of all ages, comparable
only to the influence exerted on their followers by the founders of the
great religions.'[1]

In his medical teachings, Hippocrates rejected all the beliefs
in the supernatural origins of disease, and taught that it was
caused only by a breach of natural laws. He prescribed, not from
books, or teachings, or dreams, but as the result of his own observations of the patient. He is reported to have spent hours by the
bedside of his patients, noting the symptoms and course of the
disease, and the effects of the treatment given, faithfully recording his failures as well as his successes. He travelled to Thessaly,

[1]*Greek Biology and Greek Medicine*, p. 90 (Clarendon Press, 1922).

to Thrace, and to Macedonia. He is reported to have died at Larissa, having attained a great age.

Instruction in Nursing Duties.

His instructions to his disciples on the cleansing of the hands, the care of the nails which 'should be neither longer nor shorter than the points of the fingers', the use of boiled water or wine in the cleansing and dressing of wounds, and in the detail of all that we now call 'nursing technique' show that the patients were nursed intelligently; but he makes no mention of women nurses as such. Was this the work of the temple attendants and priestesses or were all intelligent women of that age expected to nurse the members of their families and their households when the need arose? The latter seems the most probable, and it may have been so taken for granted by the men who wrote history that they did not consider it necessary to record such work, for after all, illness is such an everyday occurrence.

Hippocratic Literature.

The books attributed to Hippocrates include the Aphorisms, which are a kind of clinical jottings, numbering about 420 in all, the Prognostics, consisting of 47 chapters, treatises on Diet in Acute Diseases, Wounds of the Head, Dislocations, Fractures and Ulcers, and the Epidemic Diseases. The Prognostics are based on thorough observations of the patient's condition, including posture, colour and peculiarities of the skin and mucous membranes, facial appearance, pulse, temperature and respiration, excreta, localised pains, the shape and movements of the thorax and abdomen, and the movements of the limbs, including those indefinite and purposeless movements of clutching at the air and picking at the bedclothes which are associated with a low, muttering delirium; and there is the well-known clinical picture to which the term 'facies Hippocratica' has ever since been applied. The patient's temperature was taken by placing the hand on the skin, and the condition of his heart and lungs

F   65

ascertained by closely pressing the ear against the patient's thorax.

In the treatise on Fractures, explicit instructions are given with regard to the application of bandages, from which one might quote the following:

'There are two views of bandaging, that which regards it whilst doing, and that which regards it when done. It should be done quickly, without pain, with ease and with elegance; quickly, by dispatching the work; without pain, by being readily done; with ease by being prepared for everything; and with elegance that it may be agreeable to the sight. By what mode of training these accomplishments are to be acquired has been stated. When done it should fit well and neatly.'

'The bandages should be clean, light, soft and thin. One should practise rolling with both hands together and with either separately. One should choose a suitable bandage according to the breadth and thickness of the part.'[1]

Then follow many details with regard to the application of bandages for special purposes.

With regard to the general conduct of physicians there is a Book of Decorum attributed to Hippocrates, although many authorities do not consider this to be his work. An extract from that is translated thus:

'Let one of your pupils be left in charge to carry out instructions without unpleasantness, and to administer the treatment. Choose out one who has already been admitted into the mysteries of the art, so as to add anything that is necessary and to give treatment with safety. He is there also to prevent those things escaping notice that happen in the intervals between visits.' (Translation by W. H. S. Jones.)

The standards of personal conduct set by Hippocrates for his followers was extremely high, but pre-eminent among the ethical writings attributed to him is the famous Oath, which was taken

[1] *Genuine Works of Hippocrates*, translated by Francis Adams, published 1849.

66

by every physician upon qualifying, and which is still adopted as the standard of medical conduct. The following is the translation of the Hippocratic Oath given by Dr Charles Singer in his *Greek Biology and Greek Medicine* (Clarendon Press, 1932).

'I swear by Apollo the healer, and Æsculapius and Hygieia, and All-heal (Panacea) and all the gods and goddesses . . . that, according to my ability and judgement, I will keep this oath and this stipulation —to reckon him who taught me this Art as dear to me as those who bore me, . . . to look upon his offspring as my own brothers, and to teach them this Art, if they would learn it, without fee or stipulation. By precept, lecture, and all other modes of instruction, I will impart a knowledge of the Art to my own sons, and those of my teacher, and to disciples bound to me by a stipulation and oath according to the Law of Medicine; but to none other. I will follow that system of regimen which, according to my ability and judgement, I consider for the benefit of my patients, and abstain from whatever is deleterious and mischievous. I will give no deadly medicine to any one if asked, nor suggest any such counsel; nor will I aid a woman to procure an abortion. With purity and holiness I will pass my life and practise my Art. . . . Into whatsoever houses I enter, I will go there for the benefit of the sick, and will abstain from every act of mischief and corruption; and above all from seduction. . . . Whatever in my professional practice—or even not in connection with it—I see or hear in the lives of men which ought not to be spoken of abroad, I will not divulge, deeming that on such matters we should be silent. While I keep this Oath unviolated, may it be granted me to enjoy life and the practice of the Art, always respected among men; but should I break or violate this Oath, may the reverse be my lot.'

This, then, was the state and standard of curative work in Greece in the fourth century B.C.; and towards the end of this century there began to flourish the great Medical School of Alexandria.

67

CHAPTER IX

THE SCHOOL OF ALEXANDRIA

Decline of Athens—Foundation of Alexandria—Anatomical research— Alexandria the great centre of pre-Christian learning—Waning of Alexandrian power

Decline of Athens.

IN the fifth century B.C. Athens easily held the supremacy in the science and art of medicine, as in all other branches of learning; but after the war with Sparta, which began its downfall, one of the most deadly epidemics recorded in history raged in and around Athens. This was about 430 B.C. when Hippocrates was about 30 years of age, and yet he appears not to have known about it, although Thucydides wrote a most lucid description of it; having himself had the disease and recovered. It is known in history as the great plague of Athens, and authorities differ in assuming it to have been anthrax, typhus, or malignant scarlet fever. Whatever the malady was, its occurrence hastened the waning of Athens as a centre of learning at that time; and with the consolidation of the Roman Empire Athens lost her independence as a city state.

Foundation of Alexandria.

In the fourth century B.C. Alexander of Macedonia, after having subdued Egypt and Persia, founded the city of Alexandria in Egypt. For a short time he reigned as Pharaoh, and was succeeded by one of his generals—Ptolemy I.—who founded the great school of Alexandria in 331 B.C. This was established in cloisters adjoining the palace, and was, in effect, the first univer-

68

sity in the world. It was dedicated to the services of the Muses and was therefore called a Museum. It became the centre of Greek learning although it was in Egypt, and it exercised a great influence upon medical development of that age. The school contained libraries, laboratories and clinics; and the fresh, eager intellect of the Greek plunged into the traditional learning of the Egyptian, and emerged with much that was valueless as well as with stores of precious knowledge. The possibility of intellectual progress apart from religion had not as yet been foreseen; but this school was religious only in form, and, although its scientific scintillations lasted little more than a century, its students and learned professors have influenced educational bodies and their pupils ever since. It was here that Euclid enunciated his theorems, that Eratosthenes calculated the size of the earth to within fifty miles of the figure given by twentieth century scientists, Hero devised the first steam engine, Archimedes formulated the law we all learnt by his name in our schooldays, Apollonius worked out conic sections, and Hipparchus marked out the stars in order to check their changes. All these were among the galaxy of Alexandria, and it was the Alexandrian Medical School from whence came the beginnings of scientific anatomy.

Anatomical Research.

Herophilus and Erasistratus were the originators of dissection at this centre. They probably derived their medical knowledge from Greece, not from Egypt, and the Egyptian environment stimulated them to make the enquiries that led to their discoveries; for they not only consolidated the work already done on skeletal anatomy but they investigated the nervous system and distinguished sensory and motor nerves, although they confused the latter with tendons. Herophilus described the fourth ventricle of the brain, and many other specialised structures in the body. He recognised the brain as the centre of the nervous system and the seat of intelligence. He counted the pulse, and noted its variations in rate and rhythm. Erasistratus observed that every organ had a threefold system of vessels—arteries, veins and nerves—but he thought that minute divisions of these were plaited together to form tissues. He considered that the chief cause of disease was excess of blood—plethora—and therefore blood-letting became an habitual treatment, although neither he nor Herophilus favoured it. They considered that purgation and enemata had the same effect as venesection, in that these treatments decreased blood pressure. They prescribed fasting and abstinence, together with mild laxatives, barley water and vapour baths.

The stories told of Herophilus—the greatest of the Alexandrian anatomists—are appalling in their account of the callous and inhuman cruelty of his search after knowledge. It is said that he bought slaves in the market place for living dissection in his laboratories, and that he vivisected condemned criminals. Small wonder that the study of anatomy was opposed by other sections of research workers, who turned their attention to discovering the nature and uses of drugs.

Erasistratus complained that very few physicians of his time were interested in hygiene, so he wrote a treatise on the subject which was intended to show that hygiene was a means of substituting prevention for cure, and that health consisted in balance and stability of function.

Alexandria, the Great Centre of Pre-Christian Learning.

The commingling of cultures which took place during the Ptolemaic period is of great importance in this history, since it forms the connecting link between the old Egyptian and the new European civilisations. All the learning of the known world found its centre in Alexandria; and in the third century B.C. its medicine was introduced into Mesopotamia, and thence into Syria on the one side and Arabia on the other. It was also the greatest trade centre in the world during the four centuries before Christ. It lay on a strip of flat, sandy land that separated Lake Mareotis from the Mediterranean. On the one side was the lake harbour connected with the Nile, and on the other were two harbours sheltered from the open sea by the long and narrow island of Pharos—a magnificent position for commerce. The great library of Alexandria was the wonder of the world. If any stranger brought an unknown book into Egypt he had to have it copied for the collection, so a large number of copyists were kept continually engaged, and the library became encyclopædic.

Alexandrian scholars made a Greek version of the Old Testament for the benefit of Alexandrian Jews in the third century B.C. The sixty manuscripts of the Hippocratic Collection were brought together and edited by a group of Alexandrian scholars at the request of the reigning Ptolemy. But from this time until the time of Celsus in the first century A.D.—a matter of some 400 years—there are no new medical writings to hand. Consequently, the only information we possess of the Alexandrian period is what we are able to gather from the writings of Celsus and his successors, Oribasius, and Paul of Egina.

The library is said to have contained 700,000 rolls of manuscript, most of which are now lost, although their precise fate is unknown. Neglect, repeated religious riots and the accidents of war all contributed to their destruction. After the burning of Alexandria by Cæsar, Mark Antony is said to have given Cleopatra 200,000 rolls for the great school of Pergamum in Asia Minor, which rivalled the Alexandrian school, and which at that time seemed to be a refuge for the crashing cultures of the eastern Mediterranean. And under its princes Greek art and learning flourished again for a time.

Waning of Alexandrian Power.

The study of medicine flagged and reached a state of stagnation long before the other sciences began to languish. With the absorption of Egypt into the Roman Empire, about 30 B.C., there seemed to be a dearth of originality in any studies; and although the Alexandrian school continued its existence for several centuries after this, intellectually it was too subordinate to Rome to be of any power in the scientific world. From the time of Galen —second century A.D.—until the appearance of Vesalius in the sixteenth century, all progress was arrested, and the relaxation of intellectual fervour which followed the consolidation of the Roman Empire and the spread of Christianity led to a revival of miraculous medicine. This rapidly gained in strength and popularity, and the combination of faith healing and mysticism induced a serious decay in rational curative work. By the fourth century A.D. the great library had completely disappeared, and Alexandria was finally sacked by the Arabs under the Caliph Omar ben Khattan in A.D. 640.

During the previous century Justinian had closed the school at Athens, and, about the time that the Alexandrian school came to an end, Leo the Isaurian—a usurper Emperor—closed the Academy at Constantinople (Byzantium), thus completing the plunge of Europe into the 'dark ages'; through which the cure of disease once more passed into the hands of medicine-men and priest-physicians, the former practising magic for the most part, and the latter disdaining the aid of science and relying on faith to abolish disease and death from off the face of the earth.

CHAPTER X

PERSIA

Persian literature and religion—Persian medicine—Fees for medical attention—Later history of Persian medicine

Persian Literature and Religion.

AFTER Cyrus the Great had conquered Babylonia in the sixth century B.C., the Persians became the leaders in all affairs of the civilised world from India to the Mediterranean. They conquered and held Egypt for a time. The knowledge we have of their medical work is derived from the Zend Avesta, a collection of the teachings ascribed to Zoroaster, who founded a religion of Aryan origin which can be traced back to the Indo-Iranian people before they split up into Hindus and Persians. We know nothing of the age in which Zoroaster lived. Some authorities contend that he was contemporary with Buddha and Confucius (sixth century B.C.), others that he lived as long ago as 1000 B.C.; but we do not know the place of his birth or his exact nationality. The religion he taught was a monotheistic one. The heaven-deity was Ahura Mazda, or Ormuzd, the maker and upholder of the universe, the god of light, order, truth and purity, against whom were pitted all the forces of Ahriman, who was the personification of wickedness. The struggle, however, was not to be an eternal one, for eventually good would overcome and exterminate evil. This teaching became exceedingly popular, and even at the time of Constantine the Great—nearly a thousand years later—it was the only serious rival of Christianity; but it is no longer an important influence in human affairs. The last surviving Zoroastrians are the Parsees of India, who preserve

73

very carefully all that remains of the Zend Avesta. This literature is said to have consisted of twenty-one books, containing no less than 2,000,000 stanzas, and to have been written on 1,200 cowhides.

Persian Medicine.

Pliny declares that the religion of the Persians was founded on their medicine—rather a reversal of the usual order of things. We find that their medicine somewhat resembled that of the Babylonians with regard to the demonic origin of disease and the exorcism of the evil spirits; although taken as a whole, it bore a closer analogy to that of the Hindus. If we are to accept the authority of the Zend Avesta as reliable it would seem that the art of medicine reached much the same level of culture in Persia as that of Egypt at the time that the Ebers Papyrus was compiled. The only complete book of the Zend Avesta which has survived to this day is the nineteenth, a code of purification known as the Vendidâd, or 'Law against Demons'. This also fixes the amount of medical fees, as did the Code of Hammurabi, and it refers to three classes of physicians—knife-doctors, herb-doctors, and word-doctors—probably surgeons, physicians and magicians. Thrita, the divine physician of Persia, represented all three, for from Kshathra-Vairya, the god of metals, he was given a knife, the point and base of which was set in pure gold, from Ormuzd he obtained the 10,000 herbs that grew around the tree of everlasting life, and his divine nature enabled him to wage successful warfare against the disease demons of Persia, of whom there were 99,999, all created by the evil eye of Ahriman. Thrita was really a Vedic personage—the counterpart of Dhanwantari—and all Persian physicians were exhorted to follow in his footsteps, and to fight valiantly against the demons of impurity and disease.

One or two ideas that were new to Asiatic medicine were added—for example, it was held that the touching of a corpse produced a special contamination, and this belief naturally interfered with the study of anatomy. Surgery seems to have been left severely alone in spite of the gift from the god of metals; and there were no physicians of importance among the Persians. The Persian kings entrusted themselves neither to their own countrymen nor to the Chaldeans, and both King Darius I. and King Cyrus were obliged to send for Egyptian physicians when needing treatment—the former for an injured ankle, and the latter for an ophthalmic condition.

Fees for Medical Attention.

These, as arranged in the Vendidâd, varied with the rank and wealth of the patient, as did those of the Babylonians. A priest was expected to give no return but his blessing; the head of a house, village, or town gave the price of an ox of varying value according to the means at his command; whilst the lord of a province gave the price of a chariot and four. The physician must also treat animals, and his fee for this was the price of the animal next in rank—the dog ranked the highest and the sheep the lowest on this scale.

Later History of Persian Medicine.

The Persian link with modern medical development was forged in later centuries when European learning was meeting with such opposition from the Christian churches—in the fifth century A.D. The Persians then gave shelter to the medical knowledge of the Greeks, and to classical culture as a whole. They handed it back to the conquering Arabs, who in due course passed it back to our ancestors.

In A.D. 570 Mohammed was born at Mecca in Arabia. His teachings gave rise to yet another great monotheistic religion—Islam. This was pitted against the corrupted Christianity and the decaying Zoroastrianism of the seventh century; and in the Islamic Empire there then arose great teaching schools and hospitals, of which more will be told in a later chapter.

CHAPTER XI

ROME

General history—Roman religion—Social and economic conditions—Introduction of Greek medicine—The height of Roman power—Lay hospitals—Hygiene and military hospital organisation—Closing of Pagan hospitals in Roman Europe

Origin of Rome and the Romans.

ROME was an empire that was made through a republic, and it differed profoundly in its nature from those that came into being as a result of the victorious conquests of great leaders such as Sargon, Cyrus, and Alexander. Money was becoming a power, and when in the wrong hands, a danger in human affairs.

The Romans were a blend of Etruscans—who on being driven out of Greece, Asia Minor and the Ægean islands had come into Italy by sea—and Umbrians, Sabines and Dorians who had come down into the Italian peninsula from the north. They inhabited the whole of Italy above the Tiber, upon one part of which there was a ford. This ford formed a trading centre with the Latin races who occupied the territory south of the Tiber. On the seven hills near-by small settlements grew up, which later amalgamated into one city; and this was the beginning of Rome.

Northern Italy was the scene of extensive invasions by the Gauls, who took and sacked Rome in 390 B.C.; but a century later Rome commanded all central Italy. In constitution it was a democracy governed by a Senate, and there were two great classes—patrician and plebeian.

Alexander's empire was breaking up at this time, and many

76

delectable provinces were in a comparatively vulnerable state. The Roman character was warlike, and showed a combination of sagacity and aggressive selfishness. There followed the barbarous Punic wars ending with the fall and sack of Carthage; and Corinth also fell to the Romans in the same year—146 B.C. The prisoners of war were made slaves, cities were burned and the ruins were ploughed over to express the finality of their destruction.

Roman Religion, and Social Economic Conditions.

The spirit of the Roman was hard and ungracious, and the taxation levied upon citizen and conquered foe alike was exorbitant and pitiless. The patricians were haughty and rather merciless, and the Empire itself was founded upon harshly driven slavery. Rome was the land of the soldier, the peasant, and the small trader, without arts, literature or philosophies of its own. It had gods, but they were unloving and unloved deities —practical rather than idealistic. A fertile earth-goddess was the greatest, and the gods were nearly all nature gods, patrons of woods and fountains, corn and fruits. There was Mars for war, Neptune for a voyage, and Mercury for good fortune. They were worshipped with an inflexibly rigid ritual, and prayer arose from no sense of sin. As Cicero—consul in 63 B.C.—says, it was not to help the Romans to be good, it was a bargain with a competent deity for material benefits. In order that, in sickness, there might be no mistake by this deity regarding the organ to be repaired, votive offerings were made in the form of limbs, eyes, ears, or internal organs modelled in terra-cotta. In a home it was the father who prescribed in illness and dispensed the herbals and spices. The master treated the slaves when sick, but the nursing was the duty of the mistress of the household, and there is a good deal of evidence that Roman women *did* play an important part in the tending of the sick, both at this time and later. Women held an honourable place, not only in the home but in public life—the wife stood by the husband in all great affairs, as did Cornelia by Cæsar, and there was one law of sex honour for both men and women. There were great extravagances in dress and adornment, but that is so in all very wealthy societies.

Gladitorial shows had been initiated in 240 B.C., and had become the chief and most popular form of amusement; but the Romans had still no organised medicine. Pliny states that for 600 years Rome had done without physicians, it was considered a new-fangled calling and a canker in the State; and yet, in all the wars and pestilences that involved Rome her need must have been great.

Introduction of Greek Medicine.

Romans had been wont to travel to Epidauros when special treatment was needed, and the story goes that a severe pestilence occurred in 291 B.C. The Sibylline books and the Delphic oracle were consulted, but the pestilence still proved beyond human skill. Special sacred serpents had been imported from Epidauros, and whilst sailing up the Tiber one of these Æsculapian serpents sprang overboard and swam to an island. This was taken as an augury and a temple to Æsculapius was built on the site—and *that* is how Greek medicine came to Rome! For centuries afterwards, if a master refused to treat his sick slave the latter could go to the temple on the island, and if he was cured he became free. A Christian church dedicated to St Bartholomew was built on the site of this temple in the ninth century A.D., and it is still in existence.

After the fall of Carthage and Corinth the entire aspect of Roman medicine was changed by the advent of Greek science. Roman youths began to frequent the lecture halls of Athens, and Greeks were engaged as tutors to the sons of the wealthy; but Greek medicine was accepted by the upper classes only. Many of the Greek physicians were slaves—taken in war—and were the property of their less cultured masters.

78

The Height of Roman Power.

The zenith of the Roman Empire was reached during the first 200 years after the birth of Christ, but this period must be considered pre-Christian to all intents and purposes, for Rome was still pagan. These were centuries of spending rather than of creating; it was an age of road building, architecture and trade. The rich became richer and the poor more oppressed. There was much feasting, and very ostentatious forms of social entertainment; and the most remote countries in the ancient world were ransacked to supply the pomp of Rome. Furs, carpets, amber and silk found their way into the Roman warehouses.

Legislation improved somewhat, and laws were passed which protected slaves from extreme cruelty and forbade the selling of them for gladiatorial shows. Great and luxurious baths were built, some of which showed similitude to the Æsculapian temples. Of those built by the Romans in Britain the one at Bath in Somerset—the ancient Aquæ Sulis—shows that similarity quite well with regard to its position in such a healthy spot, its mineral springs, the access of sunshine and fresh air, and the deep recesses between the supporting pillars of the colonnade. The pool itself is 83 by 40 feet, lined at the bottom with Roman lead—and Bath is to this day a highly valued British spa.

Lay Hospitals.

There were lay institutions in Rome and Pompeii known as valetudinaria, supposed to have been built specially for the reception and treatment of sick slaves; but there is evidence that they were open also to the wealthy. Seneca makes reference to them, and in his 27th epistle he says, 'Let us discuss our common woe as if we lay together in the same valetudinarium.' That does not suggest that only slaves were treated. These institutions were supported mainly, but not entirely, by public funds. One of them at Pompeii was established for his own patients by a private physician, and was, in fact, a sort of 'nursing home'. But phy-

79

sicians were not of much account in Rome, although they seem to have accompanied armies in warfare.

None but citizens could serve in the Roman legions, and Cæsar's grant of citizenship to all physicians practising in Rome may have been the preliminary to the establishment of an army medical service. Soldiers appear to have been instructed in first aid, and each carried bandages and perhaps other appliances with him; for we are told, by Livy, that on one occasion a large number of soldiers bandaged various parts of their bodies and pretended they were wounded in order to avoid serving under an unpopular leader.

Livy also informs us that the wounded, when brought home, were cared for in the houses of the great, and that the Fabian family made themselves especially popular by their zeal in this work. That would infer that ladies of rank opened their houses as voluntary hospitals much as they did during the Great War of this century.

Hygiene, and Military Hospital Organisation.

Rome's greatest legacy to the medical world was, undoubtedly, her hygiene and her organised hospital system. The latter was definitely of military origin, and its general plan has been followed through all the ages since that time.

During the long campaigns permanent camp hospitals were built; and they were constructed after the plan of the valetudinaria. Excavations are revealing these. The remains of a very old one have been uncovered at Deutsch-Altenburg, about 40 kilometres from Vienna. The plan of these hospitals can best be traced in the one unearthed at Neuse (Novæsium) near Düsseldorf. This was in a fortress camp established by Tiberius on the Roman road to Cologne, and its beautifully designed hospital was arranged on a corridor plan. There were 36 wards for the sick, the larger ones accommodating 5 to 6 patients, the entrances and exits were planned to avoid draughts, and the rooms opened into quiet corridors and quadrangles. The Romans obviously did not favour the housing of the sick and wounded in large wards for 20 or more patients; and these small wards must have been a distinct advantage in the prevention of the spread of infection.

Instruments such as sounds and bronze needles were found. There was a large refectory in the centre of the building, and an administrative block at one end, including staff kitchens, apothecaries' shop, and rooms, maybe, for doctors and attendants; and there was also an *iatreium*—a sort of surgery or consulting room. Records that have been discovered show that there were strict rules for cleanliness, purification, nursing and good cooking. Near by there were large bathing houses and other sanitary provisions, and there are also traces of a central heating apparatus. In the completeness of its departments it may be taken as an example of the finest type of a first-century hospital. In the medical care of her army Rome spared no expense either in preserving the health of her troops or in curing the wounded.

Sir Clifford Allbutt in his *Greek Medicine in Rome* says, 'With the story of these Roman hospitals before us, and the default of any such institutions for the most part of a millennium of Christianity in Europe, we should be modest in our assumption that the hospital is the fruit of the Christian religion.'

With regard to hygiene, the water supplies and drainage systems of Rome show a marvel of engineering efficiency. Fourteen great aqueducts supplied the city with 200 million gallons of water daily. The plumbing reached a high degree of excellence, as the jointed pipes which remain to this day will show.

The drainage systems dealt with surface water as well as with sewage, and the large quantities of water continually flowing from the many luxurious baths and street fountains made this arrangement possible without insanitary or objectionable results. All this waste flowed into the Tiber.

Closing of Pagan Hospitals in Roman Europe.

All the iatreia, Æsculapieia and valetudinaria were closed by the decree of Constantine the Great in A.D. 335. He was the first Christian emperor of Rome, and he made Christianity the State religion. His decree commanded the closing of all pagan institutions, whether for worship, learning, or for care of the sick. And then progress stops. All the apparently enduring advances of Greece and Rome, both intellectually and materially, were broken and almost obliterated, as far as Europe was concerned, by the theological hatred of everything pagan. It is the eternal tendency of the fanatic to destroy existing organisations, because some factors in their aims and administration arouse his strong disapproval, without pausing to consider the tragedy of the hiatus that must follow before organisations more to his liking can come into operation. It has been argued that the pagan hospitals did not really amount to much, either in number or repute; but excavations and remains tell a different story; and if an Imperial decree was necessary for their abolition surely their work and influence must have been fairly extensive.

We shall deal in the next section with the efforts made to establish Christian hospitals, and the various vicissitudes through which they passed ere they reached the standard of humane and scientific efficiency of which we of this age are so justly proud.

82

Part II : A Vocation

CHAPTER I

THE INFLUENCE OF THE EARLY CHRISTIAN CHURCH

Rome in the early centuries A.D.—*Social and economic conditions— Pagan religions of Rome—Sports and entertainments—First persecutions of the Christians—The Emperor Nero—Later persecutions—Official recognition of Christianity—Formulation of Creeds—Christianity the State religion of Rome—Christian care of the sick—Women workers— End of non-Christian hospitals in the Roman Empire*

SINCE Christianity is the most powerful factor that has influenced the development of the nursing systems of this era in practically every country in the world, it may be well to devote some little time and thought to the conditions under which the great faith struggled for its very existence during the early centuries after the death of Christ. During this troublous period, and until it was itself organised, it could do little in organising the care of the sick.

Rome in the Early Centuries A.D.

At the beginning of the Christian era, as we have seen, two main types of pagan hospitals existed in the Roman Empire — the temple-hospitals of Æsculapius and the military valetudinaria. In the former, the spirit of Hippocrates still lived, though, being Romanised, it had become somewhat hard and materialistic, and the scientific advances of the Alexandrian School were, to a certain extent, overlaid with sorcery and superstition. The valetudinaria were utilitarian rather than philanthropic. Soldiers were valuable to the State and slaves were the property of their masters. Only those who were curable were considered worthy of

85

the trouble of extensive medical care, and many of those who were hopelessly ill received rather scant attention in the pagan institutions. This does not infer that there was *no* compassionate nursing of the sick in pre-Christian Rome, for nobility of mind and kindness of heart is often quite independent of creeds, and is to be met with in many unexpected situations.

For three hundred years after the death of Christ Rome remained, at least officially, pagan; although many of the educated people had become sceptical about the old gods and the myths and ceremonies that surrounded them. The republic was changing into a monarchy. The emperors were claiming to rule by divine right, and the magnificent and awe-inspiring etiquette of the court was redolent of the Pharaohs and of some of the Eastern monarchs; but the worship of the Cæsar made no appeal to the emotions, nor had it any moral value. It conveyed no spiritual message either of hope or of fear, or of a future life beyond the grave; and yet suicide was common, especially among the upper classes, and no one questioned another's right to leave this world if it pleased him to do so.

Social and Economic Conditions.

With regard to social life and manners, there were remarkable improvements under the Flavine and Antonine Cæsars. There was increasing kindness and charity, and the weak and infirm were better treated. Large sums of public money were used for the maintenance of poor children and orphans, and the education of the poor was encouraged by free schools which Vespasian and some of his successors founded. Wealthy citizens built beautiful baths and temples for the benefit of all classes.

Marriages by civil contract were easily made, and as easily broken. There were many high-born women who counted the years of their age by the number of their husbands, but the maternal instinct seems to have been at a very low ebb, for infanticide was a general practice. The married state was, however, regarded as desirable. Laws were made to encourage marriage and to discourage celibacy; and no active careers were opened to unmarried women except as priestesses and vestal virgins in the pagan temples.

Pagan Religions of Rome.

The non-Christian religions of Rome in the early centuries of this era included Stoicism and the Greek mysteries. The former —preached especially by Seneca—urged men to forgive injuries, and to 'bear and forbear'. It emphasised human brotherhood, and expressed a humble but unfailing reliance on a Divine Providence. However, this teaching influenced the educated classes only, the masses were more attracted by the 'mysteries'—the chief of which were the Orphic, which centred in the worship of Dionysius, a god of trees and vines. The worshippers met by night on a lonely mountain peak, and with torches in their hands they danced wildly to the music of flutes and cymbals, in a state of religious frenzy. Another series were the Eleusinian mysteries, woven around the myth of Demeter and Persephone. Some of the Oriental religions also had their followers in Rome, but none of these satisfied the deepest and most spiritual needs of man as completely as Christianity could do.

Sports and Entertainments.

For sport and amusement the Olympic games and contests had been replaced, to a very great extent, by the barbarous gladiatorial shows. These had originated in the Forum of Rome in 264 B.C., when Marcus and Decius Brutus included among the funeral rites of their dead father a gladiatorial contest between three couples. This set the fashion in Rome, and very soon gladiators were fighting by the hundred. It became the custom to buy and train slaves for these contests, and slaves who had offended their masters were sent to the gladiatorial schools to be prepared for the arena.

In the next few centuries the number and extent of these shows grew to enormous proportions. Wars were frequent, and they supplied a number of captives, who came with their characteristic national weapons, and provided the vast Roman audiences with a new thrill when they were set to fight for their lives in the arena. Criminals of the lowest classes were used also, and these contests became an extensive organisation of murder for sport. Thousands of unfortunate human beings were butchered to make a 'Roman holiday'.

The first century A.D. was a time of comparative peace, and there was a dearth of war prisoners to provide material for these contests. The shows were becoming too tame for the public taste, so wild animals were introduced, especially lions, tigers and bears. The character of the entertainments became infinitely more ferocious and inhuman, with a more certain issue, for what chance of survival had a *man* in such a contest? And then came the first extensive persecution of the Christians—under the Emperor Nero.

First Persecutions of the Christians.

It may be a cause for wonder why Christianity, of all the religions the world had ever known, should have aroused such a spirit of virulent and intolerant persecution in its opponents. In the first century after the death of Christ the greater number of His followers were the poor and lowly ones of earth. Christianity brought a message of hope to the oppressed, and a promise of a future life which would amply compensate for all the sufferings a human being could possibly be called upon to endure in the flesh; its teachings engendered kindness, long-suffering, truth and honesty, and accounted spiritual things of far greater value than material gain or advancement. Why, then, should it have aroused pagan opposition so strongly? It was not threatening pagan power at that time. It is easier to understand the persecutions of the third and early fourth centuries, for reasons that will be given later.

The Emperor Nero.

A possible explanation of this first organised persecution may be found in the character, ambition and crimes of one man—the Emperor Nero. That he had an artistic temperament all historians will agree. He visualised a new Rome, with wide straight streets instead of narrow alleys, and houses of good stone in place of the wooden hovels—but how get rid of the present buildings that filled his æsthetic soul with disgust? Rome needed a fire to cleanse her festering slums, and then, in place of the dirty, congested areas, he might build the most beautiful city the world had ever known!

The fire broke out on the night of 19th July, A.D. 64. The city watchmen were all off duty. With whose permission? They were a military corps, and desertion would have meant death. Men were seen to go with lighted torches from different quarters to set the city on fire. Soldiers dispatched to the scene were said to have kindled instead of extinguished the flames—which raged for six days and seven nights.

To the Christians it must have seemed that St Peter's prophecy was coming true. In his last epistle he described the 'Day of the Lord'—'In the which the heavens shall pass away with a great noise, and the elements shall melt with fervent heat, the earth also and the works that are therein shall be burnt up.'

Many Christians would have seen the fulfilment of that prophecy in the rolling clouds of smoke, and the fire which turned night into day. The calm and hopeful joy with which they awaited the expected second coming of Christ must have irritated the pagan priests, who later accused them of rejoicing in the sufferings of mankind. Many stories of Christian heroism, and of their help and encouragement to the stricken ones, are told in the history of that fire; but after it had died down there was rage in the heart of the populace as they sought to find the author of the calamity. Suspicion was pointing to the emperor himself, and in order to divert that, Nero realised that a scape-

89

goat must be found—and so the Christians were accused! Had they not sung songs of rejoicing even when the fire was raging at its fiercest? Their deeds of self-sacrificing heroism were forgotten, and Nero arose as the champion of justice, and condemned hundreds of them to die in the arena. His diabolical sense of humour found expression in the illumination of that spectacle— the Christians themselves were the torches.

But this persecution was not of long duration, for Nero himself committed suicide during the following year. It flared up again, intermittently, during the next two centuries, although there were periods of comparative peace and toleration of the new teaching; and then, under the emperors Decius and Diocletian, the persecutions reached their final height of severity, continuing with but few intermissions for eight years.

Later Persecutions.

The history of these persecutions is rather more complicated, for by this time the Christians were believed to be politically dangerous, breeders of riots and civil strife. Christianity challenged the divinity of the Cæsars, and other characteristic Roman institutions, as well as the worship of idols, and therefore it was considered to be a rebellious and disintegrating movement. The meetings of the faithful were often held in secret, and their Sacrament of Bread and Wine, with its mystical symbolism, was misunderstood. They were accused of cannibalism and other horrible rites, and they suffered the most appalling calumny. Referring to this new religion that was swaying the multitudes, the historian Tacitus says—'Christus, from whom the name of Christian had its origin, suffered the extreme penalty during the reign of Tiberius at the hands of one of our procurators, Pontius Pilatus. But this most mischievous superstition, though checked for the moment, again broke out, not only in Judea, the first source of the sedition, but even in Rome, the meeting place of all horrible and immoral practices from all quarters of the world.'[1]

[1] *Annals of Tacitus*, Book XV, Chapter 44, 4 (G. G. Ramsey's translation).

If Tacitus, with all his knowledge and culture, could have held such ideas of the Christians it is small wonder that the Roman rabble hated them, and applauded their condemnation by the Emperors.

The early Christians looked for the speedy coming of Christ and the end of the world, and therefore they did not seek temporal wealth or power. They were regarded as unsociable, as they did not appear at public feasts or entertainments, or join in the amusements of circus and amphitheatre, or send their children to the public schools. Strange stories were told of their sacrificial meal, and they were regarded as magicians who caused all kinds of disasters. Then again, they declined to support the 'official religion', and condemned it as sinful and idolatrous.

We know very little of the actual ceremonies of the Christians during the first few centuries. Creeds were not formulated, and there was wide variation in the beliefs held; but many of the followers of Christ undoubtedly carried His very spirit into their teaching and their lives. The very charges made against them show this, and the faith was spreading through all classes, for the general slackening of moral and intellectual fibre in the Roman Empire towards the end of the third century so dismayed the nobler-born citizens that they, too, turned to a creed that promised some stability to their ideals, gave them some hope of the ultimate triumph of human nature, and so restored their self-respect. The spread of Christianity among those of higher rank in the Empire made it a more formidable opponent of the idolatrous court.

Decius was the first emperor to organise official persecutions. His reign was rather a short one—he was defeated and killed in A.D. 251 during a raid by the Goths into Thrace—latterly Serbia and now Jugoslavia. Diocletian, who became emperor in A.D. 284, was the most fanatical of the persecutors. He reorganised the monarchy, abolished the last vestiges of republican constitution, and surrounded himself with an awe-inspiring etiquette and ceremonial. Christianity denied his claims. The test in the persecutions was that the Christians were required to offer sacrifices to the emperor. If they refused, their churches were demolished; and the punishment of death followed the holding of secret assemblies for the purpose of Christian worship. This was the great era of the Christian martyrs. It marked the crowning struggle of the old idea of the god-emperor against the already great and powerful organisa tion that denied his divinity.

Official Recognition of Christianity.

A few years later the Emperor Constantine succeeded to the throne, and reigned from A.D. 306 to 337; first as joint ruler, and then as sole monarch of the Roman Empire. The genius of Constantine, struggling to hold together the heaving and splitting vessel of the State, grasped the fact that even if Christianity was a rebellious and destructive force against pagan Rome, it was a great unifying power within its own community, and it provided the only hope of moral solidarity so necessary if the Empire was to hold together. Moreover, the faith was spreading to Persia and to Central Asia. Conscious of his own inadequacy as a unifying power, he turned to Christianity to supply the faith and the organisation that might prove to be the correlating factor so manifestly wanted at that time. In the fight against Maxentius at the Milvian Bridge on the outskirts of Rome in A.D. 312 he carried the Christian monogram on the shields and banners of his troops. He won a complete victory, and he claimed that the God of the Christians had fought for him.

In the following year he issued the 'Edict of Milan', which proclaimed the noble principle of religious toleration, and gave freedom to every man to choose the religion he deemed most suited to his needs; and the persecutions of the Christians were at an end. He publicly renounced all pretensions to divinity, re-organised his Empire and gave it a new constitution. He developed Byzantium as his new capital, calling it Constantinople. By its position on the Bosphorus, looking towards Asia, and commanding the entrance to the Black Sea and to the Mediterranean, it was a much better commercial centre than Rome; and later it became an important intellectual centre. Constantine laid it out with great magnificence of colonnaded streets, aqueducts, fine bridges and palatial buildings; and adorned it with treasures of art from Greece, Italy and the Near East.

Formulation of Creeds.

It was not until after Constantine had turned to Christianity that he appears to have realised the fierce dissensions of the theologians, who had become so agitated by tortuous and elusive arguments about the nature of God and Christ that the simple teachings of charity, service and brotherhood were almost obscured, although the spirit of these teachings did live and ennoble many lives. Constantine made a great effort to reconcile these differences into a uniform and harmonious teaching, and it was on his initiative that a general Council of the Church was held at Nicea in A.D. 325. Although he was not yet a baptized Christian—he was baptized on his deathbed in A.D. 337—he presided at this Council, the outcome of which was the formulation of the Nicene Creed.

Christianity the State Religion of Rome.

Christianity became the official or 'State' religion of Rome in A.D. 335, and by the fifth century Christendom was a greater and more enduring force than any Empire had ever been; and it had spread over a large part of Western Asia. Its authority was concentrated in the Bishop, or Patriarch, of Rome, who became the Pope; and with the fall of the Western Empire he took the ancient title of the quasi-divine Emperor—'Pontifex Maximus'. He became the ultimate censor and judge, being revered as the monarch of Christendom; and in this 'monarchy' was concentrated the 'unity of the Church in the whole world' for over 1,000 years. It made marriage a religious sacrament and opposed divorce. There came into being a Church organisation with a

93

beautiful and impressive ritual, and, though made up of scattered congregations, it was thought of as one Body of Christ, one people of God; and this ideal unity found expression in many ways. Christians upon a journey were always sure of a warm welcome and hospitality from their fellow disciples. Messengers and letters were sent freely from one church to another. Missionaries and evangelists went continually to those areas that were not yet Christian, and the gospels and apostolic epistles were widely circulated.

Christian Care of the Sick.

In no direction had the mighty influence of this idea of the common brotherhood of mankind shown itself so strongly as in the care of the sick, the destitute and the helpless. All the teachings of Christ stressed the brotherhood of man, and the duty of every human being to render, ungrudgingly, all the service in his power to his suffering or less fortunate neighbour, so that, from being merely a virtue, the compassionate care of the sick became a sacred and obligatory duty. By His Own actions in the healing of the sick, and by the parables in which He sought to show His disciples how they should live, He placed great emphasis, not only on the tending of the sick in their own households, but on the duty of His followers to seek out the sick strangers, and to minister unto them. No longer were such ministrations to be relegated to the slave or to the person of inferior rank—they were the duty of every Christian, and were to be limited only by the need of the sufferer.

Women Workers.

In the early Christian Church, teaching as it did the equality of all human beings, we find that women held Church office as deaconesses and men as deacons, and that the title 'diakonos', as used by St Paul, applies to men and women alike, both being ordained by a 'laying on of hands'.

Deaconesses appear to have ministered to the sick whenever

94

the need arose, in addition to carrying out their more ecclesiastical duties; and the first of these deaconesses to be mentioned by name in any records is Phœbe of Cenchrea, who lived about A.D. 60. St Paul refers to her in his Epistle to the Romans (chapter xvi) as a succourer of many, including himself. She is reputed to have journeyed to Rome—St Paul's reference to her is by way of being an introduction—and tradition credits her with having nursed in that city also.

Then Praxedis and Pudentiana, who were the daughters of a Roman senator named Pudens with whom St Paul is said to have lodged, are recorded as having ministered to martyrs in prison; but whether they gave spiritual ministration or attended to the physical needs of the martyrs is not clearly stated. Both these ladies were canonised. The church dedicated to St Praxedis is said to be the oldest in Rome, and within it is a well into which she is supposed to have flung a sponge wherewith she had mopped up the blood of many martyrs. Her relics are in this church, and she appears in art with a basin in one hand, and palms in the other. The baths of the original house of Pudens the senator have recently been discovered beneath the floor of the church. These can now be seen, and the visitor is shown, also, the oak water pipes which were those of the house.

It is extremely difficult to ascertain any definite histories or dates of Christian women who nursed the sick before the fourth century; but with the cessation of the persecutions and the official recognition and sanction of Christianity the work of women in the tending of the sick becomes more pronounced, and one can follow its continued course until the present day.

End of non-Christian Hospitals in the Roman Empire.

There were, as we have stated in a previous chapter, great military hospitals founded in many parts of the Roman Empire, and some account of these has already been given. But they were all pagan, as were the iatreia and Æsculapieia, and on that account they were all closed by the decree of Constantine in A.D.

95

335—the year in which he made Christianity the State religion of Rome. Before that time the Christians had had no freedom, or opportunity, to develop any curative work, and therefore the closing of all the existing institutions for the care of the sick left a very grevious void, not only in charitable work, but in medical science and intellectual research as a whole. This void constituted a very definite call for the services of Christian women, and a number of Roman ladies are mentioned as having devoted their lives to this work, some as deaconesses and others as entirely lay helpers; and many of these women were afterwards canonised.

CHAPTER II

FOURTH AND FIFTH CENTURY DEACONESSES AND LAY WORKERS

Formation and activities—Constantinople group: the Empress Helena, St Basil of Cæsarea, Macrina, Olympias, Nicarete, and Placilla—Roman group: Marcella, Fabiola, Paula, Blessilla and Eustochium—Syncletica of Alexandria

Formation and Activities.

THE origin and early history of the deaconesses is somewhat veiled in obscurity. In the 'Apostolic Constitutions' the deaconess, the widow, and the virgin are mentioned as distinct classes of workers; and yet it is provided that a deaconess shall be 'a pure virgin or a widow once married, faithful and worthy'. That would seem definitely to connect the three, for after all, widowhood and virginity are conditions of life, not offices or orders. From the many allusions to 'widows' it would seem that they were elderly recipients of the Church's charity, who gave what assistance they could in the various philanthropic activities of the Church. Deaconesses were mentioned as a recognised order in the Councils of Nicea (A.D. 325) and of Chalcedon (A.D. 451). There were definite references to them at many other Church councils, whose decrees sought to limit their activities. In the Eastern Church deaconesses were originally ordained simply to perform the offices of the Church in connection with the care of women; they were not priestesses in any sense of the word. Their chief duties were:

(1) To act as doorkeepers in the Church, receiving women as they entered, and conducting them to their allotted seats.

(2) To visit the women of the Church in their homes, and to minister to the needs of the sick and afflicted.

H   97

(3) To assist in the baptism of women, especially in connection with the anointing of the body, which always preceded immersion.

The deaconesses not only visited and tended the sick in their homes and, when necessary, received them into their own houses to be cared for, but they visited prisoners and gave them counsel, and carried messages for the clergy. In the Eastern Church the current oriental ideas made women missionaries necessary, and these orders of deaconesses spread into Asia Minor and Syria. In a lesser degree they extended into the west, according to some authorities, to Rome, Spain, Gaul, and even to Ireland. They were, however, never really popular in the Western Church, which disapproved of the ordination of women; and later, the abbess took the place of the deaconess.

The selection and control of the deaconesses was entirely in the hands of the bishops, and many rich and noble women were grateful for the privilege of entering these orders. At this period a deaconess might be married, widowed, or a virgin; if she so wished she might live in her own home, and she was not required to wear a special form of dress, except when taking office in the Church.

For much of our information concerning these women workers we are indebted to the writings of St Jerome, of Rome, St Basil, Bishop of Cæsarea in Cappadocia, and St John Chrysostom, Bishop of Constantinople. Some names and personalities stand out above their fellows, either because of their great wealth or rank, or because of special achievements. We may consider these ladies in two groups—the Empress Helena, Macrina, Olympias, Nicarete and Placilla from Constantinople and Cæsarea; and Marcella, Fabiola, and Paula and her two daughters—Blessilla and Eustochium—from Rome. Mention might also be made of one Alexandrian lady—Syncletica.

The Empress Helena.

The greater number of authorative writers state that Helena was a princess of Britain. She was a daughter of King Coilus, who held his sovereignty from the Romans and who built the first walls around the city of Colchester—the arms of this city still include a cross between four crowns, as a tribute to the great Empress. She married Constantius, then a soldier in the Roman army, and their son Constantine was born at York in A.D. 272. (Both H. G. Wells and Gibbon hold that she was the daughter of an innkeeper of Nish, in Serbia, and that Constantine was of illegitimate birth.) She was divorced in 292, but when her son became Emperor she received the title of 'Augusta', and was treated with great distinction.

At the age of 64 she was converted to Christianity, and in 325 she made her first pilgrimage to Jerusalem. She is said to have built two churches, one on the Mount of the Ascension and the other at Bethlehem, and to have founded the first Christian hospital at Jerusalem. A great many legends are told of her, the most famous being of the finding of the True Cross on Calvary, its hiding-place having been revealed to her in a vision during her pilgrimage. She died in Palestine in A.D. 328 whilst on her second pilgrimage at the age of 80, and her body was brought back to Constantinople for burial. She is accredited with having been associated with St Basil in the building of a great Christian hospital at Cæsarea, but the date given of the opening of this hospital is A.D. 369—over 40 years after her death.

St Basil of Cæsarea.

Basil was an aristocrat of Cappadocia, he was a brother of St Gregory and was one of the four Fathers of the Greek Church. With the aid of his sister Macrina, he founded a monastery in a very lovely spot on the banks of the river Iris, opposite to the convent over which Macrina ruled. Previously, monks had tended to build monasteries in unattractive places—in flat, treeless wastes of burning sand such as formed the home of Pachomius, the first known Christian monk.

St Basil suffered from frequent illnesses, and therefore he paid great attention to medicine, which he declared was the noblest of all professions. But he says that not all diseases are the outcome of natural causes, or even of vices and bad habits; some are sent directly from God as trials of faith, or as punishment for some forgotten sin, and the sufferer should by no means go to a physician, but bear patiently the chastening of the Lord till He sees fit to remove it. However, he did not let these theories prejudice his provision for the sick poor. He is the great 'hospital saint'; and the hospital which he built outside the walls of Cæsarea was described as 'one of the miracles of the world'. It was almost a city, with streets upon streets of well-built houses with rooms for every kind of sick and infirm person, who were entrusted to the care of deaconesses. It had dwellings for physicians and nurses, and for convalescent patients, and even schools and workshops for the care and instruction of foundlings, and of children who had been under the care of the monastery. It had a house of separation for lepers, and some authorities believe that the Order of St Lazarus, which flourished in the twelfth century, had its origin there. The hospital was called Basilias, after its distinguished founder, and this name was given to many other hospital foundations of that time.

Macrina.

This sister of St Basil and of St Gregory was brought up with great care by a pious and ascetic mother. When quite a young girl she was betrothed, but her fiancé died; and a short while after her bereavement she was ordained a deaconess. She was a friend of Olympias. Already the Christians had renounced such scientific medicine as was then available, and were accepting illness and disease as expressions of the will of God for the purification and perfection of His followers, and they were looking for miraculous cures as the outcome of their faith. In Butler's *Lives of the Saints* we are told that Macrina had a most painful cancer which was cured by a fragment of the True Cross, but that a black spot remained ever afterwards upon the part that had been affected.

She founded two monasteries upon her own estate at Thora, in Pontus, on the southern shores of the Black Sea. One was for men, and over this her brother Gregory of Nyssa ruled; but she herself ruled over the other for a time. She also founded a convent with her own fortune amid very beautiful scenery upon the opposite shore of the river Iris to St Basil's monastery. Here she gathered a community around her, and St Basil wrote their rule. St Basil died in 379, and a few months later Macrina became ill. St Gregory of Nyssa visited her, and he tells of finding her in a raging fever, lying on two boards, one for her bed and the other for her pillow.

She seems to have been the first to combine the office of deaconess with that of the head of a monastery. At that time the monastic idea was beginning to take shape in the minds of Christians as a means of breaking away from the satiating luxury and worldliness that characterised the Byzantine period of Roman history.

Olympias.

Olympias was born in A.D. 368. When a young and beautiful girl of 18 she married Nebridius, a prefect of Constantinople, who died 20 months after the marriage. Two years later she became a deaconess of an extremely ascetic type, and worked among the sick and poor for the rest of her life. She never allowed herself a bath, and she neglected her body in every conceivable way. The coarseness and shapelessness of her garments, 'surpassing that of the very beggars', drew forth a special commendation from St Chrysostom. We are told, in his letters, that she suffered severe sicknesses, which, considering her unhygienic mode of life, is not surprising. Later, she became a victim of all those diseases brought on by want of cleanliness and neglect of the ordinary rules of hygiene. One hopes that her patients were not expected to share in that asceticism. The neglect of personal appearance and of the common necessities of life, which St Chrysostom dwells upon with such admiration, was possibly her way of protesting against the reckless extravagance and luxury of her class.

She had a great power of organisation, and forty deaconesses are said to have lived a community life under her guidance.

Nicarete.

This lady was not a deaconess. She was a nobly-born virgin whom St Chrysostom urged in vain to accept ordination. She refused marriage, and voluntarily devoted her life to 'visiting nursing' and 'since she had a humane character, she also prepared a variety of remedies for the needs of the sick poor, and frequently cured patients who had derived no benefit from the skill of the physicians' (from *Ecclesiastical History*, Migne's Collection, Vol. 67).

Placilla.

She was the wife of the Emperor Theodosius, and she worked among the sick at Constantinople. In the 82nd vol. of the *Ecclesiastical History* we are told that 'she tended the bed-ridden with her own hands, taking hold of pots and tasting their broth and handing their bowls, breaking their bread and handing out vessels; washing their cups, and doing all those other things which are reckoned the work of slaves and handmaidens'. Two other deaconesses to whom St Chrysostom wrote several letters are Pentadia and Amprucla, but he makes no allusion to their care of the sick.

Marcella.

Marcella lost her husband in the seventh month of their marriage. She was the chief, and the leader, of a group of young matrons who had preserved their independent position and great wealth under the 'free marriage contract' then recognised in Rome; and she was renowned for her intellectual ability. In her early widowhood she meditated upon the lives of the ascetics of the east, and resolved to follow their example. We are told that thereafter she abstained from wine and from flesh foods, and never again spoke with any man alone. She had a following of many nobly-born virgins, who put themselves under her direction. This seems to have been the beginning of the 'conventual idea' in Rome. Her palace on the Aventine Hill was in the most exclusive part of Rome, and she received into it, not only her own followers, but also the sick and the destitute.

When the Goths, under Alaric, plundered Rome in A.D. 410 her house was entered, and she was scourged for failing to produce the treasures she had long since distributed among the poor. She escaped, and took refuge in St Paul's Church, outside the city walls, but she died from her injuries.

Fabiola.

She was a Roman lady who married a profligate husband. She divorced him and married again, also unhappily. Under the influence of Marcella she became a Christian, and made public confession in expiation of the sin of a second marriage, and, patrician though she was, she gave up her rank and wealth and spent the remainder of her life in ministering to the sick poor. She is credited with having built and opened the first Christian hospital in Rome in A.D. 390. St Jerome speaks of this as a 'nosocomium', that is, a house devoted entirely to the sick as distinct from the aged and poor. He says of Fabiola, 'How often did she carry the sick upon her own shoulders. How often did she wash the putrid matter from wounds another could not bear to look upon. With her own hands she prepared their food, and moistened with water the parched lips of the dying.' And again he says, 'There was hardly an institution that had not benefited by her charity, hardly a bedridden patient in Rome who had not felt her care, so that among the healthy poor many longed to be sick that they might experience her ministrations.'

She died in A.D. 399, and the 'society lead' which she had given to the nursing of the poor, developed, in later years, almost to a fanaticism. From Rome and Constantinople the movement spread all over Europe, and we read of saintly women not only tending the sick, but actually 'kissing the sores of their patients'.

Paula.

She was another patrician who was born in Rome about A.D. 347. She was a friend of Fabiola, and was one of the most highly gifted and learned women of her day. She became a widow at the age of 23. She was not at that time a Christian; but accompanied by her two daughters, she visited Marcella, from whom she received instruction, as a result of which they all three became Christians. Paula was a learned Hebrew scholar, and she assisted St Jerome in translating some of the books of the Old Testament; but she shared in the growing idea that there was merit in physical neglect. Blessilla died at an early age, after which Paula and Eustochium went on journeys through Syria, Egypt and Palestine. They built a monastery at Bethlehem, of which Eustochium became Abbess on the death of her mother in A.D. 404. She herself died in 419.

Paula is said to have founded a hospital at Jerusalem, and to have built hospices for pilgrims and the sick on the road to Bethlehem, 'that none should suffer for lack of a shelter on the road where Mary the Mother of Christ, found no refuge but a stable.' In one account of her we read that 'she was piteous to them that were sick, and comforted and served them right humbly; and gave them largely of such food as they asked. She was oft by them that were sick, and she laid the pillows aright and in point; and she rubbed their feet, and boiled water to wash them.'

Syncletica.

She was the sister of Pachomius, an Egyptian hermit who became a monk and founded many monasteries in Upper Egypt. She was born in Alexandria about A.D. 340. She was beautiful, but she refused all offers of marriage and founded a community under monastic rule. She is known as the 'Mother of Nuns', and she shares with Macrina the honour of having introduced a celibate conventual life for women.

104

CHAPTER III

DECLINE OF DEACONESSES, AND THE BEGINNINGS OF MONASTICISM

Decline of Orders of Deaconesses—The founding of Christian monasteries—The Order of St Benedict—Cassiodorus—Monastic Influence on medicine

WITH Christianity had come the conception that single women could hold positions of usefulness and responsibility; that was part of the Christian ideal of the brotherhood of man, which asserted the right of the individual to choose his or her own way of life, and which eventually cut at the very roots of the slavery that was so prevalent in all civilised countries. Nursing duties, however, were still not considered to be the prerogative of women. The available history of these centuries appears to show that a great share of the work was done by men, especially the priests and physicians, both as individuals and as members of religious, secular and military orders. But maybe the work of women was taken so much for granted that it was considered of insufficient importance for any definite record to be made of it. That may account for our dearth of information regarding their part of this work.

Decline of Orders of Deaconesses.

We have seen, at the end of the preceding chapter, that the Christian deaconesses were tending to become monastic. The Church issued many decrees that heralded their suppression as a Church Order. The first Council of Orange (in A.D. 441) enacts that deaconesses are, on no account, to be ordained; and

105

sixth century edicts forbade deaconesses to marry or to leave their Order for *any* reason; and after death their property was confiscated by the church or convent to which they belonged. The Synod of Orleans abolished them as a Church Order in A.D. 533 'by reason of the frailty of this sex'; but in spite of this, some women continued to be ordained in the Eastern provinces. After that time we hear very little of deaconesses, but they were, undoubtedly, the prototype of the nurse as we know her in modern times; and during all the centuries that have elapsed since the passing of these Orders, whenever there has been a wave of pure philanthropy, there has been some effort made to initiate another such order. Examples of this are the Order of Poor Clares and the Franciscan Tertiaries of the thirteenth century, the Orders of Vincent de Paul in the seventeenth, and of Pastor Fliedner in the nineteenth century; all of which have left their mark upon history. Others were comparatively short-lived— they were neither popular, nor thought to be desirable, by the clergy. As an example of the attitude of the Church in general we might consider the history of such a movement in the town of Wesel in Germany towards the end of the sixteenth century. A band of women called 'deaconesses' had been working amongst the poor, and nursing the sick, during a time of special need. The General Synod was asked, in 1581, to confirm the establishment of these deaconesses as a Church Order. They decided against it because of 'the various inconveniences which might arise from it; but in times of pestilence and other sickness, when any service is required among sick women which would be indelicate for deacons, they ought to attend to this through their wives, or others whose services it may be proper to engage.' (*Die Geschichte der Weiblichen Diakonie*, by Theodore Schäfer, Stuttgart, 1887.)

The Founding of Christian Monasteries.

The triumph of Christianity, in the fourth century, had not only freed Christians from the stimulus of persecution, but it had opened their doors to worldly habits and luxury hitherto unknown to them, and which made the practice of the higher ideals of the spirit almost impossible in the ordinary surroundings of family life. European morality needed spiritual uplift and character renewal rather than intellectual development. It was the realisation of this need that drove men into the uninhabited places and brought about the founding of the monasteries; and then the East grafted asceticism on to Christianity, teaching that matter was inherently evil, and that holiness could only be attained by withdrawal from the haunts of men. From India and Tibet came the teaching that pure mind, or soul, could be freed from the dominion of foul and corrupting materialism only by lonely contemplation; and Christianity has never completely recovered from that misconception. As a natural offspring of asceticism came celibacy, with its false conception of a higher personal purity.

The monasteries, however, gave shelter to a considerable amount of the learning of the age, and the cloistered monks and nuns rendered much service to humanity by keeping the lamp of true knowledge burning, even if somewhat dimly, within the exclusive walls of the great abbeys and priories that grew up during those centuries. With very few exceptions they were the only schools or colleges, and they seem to have done very much for architecture and for political organisation. They became the greatest single constructive force in Europe for over 1,000 years.

The Order of St Benedict.

In 529—the year that Justinian closed the school at Athens—Benedict founded the first cloister of the famous Order named after him on the site of an ancient temple to Apollo at Monte Cassino—a lonely and beautiful mountain in the midst of a great circle of majestic heights halfway between Rome and Naples; and this monastery became a great and powerful centre within the lifetime of its founder. Benedict discouraged solitary and leisurely austerity, and insisted that all his followers should spend eight hours of each day in hard work. Two of his most illustrious followers were Pope Gregory the Great—the first monk to become Pope—and Cassiodorus, who afterwards founded a monastery upon his own estates and set his community to work after the Benedictine fashion.

This was an age, not merely of war and devastation, but of famine and pestilences which swept the whole of Europe; and there was no effective sanitary organisation in any Christian country.

During the next few centuries Benedictine monasteries spread throughout Europe as centres of light; restoring, maintaining, and raising the standard of culture, preserving and multiplying books, and establishing a definite system for the care of the sick and poor. One of the rules of St Benedict required the abbot to provide, within the monastery, an infirmary for the ailing, and as a Christian duty to organise special care of them. The wording of the rule is as follows: 'The care of the sick is to be placed above and before every other duty, as if indeed Christ were being directly served by waiting upon them. It must be the peculiar care of the Abbot (or Abbess) to see that they suffer from no negligence. The Infirmarian must be thoroughly reliable, known for his piety, diligence, and solicitude for his charge.' Again he says, 'Let baths be provided for the sick as often as they need them.' This was in an age when abstinence from baths was considered a Christian virtue in those whose health was sound.

Cassiodorus.

Cassiodorus, who lived between A.D. 468 and 560, belonged to a patrician Syrian family that had settled in Italy. He had been the chief minister to the Ostrogoth Emperor, but after the overthrow of this monarchy and the great pestilence that preceded the barbaric rule of the Lombards he established a monastery at Scillace in Calabria. He was deeply influenced by St Benedict, and his rule also emphasised the care of the sick. 'I insist, brothers, that those who treat the health of the brethren who have come into the sacred places from the world, should fulfil their duties with exemplary piety. Let them be sad with others' suffering, sorrowful over others' dangers, sympathetic to the grief of those whom they have to care for, and always ready zealously to help others' misfortunes. Let them serve with sincere study to help those that are ailing, as becomes their knowledge of medicine, and let them look for their reward from Him Who compensates temporal work by eternal wages. Learn, therefore, the nature of herbs, and study diligently the way to combine their various species for human health; but do not place your entire hope on herbs, nor seek to restore health only by human counsels. Since medicine has been created by God, and since it is He Who gives back health and restores life, turn to Him.'

He appeared to foresee the coming loss of all learning, and of the ancient literature of the world, for he directed his brethren in the task of preserving and restoring valuable documents. He collected ancient MSS. and caused them to be copied. He wrote a history of the Gothic kings, a book on grammar, and a series of books on the arts. He made sundials, water-clocks and similar apparatus—a last gleam of experimental science before the gathering darkness of the coming centuries. Probably, his influence was even greater than St Benedict's in making monasticism into a powerful instrument for the restoration of social order in the Western world.

Monastic Influence on Medicine.

In the precincts of all the monasteries, not only of the Benedictine, but also of the other great Orders, there were 'rest-houses' for pilgrims, wayfarers and the destitute, many of whom were sick; and although the 'Infirmary' was obviously for the sick members of the Order and was not a public hospital, yet the monks and nuns ministered unto the needs of those who came to them for succour. They made medicines of simple herbs grown in the monastic gardens and they provided food and shelter for the needy, but there was very little scientific progress in medicine or nursing. The superstitious practices of paganism, which had been so sternly repressed by the early Christian church, were being resumed. Votive offerings were being hung in all the sacred buildings as of old, but were dedicated to the numerous saints instead of to the pagan gods. The Church took upon itself the task of curing disease by prayers and exorcisms, the laying on of hands, the use of holy water and holy oil. Living and dead saints, and their relics, were embellished with all the pomp and magnificence that a wealthy Church could bestow. Pieces of the True Cross, the bones of saints, and scraps of their clothing were venerated, and were relied upon to aid human sufferings. Plagues and pestilences were believed to be due to the wrath of God and could be turned aside only by the faithful prayers of the Church. Consequently, the very existence of lay practitioners so savoured of impiety that the condition and status of medical men and women fell into disrepute, and to call in their aid showed a lack of the complete and abiding confidence that was the ideal in religion. The Church of Christ, however, maintained her lofty principles in all those directions where humanitarianism did not conflict with dogma. Great numbers of devoted men and women spent their lives in ministering to the sick, often under such conditions of filth and general misery as beggar description; and, chiefly in connection with the monastic Orders, a very thorough building of hospitals, lazar houses and other refuges for the sick took place throughout Europe. Such organised kindliness and social pity had no parallel in previous history; but in the mediæval hospitals and lazar houses infectious diseases were permitted to rage as they pleased without any attempt at segregation, except in a fitful manner when epidemics were more than usually severe.

Many of the efficient medical practitioners within the pale of Christianity were Jews, for the monks were not allowed to pursue their medical work in peace. A series of edicts emanated from the Vatican during the eleventh, twelfth and thirteenth centuries which forbade the study of medicine or the practice of surgery; but these were not always obeyed. Previous to these edicts monks had gone forth from their monasteries to study at the great medical schools which were developing at Salerno, Montpelier and Paris. Afterwards, they copied and translated recipes, herbals and dietaries in which common sense was mixed with a good deal of grotesque magical lore; and monastic medicine became a blend of tradition, mysticism and charms. The belief in possession by devils, and in witchcraft, grew, and led to barbarous practices which lasted almost to our own day, especially in the treatment of the insane.

Many accounts of miraculous cures come down to us from the chronicles of these times, in fact, nearly every account of recovery from illness is an account of the miraculous healing of the crippled and deformed who, having borne their affliction for many years—often from infancy—so that limbs were twisted and useless, were carried to some shrine or altar, and there became whole. The blind, the deaf, the dumb, the leper and the paralytic all have their share in accounts of these miracles, but there is hardly any account of rational treatment and its results.

Nursing appears to have consisted of washing the sick and the making of beds—there was not a great deal of that—and of feeding the patients. For the rest—prayer and exhortation to suffer patiently the affliction God had willed humanity to bear, and to wait for the release of the soul from the tortured body, when all the sufferings of this life would receive their compensation in the joys of the life beyond the grave. This attitude became almost a cult of suffering, which reached astounding lengths. We read of St Dominic beating himself with an iron chain, of St Rose of Lima wearing next her skin a 'garment of horsehair garnished with sharp points and prickly thistles', so that she could not walk a step without pain, of St Ignatius of Loyola binding his waist with a cruel girdle of prickly leaves and concealing by squalor and neglect all signs of his noble birth and breeding, and of Catherine of Siena wearing an iron chain 'so hard and terrible that it sank deep into her flesh and seared it as with an hot iron'.

St Camillus de Lellis wore a rough and knotted shirt of camels' hair next his skin, and around his waist a band of tin with holes like a grater. Such practices were held to be a noble example to all who strove to follow in the footsteps of a Crucified Master, but they engendered an attitude of passive resistance towards the development of medical knowledge or of any kind of scientific curative work.

112

CHAPTER IV

EARLY CHRISTIAN HOSPITALS AND KINDRED INSTITUTIONS

Classification—Hospital of St Ephrem at Edessa—Nestorius—Constantinople—Rome—Hôtel Dieu of Lyons—Hôtel Dieu of Paris—Santo Spirito, or Hospital of the Holy Ghost

BEFORE attempting to trace out the history of these institutions the reader will need to become familiar with the various terms applied to charitable houses of the early mediæval period. We are already familiar with the valetudinaria of the Romans. The Christians built *xenodocheia*, which were homes for strangers, who might be travellers, pilgrims or merchants. These provided shelter for the homeless and foundlings, for young children, for widows, and for the aged of both sexes. They often contained separate buildings for sufferers from different kinds of diseases, for example, for lepers and for the insane; and the poor came to them for alms. The different parts of a xenodocheion were known by the following names:

nosokomeion—a house for the sick, essentially a hospital.
ptochotropeion—a house for the poor.
morotropeion—a house for lunatics.
gerokomeion—a house for aged men.
cherotropeion—a house for widows.
brephotropeion—a house for foundlings.
orphanotropeion—a house for orphans.

Some institutions had several of these departments, and some only one. There came into being, also, an Order known as the 'parabolani'. St Basil describes them as 'nurses and doctors, the

I

113

beasts of burden and the guides sent out to the people'. Their chief duty, at the time of their inception, was to go forth, look for the needy and sick, and, when necessary, bring them to the xenodocheion. They were probably a kind of stretcher-bearing organisation. They were originally both men and women who sought out the sick and often tended them in their own homes; and who, in times of pestilence, showed great courage and devotion. Later, they were men only, and they often degenerated into the body-guards of the turbulent bishops, whom they assisted in asserting or refuting theological doctrines by the physical arguments of their swords and cudgels. They were not heard of after the fifth century.

The basilias built by St Basil, and briefly described in a preceding chapter, was a typical xenodocheion. There was a morotropeion established at Constantinople in the fourth century, and one at Jerusalem in the fifth century.

Hospital of St Ephrem at Edessa.

Probably the first Christian hospital founded by 'voluntary contributions' was that at Edessa in Western Mesopotamia built by St Ephrem. He was a Syrian monk who, about A.D. 372, hearing that the poor of Edessa were starving in the streets, left his cave and rebuked the rich Christians for their heartlessness. They replied that it was not the spirit which they lacked, but an honest man to take charge of their offerings. St Ephrem at once made a collection, and with the money he established a hospital of 300 beds in the public galleries, which were almost disused at that time. This emergency hospital soon fell into neglect, and was restored by Bishop Rabboula, who added another hospital exclusively for women. Four pagan temples were demolished for this purpose. No account of these hospitals, however brief, should fail to include some mention of the great work which the Nestorians accomplished in connection with them.

114

Nestorius.

Nestorius was Bishop of Constantinople in 431, when a General Council of the Church excommunicated him and deprived him of his see for teaching that the Virgin Mary was the Mother of Christ but not of God. His followers, after his subsequent violent death, founded the Nestorian Church, which flourished for a thousand years in Persia, Mesopotamia and Syria, and even as far east as India and China. They gained control of the two hospitals at Edessa, and developed a very successful school of medicine in connection with them. They were expelled from there and their college buildings destroyed. Then they went to Gondisapor in Persia. Had they not carried Greek medicine to Persia it might never again have come into its own in Europe. There is further mention of this in connection with Islamic medicine.

Constantinople.

Two hospitals were founded at Constantinople by St Chrysostom, but there seem to have been no women in either of them. The records state that cooks and good workmen were chosen from unmarried men.

Rome.

Mention has already been made of Fabiola's hospital at Rome, in the building of which she was assisted by Pammachius, a son-in-law of Paula; and towards the end of the fifth century Pope Symmachus built hospitals in connection with the three most important churches of Rome, St Peter's, St Paul's and St Lawrence's; and shortly after the middle of the sixth century Belisarius, a general under Justinian, founded a xenodochium on the Via Lata at Rome.

Hospitals were being built on all roads of travel along the main routes and especially at points of danger. The journeyings of our forefathers were long, painful and perilous; and on the

115

roads to Rome, and throughout Europe we still find these hospices, or the remains of them, on high mountain passes, and near the passages across rivers, where one by one bridges have been built. Some of these hospices became great hospitals in subsequent centuries, and at least three of them deserve special mention, one at Rome, one at Lyons, and the other at Paris.

Hôtel Dieu of Lyons.

Another popular name for hospitals was Hôtel Dieu, or house of God's charity. One of the earliest to be known by this name was that founded by King Childebert at Lyons in A.D. 542. It was built by a bridge on the Rhone, its full name being 'Hôtel Dieu du Pont du Rhône'. It was designed to shelter pilgrims, the poor, the sick and the infirm. For 600 years it was under lay management and the nursing was carried out to a very great extent by 'penitents'. From the twelfth to the fifteenth century it was ruled by a religious order. In the sixteenth century it again reverted to lay management under a body of men called 'rectors'. Women who wished to enter into its service made application six months in advance, and then entered upon a year's probation, after which a very impressive dedication service was held and the sister took the prescribed vows at the altar. She was not a nun, she was still accountable to the secular authorities, and she could leave the Order if she wished. During this century a woman head was appointed, in order to improve the discipline. At this time sixteen sisters formed the female staff, but there were also nursing brothers. The hospital had large beds, each capable of accommodating five patients, but in 1630 the rectors decided that all patients should have separate beds.

During the eighteenth century this hospital shared in the general low standards that characterised that period throughout all Europe, and there was continual strife between the religious and secular authorities, although during the Revolution the religious orders were banished. In the early nineteenth century the strife became very acute and forty sisters left the Hôtel Dieu and formed an order known as the 'Bon Secours' which nursed patients in their own homes.

In the middle of the nineteenth century the hospital had 1,100 beds, the brothers and sisters were strong, healthy, honest young people of the peasant class who were allowed to enter between the ages of 16 and 24. There was a very small staff for such a large hospital, one nurse being allotted to 15 to 20 patients by day, but each night nurse was responsible for 100 patients.

During his visits to European hospitals about 1780, John Howard described the Hôtel Dieu at Lyons as the best hospital he had seen in France. Its wards were thirty-two feet wide and twenty-five feet high with two tiers of windows. There were three rows of iron beds in each ward and there were separate wards for different diseases, and for convalescent patients. The sisters made up all the medicines, so they must have had some training in pharmacy. He describes the dispensary as 'the neatest and most elegantly fitted up that can be conceived'. Incidentally, he described the Hôtel Dieu at Paris as one of the worst he had ever visited.

At the International Congress of Nurses in America in 1901, Dr Anna Hamilton gave an account of the Hôtel Dieu at Lyons in which she stated that the discipline was fairly good, the nurses were free to leave and to marry if they wished, but, although they were given some professional education, they had no real nursing training.

Hôtel Dieu of Paris.

This was founded by Landry, Bishop of Paris, in A.D. 651. It was built at the Petit Pont, and at first it was the Community of St Christopher. The canons of the cathedral of Notre Dame became governors of the hospital in 1097, and a century later it was removed to its present position on the banks of the Seine near the cathedral. It was frequently enlarged, but definite records of its organisation are available from the twelfth century only; and

117

in the fifteenth century it was united into a strict Order under Augustinian rule by Pope Innocent IV., who was opposed to the idea that any body of religious women should be self-governing. It is the oldest purely nursing order of nuns, and it was very strictly monastic. Once professed, the nuns renounced the world for the rest of their lives, and went out only on nursing duties, and then in pairs. They were cut off from social intercourse and from intellectual pursuits, and their work was exceedingly hard. Two centuries before this, in 1212, the bishops in Council had decreed that all members of the nursing orders should take vows of poverty, chastity and obedience, and should wear a distinctive garb, and also that, in order to economise the gifts of the charitable, just as few nurses as possible should be maintained in each hospital under their jurisdiction. There were thirty brothers and forty sisters of this order, and also forty novices, who had all the heavy work to do, for no servants were kept. Even the laundry work for the entire hospital was done by the novices and the younger sisters. The linen was washed in the river Seine, the nuns wading out into the water for this purpose. Every day in the year, whatever the weather, a 'little wash' was done, and this included the bed linen from the wards; and once in six weeks there was a 'great wash'. Hélyot, in *Les Ordres Monastiques*, says: 'No one who saw the religious sisters of the Hôtel Dieu not only do dressings, make beds and bathe the patients, but also in cold weather break the ice in the river Seine which passes through the midst of the hospital and stand knee deep in the water to wash the filthy clothes, could regard them other than holy victims, who from excess of love and charity for their neighbours hastened willingly to the death which they courted amid the stenches of infection.'

The sisters entered for a probationary period, which often lasted for many years. They then became 'white sisters' and after a further satisfactory period they might receive the hood of 'chaperon sisters'. The number of the sisters was strictly limited by the statutes, so that only on the death of a sister might a novice take her final vows. The records of this hospital give much information with regard to the internal management through the centuries, mainly because of the incessant strife between the religious and secular authorities. No mention is made of the work of the Brothers in these records. Sisters were in charge of male wards, so it would seem that the brothers, whilst they continued to serve in the Hôtel Dieu, must have worked under the direction of the sisters.

Towards the end of the fifteenth century a terrible epidemic of syphilis spread through the hospital, believed to have been brought in by soldiers from the Naples campaign. The beds held four to six patients each, half of them lying with their heads to the top of the bed and the others with their heads at the foot. These beds were of wood, having shelves at the head and the foot to hold the patients' medicines and feeding utensils, they had thick mattresses, feather beds, and bed curtains which were of white muslin in summer and red serge in winter. They were fairly generally infested with bed-bugs, and they were so close together that cleaning was almost impossible. There seems to have been no attempt to classify patients and to keep those suffering with various infective conditions isolated. Scabies, in particular, was very prevalent, and discharged patients carried it back to their homes and their families. There were also epidemics of puerperal sepsis, and there was no fumigation of clothing or bed linen.

In 1640 a new constitution was given which increased the powers of the Mother Superior, and visiting nursing stopped at this period, but this did not create such a hardship as one might be inclined to imagine, for the Sisters of Charity, organised by St Vincent de Paul, were then working amongst the poor in their homes. During the latter half of this century, the bitter disagreements between the religious and lay authorities were the subject of several Parliamentary decrees.

In 1662 paid domestic help was employed, and a century later some paid secular nurses were introduced, a procedure which proved distasteful to the nuns. The institution now included not only the hospital on the Seine, but also the hospital of St Louis for contagious diseases, which was originally built by Louis IX. in the thirteenth century, and was situated outside the city; the convalescent home of St Anne's, a country home for the sisters on retirement, a farm, and extensive storehouses and granaries.

In 1737 a terrible fire broke out in the Hôtel Dieu, thirty of the staff were injured and seven killed. In spite of all the complaints that appear in the records, of insubordination and inefficiency, we are told that whilst that fire raged, such was the discipline and organisation that the patients were all removed to a place of safety and 'in such order that the giving of medicines was delayed only two hours', a remarkable example of good 'team work'.

But there was no burying of the hatchet. The strife continued with even more bitterness. The religious exercises of the sisters had been increased, and they seriously interfered with the nursing. The clergy refused to allow autopsies, and in this the sympathies of the sisters were with the clergy against the physicians. The sisters resented new methods of treatment and objected to some of the established practices such as venesection, the giving of emetics and the use of vesicants, and they frequently countermanded the doctors' orders regarding diets and medicines.

A report on this great hospital was drawn up about 1788 by M. Jacques Tenon, a professor of pathology, in which he states that the Hôtel Dieu received cases of fever, contagious and non-contagious disease, surgical and obstetrical patients and cases of insanity at any hour; and without consideration of age, sex, country or religion. It was a building of four stories and contained twenty-five wards in which were 1,219 beds, 733 of them being large enough to accommodate four to six patients. In 1793 these large beds were abolished—a hundred and sixty years after this had been done at Lyons.

The Augustinian Orders suffered severely during the Revolution, and after this time the personnel of the hospital was not entirely religious. A law passed in 1848 controlled the constitution of the Hôtel Dieu—amongst other French hospitals. It was then placed under the authority of the Prefect of the Seine and the Minister of the Interior. Its administration was in the hands of a Director-General working under the supervision of a Council; but Augustinian Sisters continued to work in the Hôtel Dieu until 1908. Thus, for over twelve centuries the Order gave continuous service to the hospital, and this constitutes the longest history of nursing by any Order.

The Hôtel Dieu is now laicised and is one of the hospitals of the 'Assistance Publique', and as such is used by that body for the training of its secular nurses. The standards of training are the same as those for the 'diplôme d'état français'; but its origin is not forgotten, for a statue of its founder, Bishop Landry, stands at the entrance to one of the main blocks.

Santo Spirito, or Hospital of the Holy Ghost.

This was originally founded by the old bridge on the Tiber in A.D. 717 by Ina, King of the Western Saxons, as a guest house for the pilgrims of his own nationality. In 794 it was enlarged by King Offa of Mercia, and its income, at this time, was derived from properties in Britain. Twice during the ninth century it was burnt down and rebuilt; in 1077 it was sacked by Henry IV., and in 1162 by Frederick Barbarossa. In 1198 it was rebuilt by Pope Innocent III. who was then making a bold and far-reaching attempt to consolidate human interests into the organisation of the Catholic Church. With this end in view, he was establishing hospitals of the Holy Ghost throughout all Christendom. The form and plan of the Santo Spirito of Rome, as arranged by Pope Innocent, constitutes the beginning of its history as a hospital in the sense in which we understand it; and he placed Guy de Montpelier in charge of its organisation.

This Guy, or Guido, was a noble who had founded a hospital at Montpelier, with a secular nursing fraternity known as the

Brotherhood of the Holy Ghost, which became famous throughout Europe. Very little is known of the actual structure, or work, of the Santo Spirito at this time. It was an age of magnificent architecture, and as this hospital was under the direct patronage of the Pope it was probably worthy of its period.

In 1480 it was again rebuilt, as parts of it were falling, by Sixtus IV. in the form in which it remained until the present century when the structure was demolished in order to add to the vista of the Victor Emmanuel monument.

CHAPTER V

ISLAMIC MEDICINE AND THE GREAT SARACENIC HOSPITALS

General History—Arabic learning—Arabic advances in the curative arts—Chemistry and pharmacy—Hygiene—Famous physicians and hospitals

General History.

IT is generally agreed that the Arabs owed their medical knowledge, in the first place, to the Nestorians and the Arians, two persecuted sects of Christians who, on account of their heretical beliefs, had been banished into the desert, and who later gained control of the school at Edessa in Mesopotamia, with its two large hospitals; which they made an important centre for the teaching of medicine. They were driven from Edessa by Bishop Cyrus in A.D. 489 on account of their unorthodoxy; and they then went to Persia and established the famous school at Gondisapor—which is claimed to have been the starting point of Islamic medicine.

The Arabs were originally desert nomads, but they obviously possessed intellectual qualities and aptitudes which were in abeyance during the pre-Islamic period; but when, in obedience to the command of their great prophet, they went forth to conquer the world for Mohammedanism, they came into contact with the debris of many ancient civilisations. They conquered Egypt in A.D. 638, and their victorious forces rapidly spread across the provinces of Northern Africa, until in 698, under Musa Nosseyr, the Governor of Africa, they conquered Spain. Their Empire then extended from the Indus to the Atlantic Ocean.

123

Arabic Learning.

We have seen that the Nestorians initiated the Arabs into their knowledge of scientific curative work, but the development of their medicine was determined by their access to another source of learning. This came to them from the literature of the University and Library of Alexandria which had found its way into Asia Minor, as did also much Greek learning and literature when Constantine the Great suppressed the pagan institutions in his domain. The Arabs collected, copied and translated into Arabic the works of Hippocrates, Galen, Dioscorides, and other Greek teachers at a time when Christians were fanatically opposed to making any use of pagan literature. The chief of the Hindu medical books were also translated into Arabic, and there were many Hindu physicians in Bagdad and Gondisapor in the ninth century.

The Arabs put into practice the precepts of their prophet, 'Teach science, which teaches the fear of God. He who desires knowledge adores God, when he spreads it he is giving alms, he who has it becomes an object of veneration and goodwill. Science protects from error and sin, it lights the road to Paradise; it guides us through the pleasures and pains of life; it is an ornament among our friends and a shield against our enemies. The memorials of the wise alone endure, because their great deeds serve as models, and are repeated by the multitudes that follow them. Science is a remedy against the infirmities of ignorance, a comforting beacon in the night of injustice. The study of the sciences has the value of a fast, the teaching of them has the value of a prayer; in a noble heart they inspire the highest feelings, and they correct and humanise the perverted.'

With such a conception of the value of knowledge it is small wonder that they built up such marvellous centres of learning. Then again, Mohammed taught, 'God has not inflicted disease upon us without at the same time giving us the remedy,' and the Arabians set out on a zealous search for these remedies during an age when Christianity taught that suffering was the Will of God for His people, and that its great value in the perfecting of human nature should make His followers seek to suffer, rather than to find means to assuage the pangs.

For many centuries Arabic learning was greatly in advance of the Christian, and there grew up in the Moslem Empire a number of religious schools attached to mosques, and later these schools developed into universities. The first centre was at Bagdad, founded during the Abbasid dynasty in the ninth century, and Arabian physicians became the most learned in the world at that time. They continued to hold that supremacy for the next six centuries. Other important centres were at Basra, Kufu, and Cairo in the east, and Toledo and Cordova in the west, and all these universities had laboratories and rich libraries. The library at Cordova was the collection of one of the Sultans, and contained 600,000 volumes—the catalogue alone consisted of 45 volumes. The influence of Arabic learning passed by way of Spain into the universities of Paris, Oxford and Northern Italy, and the Arabs thus repaid to the Christians of the western world the services that had formerly been rendered to them by the Christians of the east; but the contents of most of the Arabian libraries have long since vanished as a result of the combined destructive energies of savages and theologians.

Arabic Advances in the Curative Arts.

In medicine the Arabs made great advances over the work of the Greeks. They studied physiology and hygiene, and their 'materia medica' was practically as advanced as that of England at the beginning of the twentieth century. Their religion forbade autopsies, so they acquired no further knowledge of anatomy. Jewish doctors, however, working in the Saracenic hospitals and medical schools, are said to have performed dissections. Many of the treatments given in these hospitals are still in use to-day, and the Arabs had a real science of medicine. Their surgeons performed some of the most difficult operations known, including many on the eye, the thyroid gland and the trachea. They used the cautery much more than the knife, having an aversion to the shedding of blood other than that of infidels; and therefore fewer ligatures were required; although they are supposed to have introduced catgut—the word is thought to be a perversion of 'kitgut', the string of an Arabian fiddle which was known as a 'kit'.

They induced inhalation anæsthesia by the use of hemp fumes; and this was at a time when surgery was forbidden by the Christian Church, which expected that cures would follow, if God so willed, the religious rites performed by the clergy.

In conservative dentistry, the Arabs not only filled teeth, and replaced those that were lost, but they also corrected deformities of the mouth and the dental arches, although such work is usually thought of as being essentially modern.

Chemistry and Pharmacy.

In chemistry, the Arabs made marvellous progress. They discovered new substances such as potash, silver nitrate, copper sulphate, corrosive sublimate, and nitric and sulphuric acid—all of which have their uses in the daily work of the hospital nurse of modern times. The Islamic pharmacopœia contained 200 new plants, a great many of which are still used for their medicinal properties. They added rhubarb, senna, cassia and manna to the laxatives already in use. From the Hindus they borrowed aconite and mercury, which were used externally for skin diseases. They introduced the use of nux vomica and camphor as stimulants, and Indian hemp, amber and aconite in the treatment of nervous conditions; and they used sugar instead of honey in the making of potions and syrups. The word 'alcohol' and the signs used to denote quantities in prescriptions are all Arabic, so also is the word 'algebra'—an improved science of mathematics. Spectacles and telescopes resulted from their study of optics.

Hygiene.

Islam attached great importance to the care of the body, and to the value of perfect cleanliness in the maintenance of health. 'Cleanliness is piety', says the Koran, and it was the reputation of the Arabs that they were the 'cleanest people on earth' in all that related to their person, dress, beds, and the interior of their houses. One of the opulent coast towns of Spain—Almeria—had no less than a thousand public baths. Hygiene was one of the foundation stones of their moral code, which ordained the uses of baths and ablutions, prohibited the drinking of fermented liquors, and made marriage obligatory in cases of seduction, thus protecting women from the caprice of men.

Famous Physicians and Hospitals.

Three great names stand out among the Islamic physicians, one in each of three centuries—Rhazes (860–932), and Avicenna (980–1036), both born in the east and Avenzoar (1094–1162), born in Spain. All three were at the head of hospitals, so they had all the necessary facilities for studying their patients. They made 'case histories', and the hospitals kept records of these in their registers. The Islamic physicians were the first to develop clinical teaching in hospitals.

The first Moslem hospital on record was founded by the Caliph Welid, at Bagdad in A.D. 707, and he made special arrangements for the blind and for lepers. In the tenth century, the chief hospital at Bagdad had a staff of 24 physicians. There were special departments for ophthalmic cases, for fevers, for diseases of women and for accidents, and the physicians were given charge of these in accordance with their special knowledge and skill. This hospital had a famous department for the care of the insane, and the Arabs were far ahead of the Christians in their kindly treatment of the mentally afflicted. Speaking of this hospital in his *Histoire des Arabes* published in Paris in 1854, Sédillot says—'What especially characterised the school at Bagdad in the beginning was the truly scientific spirit which presided over all. To go from the known to the unknown, then from effects to causes, and only to admit as true what had been demonstrated by experimental work—such were the principles taught by the masters.'

Under the Arabs in Egypt hospital organisation was very advanced. At the El-Nazuri hospital at Cairo (founded 874) all the patients were classified and nursed in the special section devoted to the type of disease from which they were suffering; these departments included a special hospital for women. All patients were attended by specialists, whilst a staff of musicians, story-tellers and singers were employed to while away the tedious hours of convalescence.

There is a description given of the greatest of the Cairo hospitals—the Al Mansur—as it was in 1284. In the building of it masons and carpenters had been brought from all parts of Egypt, and loiterers in the street and passers-by, whatever their rank, were obliged to assist in this work until, we are told, most people avoided going that way. When finished, it was a great quadrangular building with fountains playing in each of the four courtyards. It had its special wards for particular diseases, for women and for convalescents; there were out-patient clinics, diet kitchens, an orphan asylum and a chapel. It also possessed commodious lecture rooms and an extensive library. It had a staff of male and female nurses, and as was usual in these hospitals, a staff of musicians and story-tellers. When patients who had recovered left the hospital they were each given five pieces of gold—about 50 shillings—so that they were not forced to do any heavy work until they had completely regained their strength. The large endowment made this possible, as it also enabled the patients to be given every comfort whilst in hospital. This was the most famous of the Saracenic hospitals.

At Damascus, the largest and best appointed hospital was that founded by the Emir Nureddin in 1160, as a thank offering to the God of battles, after having conquered Edessa and driven back the Crusading hordes of Louis VII. and Conrad III. It is recorded that in this hospital treatment was given and drugs dispensed continuously for three hundred years, and that during that time its fires had never once been allowed to go out.

Cordova had fifteen hospitals during the most brilliant period of Arabian learning, and teaching schools were attached to the majority of them. Women as well as men were trained in these schools and hospitals to carry out all the treatments then in use. It is interesting to note that in the great days of Mohammedan Spain, Arabian women were not confined, as in the East, to harems, but appeared freely in public and took their share in all the intellectual, literary and scientific movements of their day.

A nursing treatment which appears to have originated in Spain in the eleventh century is the giving of nutrient enemata. Avenzoar, who was superintendent of a hospital in Seville, seems to have been the first to introduce it, and his apparatus for the purpose consisted of the bladder of a goat, into the neck of which a silver cannula had been fastened. The preliminary cleansing of the rectum having been carried out, a feed prepared of eggs, milk and gruel was injected. Avenzoar taught that the intestines would suck this up, and carry it back to the stomach to be digested. Strange that this treatment, based on such erroneous physiology, should have persisted even into the early years of the twentieth century.

CHAPTER VI

SOME QUEENS AND OTHER FAMOUS MEDIÆVAL WOMEN

Queen Radegunde—Queen Bathilde of France—The Abbess Hildegarde of Bingen—The Abbess Héloïse—Queen Margaret of Scotland—Queen Maud and her husband, Henry I. of England—Queen Matilda—Eleanor of Castile—Philippa of Hainault—Elizabeth of Hungary—Elizabeth of Portugal—Catherine of Siena—Catherine of Genoa—Isabella of Castile

ALTHOUGH there is a wealth of delightful stories told of the devoted ministry of many famous women during the mediæval period it is extremely difficult to arrive at any conclusion with regard to the authentic value of these stories. On the face of the evidence a number of these women have been accounted nurses, whereas, if the records are examined more closely, they are found to allude much more to miraculous cures than to actual clinical work. The miracles of Christ, shown in the healing of the sick and the cure of bodily infirmity, had led to a belief that physicians, in their difficult and disagreeable methods of treatment, were all wrong, and that the true remedial course was by prayer, fasting, faith, and the invocation of saints.

Christ had imparted to his disciples the power 'to heal all manner of sickness and all manner of disease'; and the apostolic records state that they went out 'and anointed with oil many that were sick, and healed them' (St Luke, ix. 6). This example and teaching led to the most determined efforts being made by the Christian Churches to be the sole procurers and dispensers of health to all sick people. The belief grew with the centuries until it reached a culminating point, giving rise, in its course, to a very degenerate offshoot—witchcraft; and then we find the more thoughtful men and women struggling to bring some rational, scientific light into the welter of superstitious darkness.

So that, among the galaxy of famous women whose life and work are here outlined, we shall find all stages of thought-progress and all types of ministry.

Queen Radegunde.

She was the daughter of Bertaire, King of Thuringia, in what is now Southern Germany. She was the first of many queens to become a nun. When only twelve years of age she was taken prisoner by Clothaire I., one of the Merovingian kings of the Frankish Empire. He educated her as a Christian, and when she was eighteen he married her, although he had several other wives. He proved a particularly selfish and brutal husband, and when, six years later, he treacherously assassinated her only surviving brother, she fled the court and became a nun. She visited the double monastery at Arles, which had been founded in 542, and which was presided over by Cæsarius and his sister Cæsaria. In this monastery there was strict communism with complete renunciation of personal property. No servants were kept, the monks and the nuns being responsible for all the work that had to be done.

Radegunde studied the arrangement of the life and its many occupations, and then founded a great settlement on her own estate at Poitiers—the Abbey of St Cross—for about 200 nuns. A woman named Agnes was the Abbess, the Queen working as a simple nun. It is recorded that baths were built in this monastery; an unusual procedure at this time.

The story goes that Radegunde tended the poor and was a recipient of a piece of the True Cross. We are told that she shrank from no disease, however loathsome. There is, however, no real evidence that she was a nurse, although one record states that 'she loved to serve the sick with her own hands'. She is reputed to have effected some miraculous cures, and to have exorcised devils, which were causing disease, by her prayers and the virtue of her saintliness. She died in A.D. 587 and was afterwards canonised.

Queen Bathilde of France.

Bathilde is reputed to have been an Englishwoman who was taken captive and sold as a slave to Erkonwald, mayor of the palace of King Clovis II. In A.D. 659 the king freed and married her. At that time slaves were publicly sold in the market place of St Denis, and when Bathilde became Queen she caused laws to be passed which mitigated the conditions of slaves, and later, she abolished Christian slavery.

She had three sons—Clothaire, Childeric and Thiery—and after the king's death in 656 she became Regent during the minority of Clothaire III.

Butler in his *Lives of the Saints* says that she 'filled France with hospitals and pious foundations'. She restored the monasteries of St Martin, St Denis and St Médard, and she founded the great Abbey of St Peter at Corbie. She was greatly helped by St Landry, the Bishop of Paris during her reign. He it was who founded the Hôtel Dieu, near his cathedral of Notre Dame.

Perhaps the most famous of Bathilde's foundations was the Royal Nunnery of St George at Chelles on the Marne, about ten miles from Paris, to which she withdrew in 665. Here she 'made it her greatest delight to visit and attend the sick, whom she comforted and served with her own hands' (Butler).

Hildegarde of Bingen.

She was born about 1098, and was undoubtedly one of the most learned of mediæval abbesses, but also much more subject to visions in her waking hours than any of her contemporaries. These visions first came to her at the age of five, and appeared to have continued at intervals throughout her life. Maybe there was some connection between her state of health and her susceptibility to visions, for she was subject to frequent illnesses. Most of our information regarding her is obtained from her own letters and the various books ascribed to her.

She was born of noble parents at Boeckelheim, in the province of Sponheim, and from the age of eight she spent her life in religious communities. She received her education at the Benedictine monastery at Disibodenburg, afterwards becoming a novice at this monastery, and remaining there until, at the age of fifty, she became its abbess.

Her writings, her reputation for sanctity, and her wise rule attracted so many new members to her community that it became overcrowded. So, with eighteen of her nuns, she withdrew to a new convent at Rupertsberg, near Bingen on the Rhine, and this convent became a centre for the intellectual life of the period. She became a great friend of St Bernard of Clairvaux, probably the most influential man in Europe at that time.

According to some modern writers, she is reputed to have established a school of nurses, but there is no mention of this in her letters, or in authentic biographies. Her own patients appear to have required no nursing, for she cured them by her miraculous powers; and we are told that nearly all the sick persons who sought her aid were instantly healed.

Her writings are published in Migne's *Patrolgia*—an immense French edition of all the important works of the Fathers, Doctors, and Saints of the Church. Its editor, Reuss, says, 'Among all the saintly religious who have practised medicine, or written about it, in the middle ages, the most important is, without any doubt St Hildegarde. . . . All those who wish to write the history of the medical and natural sciences must read this work' (her books) 'in which this religious woman, evidently well grounded in all that was known at the time of the secrets of nature, discusses and examines carefully all the knowledge of the time. It is certain that St Hildegarde knew many things that were unknown to the physicians of her day.'

Her books include the *Physica*, a description of the nature and medical properties of minerals, herbs, fishes, birds and animals, and also many recipes and directions for the guidance of those less highly endowed than herself with the power of miraculous healing.

She shares with her contemporary, Avenzoar of Seville, the honour of having first mentioned the 'itch-mite'; and in her dissertation on the subject of whether waters are wholesome to drink, she comes very near the truth as we know it. She says that swamp water should always be boiled and allowed to cool before drinking, so also should spring and river water, but that well water is safer. She tells us that red-hot steel weakens the force of poison in food or drink. She says, too, that fleas remain underground in winter, and come forth to plague mankind when the sun dries the soil in summer; but that one may get rid of them by heating some earth until it is quite dry and then scattering it upon the bed.

She relates that in one of her visions she heard a voice from heaven telling her that man contained in his body the images of all things; and in her medical writings she declares that the fact that the mole casts out the bad earth from its burrows in heaps is a sign that the animal, when boiled, dried and powdered, will expel evil humours from the body and cure scrofulous swellings; as well as much else of a similar nature.

Taking them as a whole, her writings form interesting pictures of medicine, botany and gardening in twelfth-century Germany, and give us many sidelights on the intellectual life of her day; but although she is stated to have cast out devils and to have cured every disease, there are no nursing details to be found therein. She died about 1175.

The Abbess Héloïse (1101–1164).

Héloïse of the Convent of the Paraclete was a contemporary of Hildegarde, and she is probably one of the best known of mediæval abbesses on account of her romantic and ill-starred love affair with Abélard, who was her father's secretary, and her tutor.

After these famous lovers had renounced each other they became the heads of separate religious houses; but throughout their lives Abélard controlled and counselled Héloïse in the government of her convent. This had no hospital, and although Héloïse was anxious to conform to the rule of St Benedict regarding the care of the sick, the destitute and the traveller, she pointed out that there were obvious objections to the indiscriminate reception of strangers into a convent for women. Even to admit those of the feminine sex might afford to the less spiritually minded of her nuns dangerous opportunities for communicating with the outside world. There was an infirmary, however, within the walls of the convent, and Abélard defined the duties of the infirmarian thus—'Let the infirmarian look after the sick, preserving them at once from sin and from want. Whatever their infirmity requires, whether in food, baths, or anything else, is to be given them. Meat is never to be withheld, except on Fridays and on special vigils and fasts. The more they think upon their death the better they will be kept from sin, and especially should they study silence and be instant in prayer, as it is written "My son, in thy sickness be not negligent, but pray unto the Lord, and He will make thee whole" (Eccles. xxxviii. 9). There must always be someone on duty to give aid when requisite, and the place must be provided with all things needed in sickness. Drugs must be obtained if necessary, and according to the opportunities of the locality, and this will be done the more easily if the presiding sister is not without medical knowledge. It is she who must attend to those that are bled, and some sister should be skilled in "bleeding" that it may not be requisite for a man to come in for this purpose. Opportunity for religious exercises must be provided, so that the patients may communicate, at least, on the Lord's Day, always with confession and penance, as far as possible. The recommendation of St James the Apostle, as to anointing the sick, must be carefully observed, especially in desperate cases. Let two elderly monks, with a deacon to carry the holy oil, come in and celebrate this sacrament, the sisters being present, but with a screen interposed. And the infirmary shall be built so that the monks may have access and regress without seeing the sisters, or being seen by them.'

This quotation is a translation from Migne's *Patrolgia*, and it is given in its entirety for two reasons. It is probably an example of the general attitude of most of the religious houses for women only, and it corrects the misleading pictures that have been drawn, by many writers, showing these nuns visiting and nursing the poor in the neighbourhood. For example, in *Science and Literature of the Middle Ages* Lacroix condenses Abélard's instructions thus—'Abélard exhorted the nuns of the Paraclete convent to learn surgery for the benefit of the poor.' When one considers the care that was taken to exclude even women visitors, and to protect the nuns from the gaze of elderly monks performing sacramental offices for the sick and dying members of their own community, it seems hardly probable that the nuns would have been permitted, much less encouraged, to use any such knowledge or skill except among themselves.

Queen Margaret of Scotland.

She was the sister of Edgar the Atheling, and about the year 1070 she married Malcolm Canmore, who afterwards became king. She is said to have 'distributed all she had for the use of the poor, to have washed the feet of beggars, and to have nursed the sick with her own hands'. Her special care was for pilgrims, and for these she established a hospital at Queen's Ferry near Edinburgh. Her daughter, Eadgyth, or Edith, became the wife of Henry I. of England in 1100, but the Normans were unable to pronounce her name, so they called her Matilda, or Maud; and as such she is known in English history.

Queen Maud and her Husband, Henry I.

Both were notable as founders of hospitals. The most famous was the Hospital of St Giles' in the fields at Holborn, especially for lepers. This consisted of a hall, a chapel, an eastern tower and a south-western tower. Queen Maud is said to have tended the lepers in the hospital and also to have visited them in their poor huts on the outskirts of villages, and in other lazar houses. She 'nursed them, and dressed their repulsive sores'.

Henry I. founded four other hospitals—those of St John the Evangelist at Cirencester, of Holy Innocents, near Lincoln, of St Bartholomew at Oxford, and of St Mary Magdalen at New-castle-on-Tyne. With the exception of St John's, these were all for lepers. His second wife, Queen Adela of Louvain, founded the Hospital of St Giles' at Wilton, or Fugglestone, in Wiltshire, about 1135.

Queen Matilda.

Queen Matilda, wife of Stephen, founded the Royal Hospital of St Katherine by the Tower of London. This was a permanent home for women and children, and it remained under the patronage of the Queen Consorts, the sisterships being given by the Queens to their ladies.

Queen Eleanor of Castile.

She was a Princess of Spain who became the wife of Edward I. She gave large endowments and grants of lands and manors to the Hospital of St Katherine, and she is the traditional founder of the Hospital of St John the Baptist at Gorleston.

Queen Philippa of Hainault.

She was the wife of Edward III., and she gave a Charter to the Hospital of St Katherine. This charter exhorts the brethren and sisters to visit the sick and infirm dwelling around the Tower and to nurse them in their own homes.

This was an age of great need for charitable work in England. The land groaned under the stern rule of the Norman kings, and when to this was added the oppression of the Norman nobles with their merciless treatment of their weaker neighbours the country was indeed in a state of helpless misery. The cause of

137

religion, also, was suffering a rude shock owing to the tyrannical exactions of the Pope and the loose and disorderly lives of many of the parish priests and monks.

Elizabeth of Hungary.

She was the daughter of Andreas II. of Hungary, born in 1207; and, when only fifteen years of age, she married Ludwig of Thuringia. This proved a very happy marriage except for continuous strife with her husband's family. Ludwig died five years later whilst with the Crusades, and shortly after the loss of her husband, Elizabeth's fourth child was born.

She is one of the most lovable and beloved of 'nursing' saints. From her earliest years stories are told of her ministrations to the sick and poor. The castle which was her Thuringian home stood upon a hill, and she built a 'hospital' just outside its gates for those whose infirmities would not allow them to climb the hill. After her husband's death she became a Franciscan Tertiary and she built a hospital at Marburg whence she retired, and for the remaining three years of her life 'she devoted herself entirely to the care of the sick, especially to those afflicted with the most loathsome diseases'. She died in November, 1231, at the early age of twenty-four, and was canonised in June, 1235.

Queen Elizabeth of Portugal.

She was born in 1271, a daughter of Peter, King of Aragon and a grand-niece of Elizabeth of Hungary. She married Denis, King of Portugal, when she was only sixteen years of age, but the marriage proved most unhappy. After her husband's death in 1325 she adopted the habit of the Third Order of St Francis but took no vows, as she wished to retain her wealth and property in order that she might use them in the service of the poor. She built a hospital near her palace, giving her services every day to the sick persons housed therein. She is accredited with having built a convent of Poor Clares at Coimbra.

In 1336 she was obliged to return to the court on account of strife between her son, the reigning King of Portugal, and her son-in-law, the King of Castile. In July of that year she died and was buried at Coimbra. Three centuries later she was canonised by Pope Urban VIII.

Catherine of Siena.

She was born in 1347, one of twin daughters of a wool-dyer of Siena. She was a bright, fearless adventurous child, and she proved one of the most efficient, clear-thinking, and courageous women of her time. She joined the Third Order of St Dominic when only sixteen years of age, and many anecdotes are told of her ministrations to the sick and to lepers. Especially during a terrible epidemic that occurred in 1371 she and her friends 'devoted themselves to the poorest of the stricken population, entering without fear the most infected quarters; they sang hymns of joy whilst wrapping up the poor discoloured corpses in their winding sheets, and many of the sisters fell, chilled by the icy hand of death' (*Life of Catherine of Siena*, Josephine E. Butler, 1894). One does not know what kind of nursing they did, but we are told that 'Catherine's prayers brought health to many sick persons'. Nearly all the stories of her ministrations to the sick are accounts of miraculous cures. As a preacher, her eloquence was marvellous, and great multitudes of people flocked to hear her. She had a powerful political influence, and she is mainly noted for the very effectual part she played in the restoration of Pope Gregory XI. to Rome after Avignon had been the Papal seat for seventy years. She died in 1380 at the age of thirty-three, and was canonised in 1461.

Catherine of Genoa.

She was born at Genoa in 1447. She was of noble family and she married, unhappily, at the age of sixteen. Five years later she separated from her husband and entered the convent of St Mary at Genoa, where she gave herself up to the care of lepers and the sick poor until her death in 1510.

139

Queen Isabella of Castile.

She married Ferdinand, King of Aragon in 1469—it was their daughter who was Henry VIII.'s first wife. To Queen Isabella seems to belong the credit of having introduced field hospitals and ambulances on a large scale. Speaking of the siege of Alora in 1484, the Spanish historian, Hernando del Pulgar, writes, 'For the care of the sick and wounded the Queen always sent to the camp six large tents and their furniture, together with physicians, surgeons, medicines and attendants, and commanded that they should charge nothing, for she would pay for all. These tents were called the Queen's Hospital.'

On the surrender of Malaga in 1487 the Spanish army, on entering the besieged city, was followed by the Queen's hospital in 400 'ambulancias'. At the siege of Granada in 1489 an eye-witness—Peter Martyr—wrote to the Archbishop of Milan, 'Four huge hospital tents, the careful provision of Queenly piety, are a sight worth seeing. They are intended, not only for the wounded, but for those labouring under any disease. The physicians, apothecaries, surgeons and other attendants are as numerous, the order, diligence, and supply of all things needful as complete as in your infirmary of the Holy Spirit, or the great Milan Hospital itself. Every sickness and casualty is met, and provided for, by the Royal bounty, except where Nature's appointed day is at hand.'

The Queen herself frequently visited the wounded, and when her courtiers hinted that this was contrary to Castilian etiquette she is said to have replied, 'Let me go to them, for they have no mothers here, and it will soothe them in their pain and weakness to find that they are not uncared for'. And the chronicler adds, 'Surely this queen deserved as much as those ancient Greek and Roman princesses that famous title, "Mater castrorum".'

Pedro Bosca records that the Queen's Hospital comprised nearly four hundred waggons with awnings, and that the wounded were not nursed by the highly improper persons who usually follow armies, but by honest and competent matrons. These waggons were called 'ambulancias'—probably the first use of the name, and the first use of a mobile ambulance service with independent transport of medical stores.

It would seem as though, at one bound, the active mind of the Queen had reached an understanding of the needs of the wounded which the rest of the world failed to appreciate until four more centuries of human suffering had passed. It is strange that this great effort should have been almost an isolated one, and with the decay of the hospital tents and the falling to pieces of the waggons it should have died, and that wounded men should again lie on the battlefields for days and nights before any succour was given. And then, in the chaos of Napoleonic wars and the European conflicts of the nineteenth century, it should be born again as the result of a Swiss traveller looking out over the battlefield of Solferino.

141

CHAPTER VII

THE MILITARY NURSING ORDERS OF THE CRUSADES

Knights Hospitallers of St John of Jerusalem—The Brotherhood of St John the Almoner—The first Crusade—Endowment of the Hospital by Godfrey and his followers, and the formation of the Brotherhood into an Augustinian Order—Papal recognition: The Order becomes monastic —Constitution of the Order—The Knights Templars—The second Crusade—Military career of the Knights Hospitallers of St John—Siege of Acre and the formation of the Order of Teutonic Knights—Christians recapture Acre—Recapture of Jerusalem, and the subsequent fall of Jerusalem and Gaza to the Turks—Warfare between the Templars and the Hospitallers—Loss of the last Christian stronghold in Syria—The Order of St John in Cyprus and Rhodes—Hospitallers capture Mediterranean strongholds—Two sieges and the loss of Rhodes—The Knights in Malta —The siege of Malta—The hospital at Malta—Decline of the Order —The Order in England—The Priory at Clerkenwell—The Priory at Buckland—Suppression of the English Langue—Later history of other Orders of Hospitallers—The Knights Templars—The Order of Teutonic Knights—The Knights of St Lazarus

The Knights Hospitallers.

THE Knights Hospitallers of St John of Jerusalem is by far the most famous and enduring Order of Chivalry the world has ever known. Its history begins in the middle of the eleventh century, but legend takes the history of the hospital itself much farther back than that. According to a seventeenth-century French writer, Louis Beurrier, the hospital was originally founded 150 years before the birth of Christ, by John Hircanus, a member of the Maccabees family, for the shelter and care of pilgrims to the

142

temple of Solomon. In the fourth century A.D. the pilgrims to the Holy Sepulchre at Jerusalem arrived exhausted by the rigours of the journey even if they had escaped the attentions of very numerous bands of marauders and had not contracted any of the endemic diseases. We know of several shelters, hospitals, and monasteries built in those early days both in the city and on the route; and Christian churches began to replace temples to pagan deities in the fourth century.

By the eleventh century the numbers of pilgrimages had become so great that the journey was often considered to be a fashionable pastime. The routes became centres of trade, often the pilgrim was himself a merchant, and the whole adventure became commercialised. Relics of Christ, and of the early saints, which were believed to have miraculous properties, were sold for large sums of money. Many of these 'relics' were false, and, to quote Erasmus, 'If all the fragments pertaining to be parts of the True Cross were collected, enough would be found for the building of a ship.' The Cross itself, which was in the custody of the Bishop of Jerusalem, was solemnly exposed to the gaze of the people on Easter Sunday, and the Bishop made gifts of small pieces to the pilgrims, which they encased in gold adorned with gems and carried away to their respective countries. It was supposed that the wood of the Cross itself possessed a miraculous power of vegetation, and that its substance, though continually broken off, still remained whole and unimpaired.

For centuries the Holy Land had belonged to the Islamic Empire, and all the Christian institutions were treated with more or less toleration by the rulers; but when, after four centuries of dominion, the Saracens were conquered by the ferocious Turkomans from beyond the Caspian Sea, the pilgrimage to Jerusalem, always a hazardous undertaking, became fraught with incalculable dangers which included hideous tortures and revolting cruelties at the hands of the barbarian Turks.

The Brotherhood of St John the Almoner.

About 1048 some rich Christian merchants from Amalfi, a seaport lying south of Naples, obtained permission to build and endow a hospital at Jerusalem for the Latin pilgrims who came to the Holy Sepulchre; and these merchants were the precursors of the Knights Hospitallers. It is uncertain whether an entirely new hospital was founded, or whether the old one formed the nucleus from which the new foundation extended. The hospital was arranged in two sections, one for men, dedicated to St John the Almoner, and one for women, dedicated to St Mary Magdalene; and all the chief cities of Italy and Southern Europe sent liberal funds for its continued maintenance as a refuge for sick and weary pilgrims. It was served by a body of men and women who called themselves the Brothers and Sisters of the Order of St John the Almoner, and who were governed by a 'Rector'; but they extended their services as freely to sick infidels as to Christians.

The persecutions of the Turks and their unspeakable cruelties to Christian pilgrims was creating a rapidly rising indignation throughout Europe, and this eventually led to the organising of the Crusades.

The First Crusade.

The first attempt, in 1098, failed tragically. A hundred thousand fighting men were led by Peter the Hermit, who, although a knight, lacked military ability and the power of generalship. His army was undisciplined and disorderly and it was completely routed. But the attempt was not altogether in vain, for the spirit of it fired the smouldering chivalry of the Latin races into an intense blaze, and in the following year an allied army of 600,000 horse and 100,000 foot, speaking sixteen different languages, advanced from Constantinople. It was an army 'whose like the world had never seen', and when, under the command of Godfrey de Bouillon, they had captured Nicea, Antioch, Tarsus and

Edessa in rapid succession, they stormed the walls of Jerusalem on 7th June and summoned the Turkoman Governor to surrender. He immediately imprisoned all the Christians in the city; including Peter Gerard, the Rector of the Hospital of St John, and then the Turks put up a resistance as stubborn as it was prolonged. The Christian hosts besieged the city for six weeks, and but for the invincible valour and resolution of their three leaders —Godfrey, Tancred and Raymond of Toulouse—they would have given up in despair. On 19th July they carried the city by storm and Godfrey hoisted his own banner on the battlements.

He was elected King of Palestine, but although he accepted the responsibility, he declined the title, saying that he would never wear a crown of gold where the Master he served wore a crown of thorns.

Endowment of the Hospital by Godfrey and his Followers, and the Formation of the Brotherhood into an Augustinian Order.

The Crusaders found the hospital of St John, and its work, fully established, and many of their wounded received the ministrations of the brotherhood; and then came a period of peace and prosperity for the Order. In appreciation of their skill and devotion in tending the wounded, Godfrey endowed them with the revenues of one of his richest manors in Brabant, and many other knights followed his example. Peter Gerard was still the Rector, and a Roman lady named Agnes was at the head of the Sisterhood which served the Hospital of St Mary Magdalene.

The Brotherhood was now very strong and important, and they formed themselves into a regularly constituted Order of Military Monks under the rule of St Augustine, who were to be clad in a black habit adorned with an eight-pointed white cross. They built branch hospitals in many of the seaports of Europe, so that Christians might find shelter and nursing attention whilst waiting for transport to the Holy Land.

Papal Recognition. The Order becomes Monastic.

The Order was formally recognised by Pope Paschal II. in 1113, and in 1118 Peter Gerard died and was succeeded by Raymond du Puy; a very distinguished French noble whose clear sighted vision enabled him to appreciate, at their correct value, the dangers which still menaced Christian pilgrims. He pointed out that it was not enough that the Hospitallers should be willing to live in the service of sick and wounded pilgrims, but they should also be ready to die in their defence if the necessity arose, and for that purpose he reconstructed the Brotherhood into an Order of Knighthood with three divisions:

(1) Knights of Justice, who were to be of noble birth, and who would carry arms and also tend the sick.

(2) Priests, who would perform the religious ceremonies.

(3) Serving brethren and sisters, who would minister to the sick and serve the pilgrims.

There were also Dames of the Order, who were required to be of noble birth. These knights and ladies were pledged to the service of mankind, and membership of the Order was an honour for which the proudest and most famous families in France, England, Italy, Spain, Portugal and Germany eagerly competed. Hospitals of the Order were founded in all those countries.

At the ceremony of initiation into the Knighthood the novice was instructed that the four arms of the white Cross represented the Christian virtues—prudence, justice, temperance and fortitude. The points indicated the eight beatitudes which arise out of these virtues, and its whiteness was the emblem of the purity of life demanded from those who fight in the defence of the Christian faith and live for the service of the poor and suffering.

Constitution of the Order.

Raymond du Puy was appointed Grand Master of the Order, and under him were seven Grand Priors, each representing a division, or Langue, of the Order. These seven were named after the most important countries from which the Knights and Dames had come, and wherein were the possessions and revenues of the Order. They were Provence, Auvergne, France, Italy, England, Germany, and Aragon which was later divided into two, giving an eighth Langue of Castile. In later years, when the property of the Order became so extensive, each Langue was divided into Commanderies in order that it might be properly administered, and each of these were governed by a 'Commander'.

The black robe with the eight-pointed white cross on the left breast was the conventional garb, but when fighting, the Knights wore over their armour a tunic of red with a large plain white cross on the breast. The same white cross on a red ground formed the banner of the Order. The Sisters wore a red dress, over which was a black cloak with the eight-pointed cross; but after the loss of the Island of Rhodes in 1522 they changed the red dress for a black one as a sign of mourning.

The Knights Templars.

About the same time as the Hospitallers were formed into an Order of Knighthood another great Order of Chivalry arose, and it has always been a matter of controversy which of these were the oldest Military Knights; but seeing that the Knights of the Temple were military from the time of their inception it would seem that they could claim that honour.

In the early years of the twelfth century a number of French gentlemen banded themselves into a religious Order of Chivalry for the purpose of giving safe conduct to the pilgrims through the mountain passes and other dangerous localities. To this community of fighting monks Baldwin of Flanders gave a part of the royal palace lying next to the temple of Solomon, from which they took their name—Knights of the Order of the Temple of Solomon—but they were known also as the Knights Templars, or the Red Cross Knights. They were not a nursing order, but owing to the dangers and privations of the journey the pilgrims

147

were often very sick men and women and therefore the Templars became, more or less, a stretcher-bearing organisation.

At the Council of Troyes in 1128 they were formally recognised as a religious order under St Bernard, and they adopted the Cistercian rule with the white habit of the Order, adding a red cross. Later, they changed the white for a black habit. Their banner was half white and half black.

These Knights of the Temple of Solomon rapidly developed into a great international Order, rivalling in wealth and power the other great order of Knights Hospitallers, and their Grand Master was a sovereign prince of Christendom.

During a great part of the history of these two Orders we find strife and bitter rivalries which eventually culminated in a pitched battle; but in all the great crises of the Crusades they forgot their enmity and presented a united front to the Turks and Saracens, rivalling each other only in valour and endurance.

The Second Crusade.

The second crusade took place in 1149, and it was organised by Conrad of the Germanic States, Louis VII. of France, and the Greek emperor Manuel Comnenus. These monarchs quarrelled over the division of the spoils they hoped to obtain, and their ignoble squabbling led to the futile sacrifice of 150,000 men and the general lowering of Christian prestige in the East. This inglorious ending of the crusade occurred but a few months after its commencement.

Military Career of the Knights Hospitallers of St John.

In 1152 the Knights saved Jerusalem from falling into the hands of the Saracens, for at this time Saladin was striving hard to regain possession of what was, to his people also, a very sacred city. In a letter to Richard Cœur de Lion he is stated to have written, 'Jerusalem is as much to us Mohammedans as it can be to you Christians. It is the place whence our Prophet made his night ascent into heaven, and it will be the gathering place of our nation at the Great Judgement.'

The degeneracy of the Christians in the years that followed is strongly denounced by a contemporary writer, Geoffrey de Vinsauf, in the following passage, 'In the year of the Incarnate Word 1187, when Urban III. held the government of the Apostolic See, and Frederick was Emperor in Germany, when Isaac was reigning at Constantinople, Philip in France, Henry in England and William in Sicily, the Lord's Hand fell heavy upon His people, if indeed it is right to call His people those whom the foulness of their vices had alienated from His favour. . . . Corruption had become so diffused throughout the land of Syria tha other nations now drew an example of uncleanness from the same source that formerly had supplied them with the elements of spiritual truth. For this cause, therefore, the Lord, seeing the land of His birth and passion sunk into an abyss of turpitude, suffered Saladin to put forth his might to the destruction of an unworthy people.'

Siege of Acre, and Formation of the Order of Teutonic Knights.

In 1187 Saladin laid siege to Acre, the chief seaport of Syria, but a night attack by the Hospitallers and Templars surprised and scattered his forces and he was obliged to abandon the siege. He then marched his troops to Tiberias, the capital of Galilee and captured that town.

Outside the walls of Acre, German knights under the leadership of Count Adolf of Holstein had converted their tents into emergency hospitals, and when the siege was over they formed themselves into yet another chivalric order—the Order of Teutonic Knights. Conditions of entry into this order were very similar to those of other Knights Hospitallers, and in addition to the usual monastic vows they swore to care for the sick, to build hospitals and to defend the faith. They adopted a black habit over which they wore a white cloak, with a black cross embroidered in gold upon the shoulder. The Knights were required to be of noble birth; but there were also serving brethren who might belong to families of lesser rank.

Surrender of Jerusalem to Saladin.

Later in the same year Saladin again attacked Jerusalem, and although the Knights fought one of the most memorable battles in their history, the city capitulated after only twelve days resistance; and after eighty-seven years of Christian guardianship the Holy Sepulchre fell, once more, into the hands of the Saracens. The beautiful church of St John was converted into a madhouse, and the Church of the Holy Sepulchre became a Mohammedan mosque. In the meantime Saladin's army had also taken Acre.

The Hospitallers conveyed their sick to Margat, a town still held by Christian forces; but many of the ladies of the Order decided to return to Europe. King Henry II. of England granted them extensive lands in Somerset, where they founded Buckland Abbey, and the Queen of Aragon gave them shelter at Saragossa.

Christians Recapture Acre.

After a siege of twenty-three months, during which 100,000 crusaders lost their lives, the Christians, with Richard Cœur de Lion as one of their leaders, recaptured Acre. The Hospitallers fought so gloriously in this attack that the town was henceforth known as St Jean d' Acre. The Knights re-established their hospital in the conquered city in 1191, and it was said to be even greater than the one they had been compelled to abandon at Jerusalem.

Recapture of Jerusalem and the Subsequent Fall of Jerusalem and Gaza to the Turks.

In the crusade of Richard, Duke of Cornwall, in 1240, the Knights Hospitallers were honourably conspicuous, as were the other two knightly orders. They wrested Jerusalem from the Saracens and began the work of repairing the ravages of the war; but before the work was half completed hordes of barbarous

150

Turks swept down from the shores of the Caspian Sea and again Jerusalem was lost; but not, this time, to an honourable foe. The Turks then turned their attention to Gaza, and although the Christian knights and their followers fought with almost super-human resolution for two days and two nights, they were finally overcome by sheer weight of numbers. Both Grand Masters were killed, and at the end of the battle only thirty Templars and six-teen Hospitallers remained alive.

Then Louis IX. of France took up the cudgels, and gathering a great army he sailed via Cyprus and Egypt, and thence by land to Palestine. He began his campaign in 1248 by the recapture of Damietta; and then he made the fatal mistake of delaying his advance, thus giving his enemies time to marshal their forces. The disastrous battle of Mansourah took place, the Christians were defeated, and the Sultan held King Louis and the broken remnants of his army to ransom for the enormous sum of 800,000 golden besants. To pay this the Hospitallers placed their entire treasury at the disposal of the French King.

Warfare between the Templars and the Hospitallers.

For many years animosity had smouldered between these two great orders of Knighthood. In 1252 it burst into flame and, to the scandal of Christendom, they fought each other, the Knights of St John being victorious; but they subsequently lost four strongholds to the Moslems in rapid succession from sheer lack of adequate forces to hold them. The second crusade of King Louis set out to enable them to regain these possessions, but its course was diverted into Africa, into the fever-breeding swamps of Tunis; where on 25th August, 1270, the King died. Without waiting for the arrival of the English army under Prince Edward (afterwards Edward I.), which was coming to their assistance, the French army made peace.

Loss of the Last Christian Stronghold in Syria.

Acre was now the centre of Christianity in the East, and it was famous for its wealth and beauty. This was an age of great building, and contemporary writers describe its magnificent architecture, its churches with their gem-like stained glass windows, its white marble palaces, its gardens and spacious courtyards, and its broad, straight streets. But it was inhabited by seventeen conflicting races, speaking diverse languages and amenable to different laws, so that, naturally, there was perpetual strife and unwarrantable acts of brigandage by both Christians and infidels.

In 1291 the Moslem Sultan gathered a great army of 160,000 foot and 60,000 horse and besieged the city. News of his approach had reached the Knightly Orders and they had sent nearly all the women and children on the galleys of their fleet to Cyprus, the nearest island of refuge.

The story of the heroic resistance of the Knights Hospitallers and Templars to the Moslem onslaught forms one of the most marvellous stories of dauntless bravery in the history of the Military Orders, but it ended in their defeat; and the remnants of the Knights of St John retreated to Cyprus, which had been captured by Richard Cœur de Lion a century before and was now ruled by a Christian King, Henry de Lusignan. He gave them the Castle of Kolossi, which still belongs to the English order, and is now preserved as an 'ancient monument'.

The Order of St John in Cyprus and Rhodes.

The branches of the Order in England, France, Spain, Scotland, Ireland, Portugal, Italy and Germany dispatched some of their strongest knights to Cyprus, with treasures and supplies to enable the Hospitallers to refound their hospital for the *fourth* time, and to consolidate their military power. Although the Holy Land was again under Moslem rule, pilgrimages continued, and a new element of danger faced the pilgrims—capture by the Barbary Corsairs. This meant a life of slavery, chained to the wooden

152

benches of the galleys, and labouring at the oars under the merciless lash of the taskmasters.

The rallied Order of Hospitallers, true to their chivalrous ideals for the protection of the weak against oppression, cruelty and outrage, developed their maritime power; and the Corsairs, who for centuries had terrorised the Mediterranean, now found their ascendancy challenged most persistently, and they discovered that the valiant knights could fight on the decks of a galley as formidably as from behind the rampart of a fortress. And when in 1310, under the Grand Master Villaret, the Hospitallers captured the island of Rhodes, they were able to harry the Turks from its famous harbour, and to make the island one of the best fortified bulwarks of the world. They won the supremacy of the Mediterranean, and the Corsairs learnt to labour in the galleys of the Hospitallers.

Hospitallers Capture Mediterranean Strongholds.

Alexandria had become a rendezvous for pirates, so that its capture was a necessary phase in the breaking of Turkish sea power. This the Hospitallers accomplished in 1365, and they then joined forces with the King of Cyprus and the Genoese republic for the recapture of Tarsus, Tripoli, Bellinas and Laodocia.

Two Sieges and the Loss of Rhodes.

For a time there was comparative peace, but in 1453 Constantinople was again attacked and conquered by the Moslems whose Sultan then called upon the Knights of Rhodes to be his vassals and to pay him yearly tribute. This they refused, and twenty-seven years later, in 1480, the Turks attacked the island with an enormous fleet and army. The Knights, under Grand Master Peter D'Aubusson, sustained one of the greatest sieges in history, lasting for many months; finally they drove back the Turks, gaining victory against such odds that it was attributed to supernatural aid from John the Baptist, the patron saint of the Order;

153

and for yet another forty years the Hospitallers continued to hold the island as their headquarters.

In 1522 Rhodes was again besieged by the Sultan—Suleiman the Magnificent—and after six months gallant defence the Knights were forced to capitulate. The triumphal entry of Suleiman into Rhodes on Christmas Day, 1522, formed the theme of several descriptive masterpieces of Arabic literature.

On the morning of New Year's Day the Grand Master Villiers de L'Isle Adams, and the Hospitallers, taking with them 4,000 inhabitants of the island, left Rhodes, which had been their headquarters for more than two centuries, defeated and homeless, but still 'strong in will to strive, to seek, to find, and not to yield'.

The Knights in Malta.

For eight years after the loss of Rhodes the Knights were homeless wanderers, until on 24th March, 1530, the Emperor Charles V. conferred upon them the 'perpetual sovereignty of Malta and Goso, and the city of Tripoli with all the castles and fortresses thereto belonging'. Malta was then a barren rock, with just a few ramparts and the Tower of Angelo, and with its entire population numbering not more than seventeen hundred; but under the wise and reconstructive rule of de L'Isle Adams, Malta became an almost impregnable stronghold. He was succeeded by one who is acclaimed the greatest of all Grand Masters, Jean de la Valette, under whom the Knights reached their highest pinnacle of moral and material prosperity. Valette had suffered captivity and slavery at the hands of the Corsairs, and at the age of twenty-eight he had taken part in the last defence of Rhodes. He was sixty-three when elected Grand Master, but his most glorious achievements were yet before him. It is quite impossible, in such a work as this, to give any account of the character and accomplishments of this 'giant among men' during the eleven eventful years of his Grand Mastership, for in this, as in all the history of the Order, there is romance and high endeavour sufficient for the making of many books.

One of the heaviest blows which befell the Order during these years was the loss of Tripoli, and this formed the opening of the last great military struggle for Mediterranean supremacy between the adherents of the Cross and those of the Crescent.

The Siege of Malta.

This siege lasted from 11th April until 7th September, 1565. Its heroic defence by the Knights remains, for all time, one of the greatest feats of arms of which history has record, and it was watched with the keenest anxiety by every power in Europe. Even Queen Elizabeth, who had recently abolished the Order in England, on account of its allegiance to the Pope, ordered prayers to be said in all the churches for these gallant defenders of Christendom. Eventually the Turks were defeated, having lost 30,000 men, whilst the defenders had lost 260 Knights and 8,000 soldiers, for whom a Requiem Mass has since been sung in Malta every year till this day; and as the bells begin their tolling one may hear the people murmur, 'It is the deliverance of the Knights.'

In the next year La Valette commenced the building of his new city on Mount Sceberras, to be called Valetta, which is practically the same to-day as it was towards the end of that century. The magnificent church of St John, built at that time, is as large as St Paul's Cathedral. It has six chapels on either side forming aisles, and in its decoration the arts of the gilder, the carver and the painter have been most lavishly expended. Its floor is an elaborate mosaic of coloured marbles with heraldic memorials of more than 400 Knights, and its roof is entirely covered with scenes in the life of John the Baptist, painted by the Italian knight, Mathias Preti.

The Grand Master's Palace was built between 1572 and 1581. In the eighteenth century its store of armoury was sufficient to equip 25,000 men. To-day it holds a collection of over 6,000 pieces of arms and armour which is of great historical value.

155

The Hospital at Malta.

This hospital was by far the largest building on the island. Its great ward was 500 feet in length. There were eleven other large halls or wards, a chapel, a library, dispensaries and quarters for the staff. Close by was a large linen store and a laundry. All the walls were very thick, as they needed to be in such troublous times, and the windows were small and high, thus differing from the architectural style of a century or two earlier. A visitor during the reign of Charles II. records in his diary that all the patients were given single beds and the linen was changed most regularly once a fortnight; a great improvement on the general European standards at that time. There were separate wards for medical and surgical cases, and dysentery and fever patients were isolated. There was a ward with a special guardian for the insane. The patients were served on silver dishes and the regulations of the hospital for the year 1725 show that the silver plate consisted of 1,140 articles weighing 1215 pounds. Slaves were served with pewter dishes and utensils. Great emphasis was laid on the proper diets for the sick. Rice, vermicelli, herbs and chicken were provided for the very sick, the more convalescent had meat, pigeon, game and potatoes. There were special supervisors, appointed by the Grand Master, to ensure that only the best was served in the hospital. Under the arcades of the courtyard was a pharmacy, a sort of out-patients' department, with rows of Majolica jars inscribed with the names of the drugs and herbs they held. Each day the blind, the leprous and the scrofulous of both sexes came for the medicines, the milk and the broths that the physicians prescribed for them. They were provided with bandages and crutches, and they were given a small sum of money daily. In these arcades there were rooms where steam baths were given. Two knights, having the assistance of four elderly women, carried food and medicines to the sick poor in the towns.

The Budget at Malta shows that the largest expense was the

156

upkeep of the galleys, which was 135,000 gold scudi.[1] Against that one finds that 25,000 gold scudi were required for the hospital, and 39,000 for the house to house care of the sick and relief of the poor in Malta and the neighbouring island of Gozo. These are the figures given in a report made for Pope Urban VIII., but another report made about a century later gives more than twice those amounts for the upkeep of the hospital and other charitable work. (A full account of this hospital is given in *The Regulations of the Old Hospital of the Knights of St John*, by W. K. Bedford, published 1725, reprinted by Blackwood in 1882.)

Decline of the Order.

With the centuries of comparative peace the military efficiency of the Order waned, and as so often happens in an age of great wealth and security, there was growing idleness, luxury and licentiousness which the succeeding Grand Masters failed to restrain. The spirit and the ideals which had made the Order so great in previous centuries seemed completely extinct by the time that John Howard made his memorable tour of inspection in 1785. In his report, given in *Lazarettos and Hospitals*, published in 1789, he gives an appalling account of the filth and general neglect in the great hospital. One cannot do better than quote from that report. He says,

'In the largest wards there were four rows of beds. . . . They were all so dirty and offensive as to create the necessity of perfuming them, and yet I observed that the physician, in going his rounds, was obliged to keep his handkerchief to his face. The use of perfume I always reckon a proof of inattention to cleanliness and airiness; and this inattention struck me forcibly on opening some of the private closets with which this hall is very properly furnished. . . .

The number of patients in this hospital during the time I was in Malta (29th March to 19th April, 1785) was from 510 to 532. These were served by the most dirty, ragged, unfeeling and inhuman per-

[1] A scudi was about 5s.

157

sons I ever saw. I once found eight or nine of them highly entertained with a delirious, dying patient.

The governor told me that they had only 32 servants, and that many of them were debtors or criminals who had fled thither for refuge. At the same time I observed that near 40 attendants were kept to take charge of about 26 horses and the same number of mules in the Grand Master's stables, and that there all was clean. I cannot help adding that in the centre of each of these stables there was a fountain, out of which water was constantly running in a stone basin; but that in the hospital, though there was indeed a fountain, there was no water.

There was a great want of room in this hospital. I requested that a delirious patient who disturbed the other patients might be lodged in a room by himself, but was told that no such room could be found. Opposite to this hospital there is a large house, which is now used only for a wash-house. A great improvement might be made by providing a wash-house for the hospital somewhere out of the city (its proper situation) and appropriating these spacious and airy apartments for poor knights and convalescent patients.

The slow hospital fever (the inevitable consequence of closeness, uncleanliness and dirt) prevails here. In the hospital for women there were 230 patients, who had all separate beds. The governess attended me through every ward, and was constantly using her smelling bottle; in which she judged very properly, for a more offensive and dirty hospital for women I never visited.'

Then came the great French Revolution with its ambitious and implacable leader, Napoleon Bonaparte, intent on ravaging Europe. Already the Order, being essentially aristocratic, had been suppressed in France, and many of the noble knights had gone to the guillotine. On 9th June, 1798, a French fleet, under the personal command of Bonaparte, arrived, and demanded entrance into the harbour of Valetta. After a few days of feeble resistance, the island capitulated without fighting. There was treachery within the gates, and some weakness of the leaders of the Order, especially of the Grand Master von Homepesch, the only German Grand Master the Order ever had.

The tragedy of the capitulation lies in the fact that, had the island held out for just a few weeks longer, Nelson and his British navy would have arrived, and Malta would have been saved. As it was, Napoleon sacked the church, the palace and the hospital, conveying the treasures of the Knights on board his flagship *L'Orient* which, later, was sunk by Nelson in the battle of the Nile. Much of that treasure still lies at the bottom of the sea in Aboukir Bay.

After the loss of Malta many of the Knights returned to their own countries, but some of them fled to Russia and besought the protection of the young Czar, Paul I., who was later elected Grand Master of the Order.

The Order in England.

There is very little to record, relevant to this history, of the Order of St John of Jerusalem in England before their suppression by Henry VIII.

Their first home in this country was at Clerkenwell, where, in 1130, one Jordan de Briset had given the Order ten acres of land whereon they built a great Priory. As all the Knights were, at least officially, celibate, and therefore had no legitimate heirs, their property passed, at their death, to the Order. Thus, its wealth and possessions accumulated until in 1338 it owned more than ninety manors in England as well as estates in Scotland and Ireland. It included the properties acquired by the Hospitallers when the Templars were suppressed, among whose possessions had been the New Temple in London. This the Hospitallers leased to 'Students of Law' shortly after its acquisition.

The Priory at Clerkenwell.

The Grand Prior was the Chief Baron of England, taking precedence of all other lay barons in the House of Lords. Many charters were given to the Order granting special privileges to its members, and freeing them from the usual duties to the State.

One of these privileges was the right to give sanctuary, in all their houses, to debtors and felons.

During the Wat Tyler rebellion the head Priory at Clerkenwell, and many other possessions of the Order, were destroyed by fire, and the rebels beheaded the Grand Prior on Tower Hill.

At the beginning of the sixteenth century the Order appears to have reached the zenith of its power and prosperity. The great Priory at Clerkenwell had been rebuilt with a magnificent tower, which, unfortunately, has since been destroyed, and a very impressive gateway which still stands. The Grand Prior, Thomas Docwra, stood high in the favour of King Henry VII., who was a frequent visitor to the Priory.

The Order appears to have been carrying out none of the functions for which it was primarily organised, but its members were loyal adherents to Papal authority.

About the middle of the reign of Henry VIII. the Knights lost Rhodes, and the English monarch was organising a visitation o the monasteries preparatory to their suppression and the confiscation of their property.

The Priory at Buckland.

When, in 1180, Henry II. presented the estate at Buckland, in Somerset, to the Ladies of the Order of St John of Jerusalem for the purpose of founding a community, only nine sisters under the Prioress Fina were housed there, but the number gradually increased to about fifty, and remained more or less at that figure. There appears very little real evidence that these ladies continued the work of their Order among the sick and needy. In February, 1539, pressure was brought upon the Prioress Katherine Bouchier by the Royal Commissioners, and she surrendered her Priory.

Suppression of the English Langue.

During the Reformation several of the Knights chose to die upon the scaffold rather than relinquish their faith; but eventually the Order was dissolved by the rapacious Henry VIII., and during this ordeal the Knights appear to have lived up to their traditions.

With the accession of Queen Mary one of her first acts was to open negotiations for the restoration of the Grand Priories of England and Ireland, as a result of which letters patent were issued by the Crown authorising the reinstation of the Order and the return of many of its properties. This has never been rescinded, and therefore, in theory, the Order has remained a 'body corporate'. The revival lasted but a short time, for after the death of Queen Mary and the accession of her half-sister, Queen Elizabeth, the Crown once more seized the property of the Order and the Knights fled to Malta, where some members of the English branch remained until driven out by Napoleon.

Later History of Other Orders of Hospitallers. The Knights Templars.

The ultimate fate of the Knights Templars was very different from that of the Knights of St John. After being driven from Palestine they appeared to have formed no plans for their reconstitution. They had great wealth and many estates, especially in France, whither the remnants of the Order retired. Philip IV. —known as Philip the Fair—feared their political influence and coveted their wealth; and he proved a most unscrupulous enemy.

The Order met with a tragic ending that was a disgrace to mediæval justice. As a result of trumped-up and unproved charges all the Templars in France were arrested, and many of them suffered torture, shame, and death, at the hands of their accusers. The entire Order was abolished by a Papal decree at the Council of Vienna in 1312, and the whole of its property that escaped the rapacity of the French King and Pope Clement V. was transferred to the Order of St John of Jerusalem.

In England, Edward II. ordered the arrest of the Templars in 1318, and their estates were placed in charge of a body known as the 'Guardians of the Lands of the Templars', all the rents and revenues being paid into the royal exchequer. The Pope objected so strongly to this that the King eventually ordered all the property to be handed over to the Hospitallers of St John in accordance with the Papal decree, but not until 1340 was this vexed question settled.

The Order of Teutonic Knights.

These Knights were almost entirely German, with their estates and revenues in Germany. Both during and after the Crusades the Knights undertook the management of many hospitals already existing in that country and built others, the more famous of which were the Hospital of St Barbara in Strasburg, and establishments at Elbing and Nuremberg. They were renowned for their strict organisation and excellent methods of administration. The Order became more democratic and less monastic in the thirteenth century and therefore escaped, to a certain extent, the paralysing effect of an indolent peace; but, although it possessed considerable political power, it incurred the jealous opposition of the clergy.

The famous castle of the Teutonic Knights at Marienburg was the most beautiful building of the middle ages in Germany. It is still one of the chief sights of the town and it attracts many of the visitors to the south-east shores of the Baltic Sea. Attached to it was an infirmary for the sick and aged brethren.

The Hospitaller Sisters of the Teutonic Order were the German equivalent of the Ursulines of France and Austria, and the Poor Clares of Italy. Their work included the visiting of the poor and the sick in their own homes, the care of lepers and the custody of the insane.

In the fifteenth century the Order suffered so severely from financial losses and other results of war that its pristine vigour was almost spent and it sank into comparative unimportance. In 1809 it was entirely suppressed, but it was resuscitated in Austria in 1840 as a semi-religious knighthood, and during the last century it has assisted with various ambulance services.

162

The Knights of St Lazarus.

This was a fourth Order of Knighthood that was working in the service of the sick during the Crusades. Its origin and early history is somewhat obscure. It is probably the oldest Order of Hospitallers. Tradition associates it with the basilias of Cæsarea in the fourth century, but there seems to be no proof of this. St Lazarus is the patron saint of lepers, and legend traces the origin of the Order to the time of Christ himself. It was active in Palestine quite early in the Crusades; its work lay especially amongst lepers and it received, as knights, many who were themselves stricken with the dread disease.

Its constitution was much on the same lines as those of the other chivalric Orders and it possessed great estates in Europe; but only lepers of noble birth were eligible for election as Grand Masters. This rule was rescinded in 1253, for so many knightly lepers had perished in the Crusades that the Pope gave permission for the election of a non-leper. The habit and insignia of the Order was not the same for all countries, especially in its colouring. The first Knights of Jerusalem wore a mantle on which was a plain cross with four arms of equal length. The French Cross of the Order had eight arms with tiny golden lilies in the corners, the cross itself being green or purplish red; whilst the Italian colours were white and green.

After the Crusades this Order had its greatest activities in France, Italy and Germany, but it had several hospitals in England. The principal one in this country was at Burton Lazars and was founded by one Mowbray, a crusading member of the Order. In 1608 Henry IV. united the French branch with the Community of Our Lady of Mount Carmel under the name of 'Knights of Our Lady of Mount Carmel and St Lazarus'. The extirpation of leprosy in Europe about this period rendered the special work of the Order unnecessary, but the French branch continued its existence until it was suppressed at the Revolution.

The Italian branch amalgamated with the Knights of Malta in

163

1490 by order of Pope Innocent VIII., but it resumed its independence under its own Grand Master in 1572, and was united with the Order of St Maurice. It seems to have had some sphere of activity in connection with the building and organisation of 'lazarettos', or hospitals for infectious diseases, but the records are very indefinite. By 1830 the Order had apparently become extinct.

164

CHAPTER VIII

RECONSTITUTION OF THE ORDER OF ST JOHN OF JERUSALEM

The St John Ambulance Association and Brigade—The hospital at Jerusalem, its capture by the Turks during the World War—The new hospital and its constitution—Twentieth century development in Europe —Conclusion

Revival of the English Langue of the Order of Knights Hospitallers of St John of Jerusalem.

ALTHOUGH, by the end of the eighteenth century, the fraternity in Malta had sadly fallen away from its traditions, the Grand Prior of France had been conspicuous for his dauntless fidelity to his Order and the ideals for which it stood; and from this country came the first attempt to recreate the Order on a secular basis. It could never again be military, nor could it be an order of celibate monks and nuns, but its work in the care of the sick and injured was still necessary. The French Knights sent their representatives to the Congress of Vienna in 1814, and again in 1822. They realised that in Republican France no revival of an Order so essentially aristocratic was possible, and in 1826 they suggested that the English Langue of the Order might be revived with the modifications necessary to meet with the views of the Protestant Church; and the French Catholic delegate, the Chevalier de Chastelain, worked assiduously for this new formation.

In 1831 the English Order was reconstituted with its Titular Grand Prior and sub-Prior, its Knights and Ladies of Grace, its Prelates and sub-Prelates, its Bailiffs and Commanders, and its Serving Brothers and Sisters. Its main object was to alleviate the sufferings of the injured, the sick and the helpless.

A few years later, difficulties began to arise owing to the fact that the English Langue was non-Catholic. Negotiations were opened on several occasions, but no satisfactory decisions were made. The authorities at Rome continued their refusal to recognise the legitimacy of the English Order until, in 1858, matters were definitely brought to a head and the Order became purely national with no other head than its own Sovereign. It was styled 'The Order of St John of Jerusalem in England', and the Maltese Cross, which had been surmounted with a crown and ornamented with lions and unicorns, had its embellishments removed, and the plain eight-pointed white cross was adopted as the insignia of the Order. About this period the Order acquired all that was left of the old Priory at Clerkenwell, including the old gatehouse.

St John Ambulance Association and Brigade.

In no direction has the work of the modern Knights been so conspicuous than in the formation and development of the Ambulance Association and Brigade. The genesis of this movement is connected with the Red Cross organisations, which were so actively progressive during the 'sixties'. The Order of St John sent representatives to the International Conference of Red Cross Societies held in Berlin in 1869, and in the following year many members enrolled themselves under the newly formed British Aid Society (later the British Red Cross Society) for service during the Franco-Prussian War. After this war it was realised that no Red Cross Society could be really effective during war unless its members received tuition and training during peace, and so organised its equipment and personnel that its resources could quickly be mobilised into a really efficient adjunct to the army. With the rise of industrialism and the speeding up of travel by the introduction of steam engines, there was a great increase in the number of accidental injuries among the civil population, and a consequent need for a reliable 'First-aid service'.

In 1872 a member of the Order gave £100 towards a fund for

establishing an Ambulance Service in the mining and pottery districts where accidents are of such frequent occurrence. This was followed by the purchasing, from Berlin, of two litters similar to those used by the Prussian army, and these were sent to Wolverhampton and Burslem. Private individuals and public bodies undertook to defray expenses and to superintend the management, and so, in a very short time, a large number of these litters were purchased for different centres, and also for the use of the Metropolitan Police.

In 1874 Surgeon-General Thomas Laymon, C.B., read a paper at St John's Gate on 'Observations on the preliminary care and attention necessary for accidental bodily injuries and mutilations occurring in mines and establishments where many work-people are employed'. Other papers followed this, laying down definite lines of first-aid treatment. Two years later, there was protracted war in the East and the Committee of the Order of St John passed the following resolution—'That there being no organisation in existence for giving relief, irrespective of political aim and object, a Committee should be formed of members of the Order, and others, for the purpose of affording such aid as was possible to the sufferers in the conflict raging in the East'. At this meeting the Eastern War Fund and the Wounded Relief Fund came into existence; both of these being subsequently merged into the British National Aid Society.

During the Turko-Russian War the Order organised and directed nine hospitals in European Turkey and Asia, supplying field ambulances, a sanitary service, and railway transport.

Meanwhile, the Ambulance movement was spreading throughout Britain, courses of instruction were being arranged which included a minimum of five lectures followed by an examination, and advanced classes were formed for women at St Mary's Hospital, and for men at King's College and Westminster Hospitals.

In 1879 the first manual of instruction in first aid was published and over 26,000 copies were sold at once. There were improvements in stretchers, bandages and general equipment, and

167

English firms began to supply these needs, thus adding a new industry to the country.

This work had now captured the imagination and awakened the enthusiasm of the people of all ranks. It was spreading throughout Europe, as was also the Red Cross movement, and in spirit if not literally, there was a return of the chivalric zeal which animated the original Order and which led the nations of the West once again to combine in a Crusade for the purpose of lessening the sufferings of humanity in the accidents both of peace and of war. They established a Transport Corps, and to this was added a Nursing Corps of women who had received instruction in first aid and sick nursing. Very soon, Ambulance stations were organised at national and international exhibitions, and at all places where large crowds assembled. These were in charge of a paid attendant, usually an ex-service man from the Army Medical Corps, assisted by voluntary workers, with a local medical man 'on call', who could be summoned in case of serious injury or illness.

No rank or grade of society was unrepresented in this great national work—from the Royal family to the humblest of manual labourers—and in 1888 the Prince of Wales (afterwards King Edward VII.) as Grand Prior of the Order, presented to Queen Victoria the humble petition of the Knights of St John that she should grant them her Royal Charter of Incorporation. This she did, with her own royal hand, graciously becoming its Sovereign Head and Patron. The reception of this Charter was the great landmark in the history of the modern Order, which in it is designated as 'The Grand Priory of the Order of the Hospital of St John of Jerusalem in England', the St John Ambulance Association being incorporated with it as one of its principal activities; and thus opened a new era in the history of the English Hospitallers.

The Hospital at Jerusalem.

In 1882 a hospice and ophthalmic dispensary was founded in Jerusalem on the Bethlehem road, not far from the Jaffa Gate and overlooking the valley of Hinnon. It was strictly non-sectarian, all races, ranks and creeds being treated according to their need; and in this country, where diseases of the eye are so prevalent and lead to such terrible results, its work increased stupendously. Within the first six months from its opening 1,952 patients were treated, whilst the total number who received advice and medicine was 6,138, and on many days upwards of 140 patients were in attendance.

Year by year these numbers increased and the fame of the hospital spread so far and wide that patients journeyed to it on foot from the furthermost parts of Syria and Persia in the hope of being saved from the horror of blindness.

In 1891 two trained nurses were sent out from England, and a new out-patient department was built in honour of General Gordon. In 1914, soon after the commencement of the Great War, the hospital was captured by the Turks, who, being short of hospital supplies, stripped it of almost everything it contained, and in the following year, turned it into an ammunition depot. It was used for that purpose until Lord Allenby made his victorious advance upon Jerusalem on 4th December, 1917, when the Turks blew up the hospital before evacuating the city. It was not completely destroyed, however, and after the War the Order undertook its restoration, at the same time carrying out some necessary improvements.

The New Hospital and its Constitution.

The newly constructed hospital was opened by Lord Allenby on 26th February, 1919. Every nationality, creed and institution in the Near East was represented at this official ceremony, and the Grand Prior of England, H.R.H. the Duke of Connaught, sent the following telegram—'I rejoice at the opening of our hospital at Jerusalem, and I trust that it will be able in the future to continue the good work it has done in the past—Connaught.'

In the year 1921 the Chapter-General decided that the Christian nursing staff of the hospital, so long as they continued to act in that capacity, should be members of the Order of St John of Jerusalem in the grade of Service Brethren and Sisters, that the Medical Superintendent should be known as the Warden, the second surgeon as the sub-Warden, and the third as the Registrar; and that these officers should be invested with the insignia mantle and cap of the Order.

For a few years things went smoothly, and then in 1927 the hospital suffered severely as the result of an earthquake. In the following year the work of restoration was commenced, and again improvements and additions were made, the out-patient department was remodelled and enlarged, and an annexe was built in which the patients could rest between their treatments. Very frequently it has been found, however, that women and children are left in the Annexe without either food or money, the husband and father having returned to his native village. Then the hospital must provide food, or the ophthalmic treatment will be of no avail.

One of the major problems which this hospital has to face is the scarcity of water. For six years after its rebuilding Palestine endured exceptionally dry winters, the springs upon which the country had learned to depend completely dried up, and this water famine rendered the taking of the usual number of in-patients quite an impossibility; only emergency cases could be admitted.

In addition to the work at Jerusalem the hospital has been responsible for superintending six ophthalmic clinics attached to Government hospitals at Acre, Beersheba, Gaza, Nablus, Ramleh and Tulkesham. A seventh was added, in 1932, at Jaffa, and three more in the following year. These clinics are staffed with trained male orderlies. There is now a scheme in operation for the training of Arab girls in the elementary principles of hygiene, home-nursing, sanitation and first aid, after which it is hoped that they will be able to assist with the work of the hospital and the clinics.

The Order also supplies First Aid boxes for the use of its staff when travelling; and in such a country one can well understand the necessity for this.

For the past few years the number of new patients annually has been over 20,000, and the actual operations each year has been between three and four thousand, about 60 per cent of which have been for the relief of trichiasis.

And thus, in Palestine, this great Order continues its ministrations to the needs of humanity. The days of armoured knights have long since passed, the lances and swords have given place to bombs, machine-guns, poison gases, and all the other impedimenta of twentieth-century warfare; but the spirit of knightly chivalry still glows in human hearts as brightly as in those long dead centuries, although in the security of modern civilisation it finds expression in quieter and more systematic, even if less spectacular, endeavours.

Twentieth Century Development in Europe.

By the end of the nineteenth century practically every town in England had its branch of the St John Ambulance Association, which arranged courses of instruction in First Aid and Home Nursing, held examinations and gave certificates to those who satisfied the examiners. It was soon realised, however, that a large number of those who gained the certificate quickly forgot all they had learned from want of practice, and so facilities were provided for the holders of certificates to be re-examined twelve months later, and if satisfactory, to receive a medallion. Up to the present time nearly a million certificates and half a million medallions have been awarded. Thus, knowledge is taken into the homes of the people, and every thoughtful member of the general public is fully aware of the inestimable services rendered to humanity by such an organisation, not only in England but throughout the world; quietly and inconspicuously during times of peace, but providing and equipping hospitals, training stretcher bearers, orderlies and nurses for emergency work in war, and sending out contingents of efficient helpers, fully equipped to contend with any accidents or sudden illnesses that may occur on public occasions.

Such was the training and organisation, that in 1914 thousands of nurses and orderlies were ready to help with the stupendous task of tending our wounded, not only with the British forces but also with the Canadian, the Australian and the South African.

In October, 1914, the Order of St John joined forces with the British Red Cross Society, forming the Joint War Committee— the greatest single organisation of voluntary aid the world has ever known for the relief of human suffering. It embodied the true spirit of chivalry as unmistakably as did the Knights of eight centuries ago, working on every battlefield and in every clearing station, and organising transport with such efficiency that thousands of wounded men were transferred to home hospitals within a few hours of being picked up on the battlefield. In addition, it equipped and staffed its own hospitals and assisted in the work of both military and civilian hospitals under other organisations.

Malta, so rich in the memories of the Knights, again became a hospital base with a bed accommodation in April 1915 of 825. In May, the wounded arrived in great convoys from Gallipoli and the number of beds rose in that month to over four thousand. In June they reached seven thousand, in August eleven thoussand, and in December the total was 11,109. All the available public buildings were utilised, and, as in England, many private houses were given up for emergency hospitals.

In 1916 hostilities in Salonika resulted in the transport of many thousands of wounded to the island, as did also the epidemics of malaria and dysentery. Altogether some 200,000 soldiers of all ranks were treated in the hospitals of Malta.

Conclusion.

It is surely unnecessary, in a work such as this, to give any further account of this great and historic Order. Can we envisage our twentieth-century England without its ministrations? It is so very much a part, not only of our national life and of life in all the far-flung outposts of Empire, but also of many countries belonging to other nations. The realisation that practically all of this great work is entirely voluntary, that men and women of all ranks, in their tens of thousands, are still quietly and unostentatiously giving of their leisure and their substance to aid those who are sick and injured, must surely bring with it a renewed and refreshing faith in the innate qualities of compassionate selflessness in human nature.

173

CHAPTER IX

SECULAR NURSING ORDERS

European conditions in the early mediæval period—Secular Orders as an outlet for women's activity—Pre-Reformation Secular Orders—The Antonines—The Humiliati or Hospitallers of the Observance—The Oblates of Florence—The Misericordia—The Béguines of Flanders—The Franciscan Tertiaries and the Minoresses of St Clare—The Order of the Holy Ghost and the Medical School of Montpelier—The Grey Sisters— The Alexian, or Cellite Brotherhood

European Conditions in the Early Mediæval Period.

FOR more than a thousand years after the crash of the Roman Empire the progress of civilisation throughout Europe was exceedingly slow. Vast tracts of country were wild and uncultivated, abounding in primeval forests, dark marshes and desolate moors. Journeys were dangerous, men went forth armed and accompanied by a retinue, whilst women were sheltered within the guarded castle, or cloistered within the convent walls. Passions were intense and social customs were brutal and violent. Luxury was practically unknown, for even the nobles lived hard, bare lives, their homes were cold and gloomy, their food was coarse, heavy, and usually much too abundant. Nature appeared to share in the harsh cruelty of mankind during this period, for there were an unprecedented number of cyclones, earthquakes and floods, destroying vineyards and harvests, demolishing homes, and killing or injuring the occupants. People lived with terror in their hearts, knowing neither how to account for, or how to meet, such disasters. Flood and famine brought pestilence in their train, and epidemics ran an unobstructed course amongst

174

the squalid and anæmic people, for hygiene had reached its lowest level in the unpaved and undrained cities, where most of the houses were leaky hovels and the streets were veritable sewers. The 'Black Death' of 1348 was undoubtedly the most destructive of these pestilences, for whole districts were depopulated; and historians estimate that one-third of the population of Europe perished during this epidemic alone.

Most of the practice of medicine during this age was carried out in the monasteries, and they were the chief refuges for the homeless and the sick.

Secular Orders as an Outlet for Women's Activity.

From the eleventh to the thirteenth centuries woman's activity in the field of charity developed greatly in advance of man's, and strove to set itself free from monasticism. This was the age of the Crusades, and some women went forth with their loved ones to the wars, whilst many others entered convents to await their return. These latter were, naturally, not seeking to live the celibate life of the cloister, or to bear all the austerities of the monastic life. There was, too, at this time, a growing feeling that the monasteries were becoming far too rich and powerful, and there were abuses creeping into the cloistered life which alienated the sympathies of the lay mind. Meanwhile, the sick and the destitute in the world outside the monasteries were not being ministered unto according to the teachings of Christianity. They needed much more help than was being given, and, in response to this need, there arose many uncloistered Orders. Some were for men only, but many included, or were entirely composed of, women. Quite a number of these have survived the many vicissitudes of religious thought, social order, and government organisation that have occurred since their inception, and are still to be found actively carrying out some type of charitable work in the world to-day.

As the Crusades went on, with their inevitable toll of human life, the number of desolate women in Europe increased rapidly,

175

and doubtless many of these became attached to the new Orders that were springing up, finding solace in the various activities which the work demanded from them.

Pre-Reformation Secular Orders. The Antonines, or Hospital Brothers of St Antony.

This was an Order founded about 1095 by a certain Gaston de Dauphiné in thanksgiving for a miraculous cure from a disease which was very prevalent at that time and was known as St Antony's Fire. It was probably the condition we know as erysipelas, and the members of the Order devoted their energies exclusively to the nursing of sufferers from this disease. The brothers built a hospital that became the centre of the Order, and very shortly afterwards they initiated a Branch Order for women. During the next few centuries they built special hospitals for erysipelas throughout Europe and undertook all the required nursing, but they neither admitted patients with other diseases nor nursed them in their own homes. Apparently this indicated a recognition of the contagiousness of erysipelas, and it was, to all intents and purposes, a segregation of those suffering from it; for undoubtedly the existence of such special hospitals made it possible to control many of the epidemics that occurred.

At first the Antonines were a lay Order, but the brothers and sisters received monastic vows under the Rule of St Augustine in 1297. Among their privileges was that of arranging a special branch to care for the sick in the Papal household, and this appears to be the only instance of the Antonines undertaking the nursing of diseases other than erysipelas. After the suppression of the religious Orders in England these special hospitals disappeared, and erysipelas came back to be a very serious scourge in the general hospitals, especially among surgical cases and parturient women, for the contagiousness of it was not generally recognised until less than a century ago.

The Order was canonically united with the Knights of Malta in 1777, but it was suppressed during the French Revolution.

The Humiliati, or Hospitallers of the Observance..

This was a penitential Order formed in the twelfth century, and its members were principally Lombard nobles who had been taken captive to Germany, but were given their freedom. The men of the Order formed trading associations, and played an important part in the civic life of every community in which they were established. The first women of the Order belonged to some of the principal families in Milan, and they formed a community under the leadership of Clare Blassoni, devoting themselves to the care of lepers in neighbouring hospitals, especially in Florence. There are still, in Italy, five independent houses of the Humiliati, the sisters are known as 'Barretines' and wear a grey dress.

The Oblates of Florence.

This was a group of Orders that arose during the twelfth and subsequent centuries—an oblate being a secular person working in connection with a monastery but not under its vows. The group included both Brotherhoods and Sisterhoods, some of the most famous being the Humiliati, the Order of Santa Maria Nuova, and the Misericordia. The second of these is still in existence and its members live in the Convent of the Order which stands opposite the Hospital of Santa Maria Nuova. They visit the hospital each day. Their duties are to direct and supervise the housekeeping and to give food and medicines to the patients, but beyond this they do not undertake any nursing work.

The Misericordia.

The Misericordia were a kind of ambulance brotherhood founded in 1244 who did volunteer work in Florence and other Italian cities. They were sometimes known as the 'Masked Brotherhood'. It is difficult to find definite details of their work, but the spirit of it is exemplified in the following poem about a

porter of a city gate in the middle ages when plague and leprosy
were rife.

'Piero Luca, known of all the town
As the grey porter by the Pitti wall,
Where the noon shadows of the gardens fall,
Sick and in dolour, waited to lay down
His last sad burden; and beside his mat
The bare foot monk of La Certosa sat.

. . . .

Unseen, in square and blossoming garden, drifted
Soft sunset lights, through green Val d'Arno sifted;
Unheard, below, the living shuttles shifted
Backward and forth, and wove, in love or strife,
In mirth or grief, the mottled web of life.
And when at last came upward from the street
Tinkle of bell, and tread of measured feet,
The sick man started, strove to rise in vain,
Sinking back heavily with a moan of pain.
And the monk said, "'Tis but the Brotherhood
Of Mercy, going on some errand good;
Their black masks by the palace wall I see."
Piero answered faintly, "Woe is me!
This day, for the first time in forty years
In vain the bell has sounded in my ears,
Calling me with my brethren of the Mask,
Beggar and prince alike, to some new task
Of love or pity—haply, from the street
To bear a wretch plague-stricken, or with feet
Hushed to the quickened ear and fevered brain,
To tread the crowded lazaretto's floor
Down the long twilight of the corridor:
Moist, tossing arms, and faces full of pain.
I loved the work—it was its own reward.
I never counted on it to offset
My many, many sins, or make less my debt
To the free grace and mercy of our Lord.

178

But somehow, father, it has come to be
In these long years so much a part of me
I should not know myself if lacking it;
But with the work, the worker too would die,
And in my place some other self would sit,
Joyful or sad—what matters, if not I?
And now, all's over. Woe is me!" "My son,"
The monk said, soothingly, "thy work is done,
And no more as a servant, but the guest
Of God, thou enterest thy eternal rest.
No toil, no tears, no sorrow for the lost,
Shall mar thy perfect bliss. Thou shalt sit down
Clad in white robes, and wear a golden crown
For ever and for ever." Piero tossed
On his sick pillow. "Miserable me!
I am too poor for such grand company.
The crown would be too heavy for this grey
Old head; and God forgive me if I say
It would be hard to sit there night and day
Like statue in the Tribune, doing naught
With these hard hands, that all my life have wrought
Not for bread alone, but for pity's sake.
I'm dull at prayers. I could not keep awake
Counting my beads. Mine's but a crazy head,
Scarce worth the saving if all else be dead.
And if one goes to Heaven without a heart,
Surely he leaves behind the better part.
I love my fellow men. The worst, I know
I would be good to. Will death change me so
That I shall sit among the lazy saints
And turn a deaf ear to the sore complaints
Of souls that suffered! Why, I never yet
Left e'en a dog in danger hard beset,
Or ass o'erladen. Must I rate man less
Than dog or ass, in *heavenly* selfishness?
Methinks (Lord, pardon if the thought be sin)
This world of pain were better, if therein
Our hearts might still be human, and desires

Of natural pity drop upon its fires
Some cooling tears."
　　　　　　Thereat, the pale monk crossed
His brow, and muttered, "Madman, thou art lost"
Took up his pyx and fled. When left alone
The sick man closed his eyes with a deep groan
That sank into the prayer, "Thy will be done."
And when he looked, lo' in the stern monk's place
He saw the shining of the dear Christ's Face.'
　　　　　　　　　　　　　　　　(Author unknown.)

The Béguines of Flanders.

This was the first of the more important secular Orders. It is
believed to have been founded about the year 1184 by Lambert
le Begue, who was a priest of Liège. Its members were widows or
unmarried girls who, without renouncing the society of men, or
vowing poverty, perpetual chastity and absolute obedience, led
a life of labour and service for their fellows.

The first Béguinage, which was dedicated to St Christopher,
the patron saint of travellers, was founded principally as a home
for widows and orphans of crusaders. The women of the Order
lived in small communities of two to five in a house of their own,
and their buildings included a chapel, a hospital, and an infirmary for the sick sisters which was quite distinct from the
hospital itself. Each Béguinage, therefore, formed a complete
community or village.

A branch of the community was established at Tirlemont in
1202, another at Ghent in 1235, and before the end of the thirteenth century there was an important Béguinage at Bruges. The
members of all the communities lived very simple lives, but all
classes of society were represented in the Order, and there were
many points of resemblance between the Béguines and the Tertiary Orders of St Francis and St Dominic.

There was essential antipathy between the free fellowships and
the monastic Orders, and Council after Council denounced the
Béguines as heretical, so also did two bulls of Clement V. in the

180

year 1311, and one of John XII. in 1317. But the sisterhoods had spread into Germany, Switzerland and France. They were far too numerous and useful to be exterminated by a Papal bull, or by the canons of a Council. They were, moreover, definitely in harmony with the spirit of the age, and very deeply rooted in the affections of the people. So we find, that a few years later, bulls were issued giving protection to the orthodox Béguines of Tuscany and Lombardy, and all Béguines were finally absolved from censure by the Council of Constance in 1414. About that time it was estimated that the Order numbered 200,000 members.

The hospital at Chalons-sur-Saône—a very beautiful building —was originated by Béguines, and became the home of a special branch—the Sisters of St Martha of Burgundy.

The Béguines have always been self-supporting. They not only nursed the sick in their own homes, but they helped in hospitals, undertook teaching and developed lace-making, spinning, and other handicrafts. They lost their property in Germany at the time of the Reformation. Hélyot relates that Béguinages existed in France until the early seventeenth century, and that in the first half of the eighteenth century there was a flourishing one at Malines, with a membership of 1,500 sisters. This was probably the largest settlement of the Order.

During the war that culminated in the battle of Waterloo in 1815 they turned their buildings into hospitals and gave their services to the utmost, not only to the soldiers, but also to the civilian population. In the many cholera epidemics that raged during the middle of the nineteenth century they worked in hospitals and in the homes of the patients. In all times of acute industrial distress, after fires and floods, and in times of famine they were ever ready to give immediate help until other charitable measures could be organised. Many Béguinages adopted the Third Rule of St Francis. There are surviving branches of the Order at Ghent and Bruges; and also at Mechlin, Louvain and Amsterdam, although there are now very few outside Belgium.

181

The Franciscan Tertiaries, and the Minoresses of St Clare.

St Francis is probably the best known of all the 'nursing' saints. He was born in 1182, the son of Pietro Bernardone, a wealthy cloth-merchant of Assisi. As a young man he fought in the wars between city states, was taken prisoner, and by the time he re-gained his liberty he was suffering from a malady that was to revisit him for the rest of his life and somewhat hamper his head-long career. There are many stories told of his thoughtless and irresponsible youth; but whilst still young he began his long vocation of ministry among lepers. In this he was joined by two companions, Bernard of Quintavelli and Peter, a canon from a neighbouring church. They built themselves a rude hut adjoin-ing the leper hospital outside the city walls, and there others joined this small group in their ministry to lepers and ragged mendicants. The community grew, and Francis took steps to regularise it. He did not call his followers monks—they were to him the 'little brothers', and the name he gave them is generally rendered into English as the 'Friars Minor'. They took the usual vows of poverty, chastity and obedience, but added a fourth— joyfulness. No monastery enclosed them or provided them with the necessities of life. They were almost nomadic, they mingled with the world and found their work amongst the sick and the poor. A man who became a Franciscan friar had to take his chance of sleeping under a hedge or on a doorstep, of eating berries in a lane or begging a crust from a kitchen; and for cloth-ing he wore a coarse and shapeless brown cloth garment girdled with a piece of rope. A fanatical sort of Order, and yet, requiring no funds or buildings, it grew more quickly than any other, and it has lived for over 700 years.

The Second Order.

The Second Order formed by St Francis was the Order of Poor Clares—also called the Minoresses. This owed its inception to the beautiful friendship of St Francis with a girl belonging to

182

one of the noble families of Assisi. Her name was Chiari Scifi, and she was born in 1194, twelve years after St Francis. When she was only seventeen years of age he helped her to escape at night from her home, in order to join in the work of his community. She attracted a number of other young women, and they lived at the little hermitage of St Damian, among the olive groves.

The Third Order.

The Third Order of St Francis or the Franciscan Tertiaries, was formed entirely as a lay Order; and in the centuries that followed many famous men and women became its members, including St Louis of France, St Elizabeth of Hungary, Dante, Galvani—the 'father of electricity'—Vincent de Paul and Roger Bacon.

Towards the end of his somewhat short life—he died at the age of 44—St Francis suffered from some disease of the liver, from indigestion and from inflammation of the eyes. He was brought to a small rat-infested hut near St Damian's, where Clare and her nuns nursed him for forty days. It is said that the rats made sleep impossible during the nights, for they ran about the hut and over the table and bed. He recovered sufficiently, however, to go to Tuscany in search of health, but very soon afterwards he died —in 1226. Clare survived him for 27 years.

There are an immense number of legends and anecdotes about St Francis, and the majority of them have to do with his great and compassionate love for his fellow men, and for birds and animals. But, although he is loved and revered as one of the greatest of the 'nursing saints' yet, during some parts of their history, the Friars Minor have not been specially noted for the care of the sick. After the death of their leader they seemed to fall away from the ideals he had set them. They kept the carefree spirit of their founder, but not his asceticism. They became lazy and overfond of the pleasures of the table, until as dirty, degenerate mendicants some groups of them were regarded as a nuisance in all the cities of Europe. Not all of them gained such

183

an undesirable reputation, however, for in Meiklejohn's *History of England* we are told that during the thirteenth century 'the Friars came as a blessing to this country. Wherever there was work neglected or to be done, thither came the Friars to pray with the sick and the dying, to tend those who were afflicted with the dreadful disease of leprosy, and to work among the horrible poverty that prevailed in the suburbs of the larger cities. These Friars had no clothes and no food but what the people chose to give them. Barefoot they walked through deep snow and over the roughest roads, and they were weak with fasting and the different penances they imposed on themselves. The clergy loathed them, and the very people whom they came to tend mocked at them as foreign beggars. But their work was to help the sick and the needy, and they did it, and gave to the world the much-needed lesson of absolute self-sacrifice and self-denial.'

The Clares became an enclosed Order. A branch came to England about 1293, and their first and most important foundation in this country was in London, in a street near Aldgate which is still called the 'Minories'. Their Abbey was on the east side of the street leading from the Tower to Aldgate.

Nearly all the convents of the Minoresses in England were suppressed during the Reformation and their property confiscated by the Crown. One, the convent of Brusyard in Suffolk, obtained a Royal grant to remain undissolved, but we find that two years later—in 1539—it was surrendered to the Crown.

Towards the end of the eighteenth century, as a result of the French Revolution, some French branches returned to England, but many went to Canada and the United States.

From the *Rule of the Order of St Clare* we read: 'The abbess is strictly bound to make compassionate and charitable provision for the sick according to the possibilities of the place, and to make enquiry as to what utensils, food, and other necessaries their infirmities require. Because it is an obligation on all sisters to serve and care for the sick as they would themselves wish to be cared for if they were taken ill. . . . The sick are permitted a mattress of straw and a feather pillow for the head, and those that need woollen coverlets may have them.'

'The surgeon, doctor and barber must be Catholics, and mature and spiritual persons, and must not be introduced into the convent except in cases of manifold necessity or serious illness, . . . and should it happen that one of the sisters should have some infectious or lasting disease, such as leprosy and other serious illnesses, on account of which she may not be with others without danger, there shall in that case be provided for such a one a room apart within the convent, where she may be attended to as her sickness requires.'

One of the best known hospitals in the United States—St Mary's of Rochester, Minnesota—has always been under the charge of Franciscan Sisters. It is the hospital at which the famous Mayo brothers attracted world-wide attention for their magnificent work in surgery, and it claims to be one of the best equipped and organised hospitals in the world to-day.

The Order of the Holy Ghost, and the Medical School of Montpelier.

This important Order was founded at Montpelier in Southern France towards the end of the twelfth century in connection with the famous Medical School of that town. It is not known definitely at what date the school began—probably in the eighth century. According to the *Catholic Encyclopædia* it was founded by a graduate of the Spanish Medical schools. It was proclaimed as a Faculty of Medicine in January, 1180, and received its statutes from Cardinal Conrad d'Hurach, the Legate of Pope Honorius III. The essential provisions of these statutes remained in force for over five and a half centuries—until a law of 12th April, 1792, brought about the 'legal death' of the school. The greatest period of its history was the thirteenth and fourteenth centuries.

However it was founded, the fact remains that Arabian influences appeared to be much stronger at this school than at Salerno. It was essentially a lay school, but many of its greatest men were Franciscan Minorites. The renown of its physicians

185

spread all over Europe. It was situated in a very beautiful and healthy spot not far from the sea and near several mineral springs; and patients flocked to Montpelier in the hope of being cured. It had a botanical garden which for many years was reputed to be the finest in Europe.

Anselm of Havelburg, writing in 1137, says, 'Montpelier offers to medicine both a home and a temple. Here both doctrines and precepts are taught by physicians who, meditating upon the force of things, teach hygiene to the healthy and obtain the cure of the sick.' One of the greatest of its students was Guy de Chauliac (1298–1368). He is considered to be the 'Father' of modern surgery.

But it was another Guy who initiated the Order of the Holy Ghost. He was a noble knight known as Guy de Montpelier, and the Order included both Brothers and Sisters in its ranks. They nursed among the poor and in the large hospitals. They took over all the nursing at the Santo Spirito Hospital in Rome in 1204; and during the next two centuries they nursed in many hospitals, not only in Italy, but also in France and Germany. Especially did they care for lepers and sufferers from other infectious diseases who were housed in the shelters that were built outside the towns.

In 1446 the Order became monastic under Augustinian rule. Its French branches were abolished during the seventeenth century. The few remaining branches of the Order still nurse in some of the Italian hospitals, but they devote themselves chiefly to the care of foundlings.

The Grey Sisters.

This was an Order of uncloistered nuns founded in 1222. They resembled the Béguines in many respects, and they reached the height of their fame during the fourteenth and fifteenth centuries, mainly because of their association with the Alexian Orders that were founded in the fourteenth century for the purpose of nursing those stricken with plague. The work of the Grey

Sisters was 'to receive the poor and miserable persons into their hospitals, and exercise other works of charity according to their power, that is, visit the sick, keep and nurse them in their sickness when haply required to do so'. They also tended the sick in their own homes, and they chose St Elisabeth as their patron saint, therefore they were often called 'Elisabethinerinnen'. When, in 1696, the Bishop of Nancy tried to compel their cloistration they appealed for help to the civil powers, as the Béguines had done three centuries previously. They received the support they asked for, and continued to live their free, uncloistered life, serving the community in which they lived. They undergo a novitiate of from one to three years before the fitness to be a Grey Sister is held to be proved. The Order is still in existence in considerable numbers to-day, although it suffered terribly during the French Revolution, some of the Sisters being massacred and others guillotined.

The Alexian, or Cellite, Brotherhood.

This had its origin at Mechlin, in Brabant, about the year 1348, during the terrible ravages of the 'Black Death'. Laymen, under the guidance of a man named Tobias, banded together to succour the plague-stricken without taking any vows or adopting a definite rule. They also undertook the burial of plague victims, and were therefore called 'Cellites', from the Latin word *cella*, that is 'a grave' or 'a cell'.

In 1431 they became an organised body of religious nurses and adopted the Augustinian Rule, taking vows of chastity, poverty and obedience. They chose Alexius as their patron saint. He was the son of a Roman noble who lived during the fifth century A.D. and he served for many years at the hospital of St Ephrem, at Edessa in Syria.

The Order is still active in hospitals, mental homes, and homes for the aged and infirm. The Alexian brothers have houses in Germany, Belgium, Switzerland, Bavaria, England, Ireland and the United States. They built four hospitals in the United States

187

during the nineteenth century—one at Chicago in 1866, one at St Louis, 1869, with departments for the insane, for nervous diseases and for inebriates. A third was built at Oshkosh, Wisconsin, in 1880, and the fourth at Elizabeth, New Jersey, some years later. Competent physicians and surgeons attend the patients, but the brothers are the nurses, and also do all the housework of the hospitals.

A branch of the Order came to England in 1875, at the invitation of Cardinal Vaughan, then Bishop of Salford, and established an institution for the aged and infirm at Newton Heath, Manchester. In 1902 the Brothers purchased the beautiful Manor House and grounds of Twyford Abbey, Willesden, London, which they have greatly enlarged and improved, making it an ideal Convalescent Home, and a place of rest for retired gentlemen.

More recently a house has been opened at Shillington Hall, York, and another at Warrenpoint, Co. Down. Here aged and infirm men are cared for, but no asylums for the insane are attached to the English houses, as is the case in Germany, Belgium and America.

The English Novitiate of the Order is at Twyford Abbey, where suitable candidates are accepted, not only for nursing the sick, but also for the domestic work of the Home and for the work of various trades.

Alexian nuns were affiliated to the Order early in the fifteenth century; but living in separate institutions under their own rule and doing a similar work for women. They were also known as 'Black Sisters'. At present they have their Mother-house at Cologne, but they take no part in the work of the brothers either in England or the United States.

The Alexians claim to be among the pioneers of organised nursing in the hospitals of Europe. They still live under definite rule and ecclesiastical authority, and all the members are bound by vows.

CHAPTER X

MEDIÆVAL SURGERY AND MEDICAL EDUCATION

The School of Salerno—Nursing conditions at the end of the mediæval period—Reliance on supernatural aid—Ecclesiastical limitations of medicine—The woman-healer and the growth of witchcraft—The misuse of hospitals—Relation of hospitals with monastic life—Deterioration and suppression of the monasteries

The School of Salerno.

SOME account has already been given of the Medical Schools in the countries belonging to the Arabian Empire, particularly those in Spain, and also of the school at Montpelier, but there was another very famous centre of medical research and education at Salerno which is still considered to be the most ancient university in Europe, for it antedated the school at Montpelier. It was beautifully situated on the Italian coast about 30 miles south-east of Naples and many authorities believe that it was founded by Benedictine monks, whilst others hold that it was never founded—it just grew. At first it was a port of call for Mediterranean shipping. By the ninth century it was a hospital centre, a century later it was famed for the skill of its physicians, and in the eleventh century it was the most celebrated medical school in Europe. From being a trade centre it became a spa because of its beautiful and healthy position and its mild climate, and a place of sojourn for pilgrims, crusaders and invalids, who flocked there from many countries.

It was first mentioned in A.D. 924, but no definite authentic history is available before A.D. 1000—from that date numerous great names and famous documents are associated with it. Its

189

medicine at that time was independent, based upon Latin and Greek works and having borrowed nothing from the Islamic school. Later, Arabic elements were introduced, particularly by Constantine the African, and the Arabian poly-pharmacy that developed was opposed by some of the teachers at Salerno as being a serious hampering influence on medical advancement at that time. From the writings of the masters of this school we learn that there were many women physicians who were held in high esteem. They were allowed considerable scope, and were greatly sought after by patients, but there is still no reference to 'nurses' as such. Nursing was evidently not separated from medicine, and one is forced to think that all the important nursing treatments were carried out by physicians, of both sexes, and that the toilet of the patient was attended to by lay helpers. In 1134 laws were made governing the practice of medicine and surgery in order to eliminate charlatans and, although during the following century most of the medicine of Salerno was derived from Islamic sources, from about 1230 its surgery made rapid progress, mainly owing to the work of Robert of Parma.

Women often assisted at dressings and operations, and were known as medical attendants. In his *Short History of Medicine*, Dr Charles Singer shows a picture of a surgeon at work in a siege of Salerno assisted by two women bearing drugs and dressings. We have been so accustomed to think that European surgery was a development of recent times, and that its ultimate success was made possible by intelligent post-operative nursing, that it is rather a shock to modern complacency to find that there was a period of magnificent surgery, with 'first intention' healing in twelfth and thirteenth century Italy. The mediæval surgeons successfully performed operations that nineteenth century surgeons, before the time of Lister, refused to attempt because they were so likely to be followed by the death of the patient. In order to induce anæsthesia a sponge was soaked in a mixture of opium, hyoscyamus, hemlock, mandragora and ivy. This was then dried, and when required it was moistened with water and placed over the mouth and nose of the patient—the inhalation producing unconsciousness. They washed wounds with wine that quickly evaporated, and then they brought the edges together taking scrupulous care to remove every foreign particle. For dry dressings linen cloths were steeped in very strong wine and then applied to the wound. The wine itself and the evaporation process not only left the dressing quite dry but also killed any microbes present. Actually they were practising antisepsis and asepsis although these terms had not been invented and bacteria were still undiscovered. Such development might seem quite incredible were it not that we have the documentary history of it, and our knowledge is not based on tradition.

Beauty culture obviously had almost as great a vogue then as now, for the lady physicians of Salerno had a prescription for an ointment that was a remedy for sunburn, another to keep the hair soft and silky, and a number of formulæ for definite beauty treatments, but they followed many superstitious practices also. For example, as a cure for melancholia a herb was to be plucked at 3 o'clock on the morning of Ascension Day whilst a paternoster was being said.

The most famous of these ladies would appear to be one Trotula, the wife of John Platearius the Elder, who lived about the middle of the eleventh century. She passed into literature as the 'Dame Trot' of the fairy tales. In a treatise ascribed to her she advises patients to take sand-baths on the seashore in order to reduce flesh—the 'slimming' being accomplished by the perspiration induced by the heat. There is a chapter on the care of the newly born, one on the choice of a nurse, and another on the hygiene and feeding of infants. Particular instruction is given regarding dentition and teaching the child to speak correctly. All her doctrines are practical rather than theoretical, but as the works ascribed to her deal specially with gynæcology and child welfare some authorities believe that 'Trotula' was a generic term for womankind, and not the name of a real person, others that it may have been a name given to a collection of recipes and prescriptions; but, however that may be, Trotula is frequently quoted by other Salernitans.

Nursing Conditions at the End of the Mediæval Period.

Men and women had withdrawn from the world into the great cloistered houses in order to save their own souls, and they did what they could to help each other when sickness or other affliction came upon them. Wayfarers claimed, and received, their hospitality, sympathy and help, and the clinical experience thus gained caused their fame as healers to spread abroad, so that the halt and the maimed flocked to their gates from the surrounding country.

Medicine was taught at this time in the universities, but it was mostly theoretical, not clinical, medicine.

If we wish to know something of the type of poorer patients in the fourteenth century we may refer to some of the drawings in mediæval manuscripts, such as the Luttrell Psalter.

These drawings show unkempt figures clad in long loose gowns of homespun cloth with loose sleeves and no fastenings. When active work had to be done the skirt was pulled up and tucked into a belt or cord around the waist. For headgear they wore felt hats shaped like a pudding basin. The very poorest had literally no other garment, and when on tramp it is unlikely that the gown was ever taken off, so that it must have become indescribably filthy and verminous. Those who were a little better off added a shirt, hose and shoes, with a hooded cape for bad weather, which fitted closely round the head, leaving an oval opening for the face.

Reliance on Supernatural Aid.

The legacy of pagan superstition which had lingered through the early centuries of Christianity had gradually come to assume a kind of orthodoxy in that the aid of saints was invoked in order that relief might be obtained from pain and disease. Hence, young expectant mothers were admonished to repeat the 18th

Psalm and reflect upon the wonderful deliverance of St Margaret of Antioch, or to appeal to St Dorothy, who, in the agony of her martyrdom, had prayed that women in labour might be speedily relieved by calling upon her name.

St Antony was specifically invoked for the cure of scorbutic diseases, St Apollonia for toothache, St Clare for ophthalmic diseases, St Erasmus for abdominal complaints, St Lawrence for burns and scalds, St Petronilla for fevers, St Vitus for nervous diseases, St Fillan for insanity, and St Roche and St Sebastian for protection from, and cure of, plague.

Ecclesiastical Limitations of Medicine.

The study and practice of medicine and surgery by those living within the cloisters was controlled and hampered by a series of decrees, for in 1123 the Lateran Council passed a decree forbidding monks and priests to go to the bedside of the sick other than as ministers of religion. In 1131 the Council of Rheims prohibited monks from frequenting schools of medicine, and directed that they confined their practice within the limits of their own monastery, the reason given being that—'An unchaste eye is the messenger of an unchaste heart, and whatsoever things are shameful to speak of, an honest priest should not meddle with.'

These decrees were, obviously, not unquestionably obeyed, for in 1139 the Lateran Council threatened monks and priests with severe penalties and suspension from ecclesiastical functions if they practised medicine. In 1163 Pope Alexander III. threatened monks and priests with excommunication if they persisted in studying medicine, and in 1215 Pope Innocent III. directed an anathema against surgery—no priest was to perform any operation where steel or fire was used, and any who did so were to be refused benediction.

Monastic Nursing.

No doubt nuns nursed each other, and also their boarders, some of whom must have been old and ailing. The nuns of Rom-

o   193

sey had a hospital attached to their convent in which to receive any of the nuns' parents and relatives who were poor and ill; but this does not prove that they nursed them. There were, however, special sisters whose duty it was to serve in the 'spitals'. There is no real documentary evidence that nuns spent their time in nursing. Some were, possibly, skilled in the preparation of herbs and in simple forms of home nursing, medicine, and surgery, and probably their knowledge was first acquired in their own homes, for it was the function of the lady of the manor to know something of these things. Girls educated in the nunneries often acquired an elementary empirical knowledge of nursing, as well as of needlecraft, domestic arts and management. If, however, a woman practised this knowledge outside the limits of her own home and claimed to possess something more than the skill of an amateur there forthwith arose an outcry against her as a witch.

The country housewife, also, was expected to be able to look after the physical needs of the members of her household in sickness as well as in health, and to have a certain skill in nursing, medical, and surgical procedures. Mediæval romances teem with instances of ladies physicking and patching up their knights, and recipes and remedies were handed down from mother to daughter, together with those for puddings, cakes and jams.

The Woman-Healer, and the Growth of Witchcraft.

As we have seen, with the scarcity of doctors, women sought the healing herbs of the fields in the hope that preparations of them might mitigate the sufferings of their friends and neighbours; but only within the definite limits of their own homes might they practise their arts, for the Church denounced the woman healer as a witch and singled her out for the most exquisite tortures, until 'witch-finding' became almost a profession. For nearly two centuries this fearful mania of witch-hunting ravaged the homes of the poor and helpless throughout Christendom, and even invaded the higher social circles and courts. It appears to have begun in the first half of the fifteenth century.

The records show that during that fifty years alone 7,000 witches were put to death at Trèves, 1,500 at Bamberg, and 800 at Wurtsberg. When the persecution reached Geneva 500 were killed within three months. A century later, in one year—1524—a thousand perished by fire in the diocese of Como, and 900 were burnt in Lorraine. England and Scotland added their dire quota to this multitude, and it is estimated that altogether over 30,000 human beings were tortured and killed before the folly and wickedness of this persecution dawned upon either the authorities or the people, and the element of insanity in both the witch and the bewitched became recognised.

The Misuse of Hospitals.

This was evidently a serious problem a century before the Reformation. A statute passed in 1414 sets forth the need for a thorough reorganisation of the hospitals in the country. Patrons and official visitors were using the hospitals not only as places of residence for themselves but also for their retinue, thus crowding out the sick and the poor. By order of the kings or bishops they had often to receive, and maintain for life, those servants of the state or church who were poor and unable to work. Unwanted and elderly relatives were too often dumped upon the hospitals, and all this constituted a grievous burden upon them. The same thing was happening in the lesser and poorer monasteries.

Added to this, there was misrule in the hospitals themselves. Many were controlled by a number of non-resident wardens, some of whom very seldom visited the hospital. Of those that did, a considerable portion were untrustworthy and generally incapable of organisation. In some cases the poor and needy were cast out and the officials converted the funds and the goods to their own uses.

Relation of Hospitals with Monastic Life.

Not all the pre-Reformation hospitals were monastic. Private patrons sometimes founded hospitals and handed them over to the monasteries for administration. In these cases the endowment of the hospital was distinct from that of the monastery, and some of the staff might be laymen or women. There were also city hospitals which had been built by the municipalities, but their methods of administration left much to be desired. They were usually in charge of a man who was not a physician and there was no matron, or woman 'head', to superintend the nursing. The religious motive was lacking, and the general want of cleanliness and the disagreeable features of the work caused it to be considered unfit for any woman of refinement.

The monastic infirmary was for sick members of the Order. Guest houses were for travellers. Some abbots and priors founded hospitals which were dependent upon the monasteries for staff, provisions and other necessities, and these were looked upon definitely as monastic hospitals; but all hospitals in the country were subject either to royal or to episcopal control.

Deterioration and Suppression of the Monasteries.

The monastery was, in its essence, a place where a number of people lived a communal life, owning no personal property but holding everything in the name of the community. The inmates of a monastery spent almost the whole of their time together, they prayed, worked and ate together, and they slept in dormitories. It seems, however, that the craving for a certain privacy of life, and for at least a minimum of private property is a deeply rooted instinct in human nature, and the attempt to eradicate it was predestined to failure, becoming one source of perpetual conflict, though not, perhaps, the greatest.

It is the history of ecclesiastical celibacy that provides the greatest tragedy of religious life. For the average man and for many women it has always been an unnatural state, and the vow was constantly being broken. Even when such vows were rigidly kept it was often at a cost which psychologists have only recently begun to understand. Visions that were at once the joy and the torture of so many mystics were sexual as well as religious in their origin, as in their imagery; resulting, as they did, from the repression of the most powerful of natural instincts, together with the absence of sufficient counter interests and employments. And then, especially in the convents for women, many had not chosen the celibate life of their own free will. It had been forced upon hundreds of girls for various reasons, especially when parents or guardians wished to be rid of them. Many were professed even before they reached their teens, and they never became reconciled to the religious life, their temperament and character being quite unsuited to its austerities. Small wonder that scandals arose, especially in the smaller communities.

In the great religious houses of the country wealth and power had accumulated until they surpassed that of the monarch himself. In 1405 they were estimated to possess a third of the property of the country, and laws were passed which aimed at limiting this accumulation. From time to time the State had confiscated lands, tenements and tithes, but often these were bestowed by the King or Parliament upon the monasteries more in favour, so that the total wealth was not lessened; and then, in the next century, with the rise of Cardinal Wolsey to power, England experienced, for the first time, supreme spiritual and secular authority exercised by one individual, and it was an unfortunate precedent. For when, a few years later, Henry VIII. assumed the spiritual headship it did not create the surprise or consternation it might otherwise have done. The King then began to look with a greedy eye upon the enormous wealth of the religious houses, but he realised that even a monarch as absolute as himself required a very plausible excuse for their open spoliation. This he found in the tales of the gross irregularities that occurred in monasteries, nunneries and convents alike; although it is doubtful whether they were any worse at that time than they had been for several centuries past; and certainly the evils placed at their doors were more than counterbalanced by their long record of charitable, literary and educational work.

A visitation was decided upon, and in 1534 the commissioners of Wolsey and of Thomas Cromwell were busily journeying through England, ostensibly to administer the oath of supremacy (of the king) to the religious, and to extract explicit renunciation of Papal power and jurisdiction. Reports on the condition and conduct of the houses were compiled into the 'Black Book'. Stories of mismanagement and disorderly conduct lost nothing in the telling, and in February, 1536, an Act of Parliament was passed which legalised the suppression of all religious houses whose income fell below £200 a year. In Burnet's *History of the Reformation* it is recorded that 376 of the lesser monasteries were dissolved during 1538–1540, and that during the latter year the larger monasteries shared the same fate. As a consequence, large numbers of helpless sick poor were left unrelieved in the streets.

Thus ended the work of the monastic hospitals in England, and the dissolution of the convents resulted in the extinction of any kind of systematic education of girls and women for a very long time.

198

CHAPTER XI

THE FIVE ROYAL HOSPITALS OF LONDON

Pre-Reformation history of the three hospitals—St Bartholomew's, St Thomas's and Bethlehem Hospitals—Bridewell Hospital—Social and economic conditions in the sixteenth century—Refounding of St Bartholomew's Hospital, and Bethlehem Hospital—Treatment of the insane—Refounding of St Thomas's Hospital—The work at St Thomas's Hospital—Bridewell Hospital—Christ's Hospital

THE five 'Royal' hospitals owe that title to the fact that Henry VIII., or his son Edward VI., is accredited with either founding or refounding them. They are St Bartholomew's, St Thomas's, Bethlehem, Bridewell, and Christ's Hospital. Most of them had originally been founded several centuries before, and had been suppressed at the Reformation, and, with one exception, the real founders were, undoubtedly, the citizens of London; the King having merely signed the Charter which authorised the work. The exception was Bridewell Hospital, and this was a Royal Palace until it was presented by Edward VI. to the City of London for beneficient purposes; but neither it nor Christ's Hospital were primarily hospitals for the sick; although they were so characteristic of the spirit of the time, each dealing with a special aspect of the social problem, that some brief account of them would seem to be justified in this narrative. The other three had been hospitals before the Reformation, and Christ's Hospital had been a convent of the Grey Friars, or Franciscans.

Pre-Reformation History of the Three Hospitals.

St Bartholomew's Hospital.—This is the oldest of the existing London Hospitals, and it still stands on the site on which it was first founded in 1123, although nothing now remains of the original buildings. One of the most charming stories of English hospital founders is that of the humbly born monk Rahere, said to have previously been a minstrel or jester at the court of King Henry I. He had a deep sympathy with the tribulations of the wretched sufferers from extreme poverty or disease, and the building of the hospital was an act of gratitude for his recovery from a very serious illness whilst in Rome.

His former master, Henry I., gave him the site at Smithfield, and he established a hospital and priory simultaneously. The two foundations remained distinct, although allied, until the Reformation, when they were both suppressed—the priory then ceased to exist. King John, in confirming the association between the priory and the hospital said, 'If any one shall separate the said hospital from the aforesaid church, and from the subjection of the aforesaid prior and canons, he and all that to him belongs, shall become the right of the King' (Chartulary 5. Johan).

The hospital was designed to give help to the needy, the orphans and the outcasts of the district, as well as to afford relief to every kind of sick person and homeless wanderer. The sick poor were to be tended until they recovered, women with child were to be provided with shelter and attention until they were delivered, and if the mother died whilst in hospital the child was to be maintained until it reached seven years of age—after which time it was considered old enough to work for its own maintenance. The staff consisted of a master, eight brethren, and four sisters. The priory had a prior and thirteen canons, who lived according to the Augustinian rule.

The master of the hospital was to 'be gentle, good-tempered, kind, compassionate to the sick and willing to gratify their needs with affectionate sympathy. Further, he ought to have a servant fit for his place, who is to stay continually in the infirmary, and wait upon the sick with diligence and care in all gentleness. He is to get their food ready at the proper time, show their water to the physician, and take a careful note of how they ought to diet themselves.'

The hospital was, at first, very poorly endowed, and the brethren and novices begged, and gathered alms by preaching.

The four sisters appointed at the original foundation were professed nuns. They had a common dormitory and refectory, and they wore a grey habit which was not to reach lower than their ankles. Their work was life-long, and no doubt many of them became skilled in the dressing of wounds and in midwifery. The number of sisters remained unaltered until the Reformation—four hundred years after the founding of the hospital. The number of in-patients varied from sixty to a hundred, but there were out-patients also to be tended. Quite obviously the four sisters could not have carried out all the nursing and many of the domestic duties of the hospital, even with the help of the eight brethren, but there are no records of their assistants.

Practically the only record now existing of the kind of treatment given to the sick at that time is contained in the *Breviarum Bartholmei*, written by John Mirfield about 1357. We find that prayers and pharmacy were intermixed. It may be that in an age which had no clocks the reciting of a certain number of prayers or verses of scripture measured the length of a treatment given, and also the time interval between the various stages of a treatment, and probably increased the patient's faith in its efficacy. For example, in the treatment of a condition which was obviously chronic rheumatism olive oil was put into a clean vessel, the pharmacist made the sign of the Cross over it and then the vessel was placed over the fire and a given number of verses of a Psalm, the Gloria, and two prayers were recited, the whole being repeated seven times. The affected parts were then rubbed with the hot oil during the recitation of further prayers. One can well imagine that the sufferer might be greatly relieved by such treatment.

Mirfield is very precise in his description of the union of fractures. He notes that the process is slower in the aged, and that a broken rib takes twenty days to unite, and a broken humerus or femur forty days. He records the treatment given to a canon who was thrown from his horse with such force on to his head that he became unconscious. The canon's head was shaved, the scalp was rubbed with oil of roses and a quart of warm vinegar, and then thoroughly bandaged with linen, the whole being covered with a lambskin. Twice a day the neck and spine were rubbed with ointment. The patient spoke, imperfectly, on the third day, was rather better on the fourth, and was given chicken broth on the sixth.

Thenceforth he grew stronger, and was given the brains of fowls and kids in order to repair the damage to his own; but it is recorded that he was never of the same mental ability and good memory as he had been before the accident.

St Thomas's Hospital.—There was a Priory of St Mary Overie —or St Mary the Virgin—on the banks of the river Thames at Southwark, outside the entry into the city where all the great southern roads converged towards London. An ancient bridge existed at this point, at least from the time of the Roman Conquest in A.D. 43. How long the priory had stood there is a matter for conjecture, but it was restored by Bishop Giffard in 1106 on the site of the present Southwark Cathedral. It was under the rule of St Augustine, and its infirmary undoubtedly became a hospital for the sick and infirm who passed along the great highway towards London. St Bartholomew's Hospital played the same part with regard to the northern entry into the city.

From the time of its restoration in 1106 until Bishop Peter des Roches separated the hospital from the priory in 1215 the former was dedicated to St Thomas the Martyr (Thomas à Becket). He (Peter) appealed for funds to restore the foundation after its evident destruction by fire. 'Behold at Southwark,' he says, 'an ancient spital, built of old to entertain the poor, has been reduced to cinders and ashes.' This was about 1215, and from that date the history of St Thomas's Hospital is continuous. One of the strongest arguments for the existence of a hospital before

1215 is that no Royal charter was granted at that time, as would have been the case had it been a new foundation.

In the fourteenth century it housed forty patients in addition to a continual stream of casualty cases from the turbulent and insanitary neighbourhood, but the records supply us with no details as to the treatments given, although we know that patients were bled on certain days. The principal conditions treated appear to have been typhus, enteric, dysentery, scurvy, tubercle rickets and malaria. Acute rheumatism was also prevalent at the time, but was not diagnosed from other fevers. The work was carried out by Augustinian canons and nuns, and as their number remained constant until the hospital was handed over to Henry VIII. in 1540 we may presume that the accommodation also remained the same. The King declared Becket to be a traitor, and no saint, and when the hospital was refounded it was known as the hospital of St Thomas the Apostle.

Bethlehem Hospital.—This hospital probably had its origin in Bethlehem during the fourth century A.D., its mother-house being called the Basilica of the Nativity—built under the direction of Paula, the famous Roman deaconess. The Hospital of St Mary of Bethlehem, which, under the rule of the Knights Hospitallers, figures so largely in the history of the Crusades, was, presumably, one of the daughter houses of the original Bethlehem Hospital.

Quite early in the thirteenth century Pope Honorius III. granted an indulgence to the monastery of St Mary of Bethlehem, Palestine, and its daughter-houses; but in 1244 the Kharasmians, a wild horde of Mohammedans from Central Asia, fell upon Bethlehem and left its convent in ruins. The brethren were dispersed over Europe, finding their way into Italy, France, England, and Scotland, forming a chain of little colonies of Bethlehemite Hospitallers.

In September, 1247, Henry III. of England granted 'protection without term' to the brethren of the house of 'Bethlem'. A month later the brethren, under the leadership of one Simon

FitzMary, founded the Priory of St Mary of Bethlehem in Bishopgate without London. Here the monks built an infirmary with a long gallery of cells for twenty patients leading out of it. Above the stairs was a dormitory, probably used for wayfarers.

In 1340 the Mayor and Corporation of the City of London took over its affairs and conduct, and by 1403 the hospital was definitely being used as an asylum for the insane, although the work was still being done by a religious community of both sexes.

A writer of the fifteenth century—one William Gregory—says, 'A church of Our Lady that is named Bethlem—and in that place are found many men that are fallen out of their wits. Right well are they cared for in that place, and some are restored to health again, and some are there for ever, for they are incurable'. And when Gregory died, in 1465, he left a legacy of forty shillings to the 'pouere sicke' people of Bethlem.

Sir Thomas More in his *Apology* (1533) tells of a man who had been 'put into Bedlam, and afterwards by healings and corrections gathered his remembrances to come again to himself; but being thereupon set at liberty and walking about abroad, his old fancies began again to fall on his head'. Of the same man the chancellor states, 'I caused him to be bound to a tree in the street before the whole town, and constables striped him with rods until they became weary.' The poor patient was probably completely exhausted and therefore thoroughly quietened, but More considered the cruel treatment quite justified, for he says, 'Verily, God be thanked, I hear no more harm of him now.'

The Royal Commission of Henry VIII. contains an account of the visitation of Bethlehem Hospital. Much suspicion and slander were in the air, so that we are not surprised to find the nuns accused of 'too much coming and going through the wicket gate', and that the prioress was ordered to 'sleep in her own bedroom', and to see that no visitors were admitted to roam about the cloisters.

Bridewell Hospital.

As early as A.D. 971 a charter of King Edgar described the eastern boundary of the vast estates of Westminster as defined by a line drawn from 'the old wooden church of St Andrews' (Holborn) 'along London fen southward to the Thames in midstream'. This 'fen' was a tract of marshy land often entirely submerged by the tides from the estuary. It is also recorded that in 1162 Henry II. ignored the claims of the Abbot of Westminster, and conferred the site on which the Palace of Bridewell eventually arose upon the Knights Templars. By this time a flourishing garden and orchard had developed, and then, when the estates of the Templars fell into the hands of the Knights Hospitallers a house, a mill and twelve gardens are also described.

The Hospitallers leased the property, under compulsion, to Cardinal Wolsey for Henry VIII., and Wolsey erected upon it the famous Palace of Bridewell for his master's occupation. Twenty-two years later Edward VI. presented it to the City for 'beneficent uses'. For a time it figured as an imperial embassy both for Spanish and for French ambassadors.

Social and Economic Conditions in the Sixteenth Century.

The dissolution of the monasteries had been followed by an influx of rogues, vagabonds, cripples and the destitute into London and other great cities. Hitherto they had lived at the expense of the indiscriminate charity of the religious houses. Now, many of them were finding shelter in the great deserted monastic hospitals by night, but during the day they begged or pilfered in the streets, lay about the fields, or spent idle hours in the alehouses. Their fraternity was greatly augmented by the smallholders of land and the farm labourers who had been driven from the countryside by the nobles and court officials who had recently been enriched by grants of monastic property.

There were changes in the type of farming then being carried out, for wool was realising a very high price in England and the easiest and most profitable form of farming was pasturage. The new landlords turned arable land into meadows for sheep, and they no longer allowed the villagers and small-holders to use the commons for grazing their cattle, as had been their wont under the monastic landlords.

The citizens of London, therefore, found themselves besieged by the destitute farm-hand with his importunate begging, the 'leper' with his bell, the cripple exhibiting his deformities, and the rogue with his plausible tales, and, moreover, the brethren, sisters and lay workers who had been expelled from the monasteries went to swell the mass of starving humanity for whom no employment could be found.

The movement for refounding some of the hospitals was not entirely an act of piety. It was, in part, a measure for the convenience of healthy citizens who disliked to see diseased, dying, and often infectious mendicants lying in the streets and market places, and often upon their own doorsteps. There was, undoubtedly, much pure philanthropy in the carrying out of the work, but it was utilitarian rather than inspired, and the activities of these five Royal Hospitals formed a fairly complete scheme for dealing with the situation, combining, as they did, two hospitals for the sick, an asylum for the insane, a house of correction for the criminal and the rogue, and a home for fatherless and abandoned children.

The few hospitals which were already the property of the municipal authorities were fairly secure, but all the ecclesiastical foundations had been thrown into the melting pot, old moulds had been broken up, and, in common with the rest of England, London was faced with the problem of reforming all its charitable institutions.

The Refounding of St Bartholomew's Hospital.

A few patients had remained in the hospital during the dissolution, therefore we may presume that someone was left in charge of them to attend to their wants, and it was the first of the hospitals to be officially reopened. Shortly after Henry VIII. had seized its revenues the citizens of London petitioned that its work might be continued, on the ground that 'there were miserable people lying in the streets offending every clean person passing by the way with their filthy and nasty savours'.

The reopening took place in 1544, and five sisters were appointed, the number being increased to twelve in 1551. One of these acted as matron, and they each received a yearly grant of six yards of cloth wherewith to make their 'uniform'. This was, at first, of russet frieze, but in 1555 it was changed to 'watchet blue'.

A master and four chaplains had also been appointed at its reopening in 1544, but they proved themselves so negligent that three years later the City authorities decided to take the matter into their own hands and to govern the hospital on lines that were, by then, proving successful with other institutions, and St Bartholomew's was added to the 'Royal' hospitals in 1557.

The new sisters were, of course, not professed nuns, they appear to have been drawn from a very different class, to have had much lower ideals and very little of the spirit of service. Their duties were clearly defined in the 'charge' delivered to them on their appointment. The matron was to 'receive of the hospitallers of the house all such sick and diseased persons as he, by his warrant signed by the almoners of this house, shall present unto you, and the same persons shall bestow in such convenient places within the house as you shall think meet'. She was to be responsible for the work of the sisters and to see that they 'did their duty unto the poor as well in the making of the beds and keeping their wards as also in washing and purging their unclean clothes and other things'. But they were to remain in the women's ward at night and not to come out of it 'except for some great and special cause, such as present danger of death or needful succour of some poor person', and they were to remain with the sick person no longer than was absolutely necessary.

By 1755 there were sixteen sisters, and in addition there were

207

night nurses known as 'watchers' who lived outside the hospital, and were employed only when their services were required. On the whole, the 'nursing staff' were characteristic of their age. Most of them were middle-aged widows not renowned for honesty or sobriety, and certainly not educated, in fact, the majority of them were too ignorant of the amenities of life, and too ill-fed, overworked and wretchedly treated to be capable of giving adequate care to the patients, or even of maintaining decent cleanliness.

The first of the great structural changes was the building of the gateway in 1702, and the hospital was completely rebuilt between the years 1730 and 1759, the cost being defrayed by voluntary subscriptions. The names of the subscribers, together with the sums they gave, are inscribed in letters of gold on the walls of the Great Hall. The three large blocks devoted to the patients contained 28 wards arranged in pairs, with a sister's bed-sitting room opening out of the front ward by a half-glass door. The fourth block was the administrative department.

In 1877 definite training of nurses was commenced, courses of instruction in both theoretical and practical work were given, examinations held, and certificates of efficiency awarded.

Bethlehem Hospital.

A deed of covenant signed by Henry VIII. on 27th December, 1546—just a month before his death—agreed to grant St Bartholomew's Hospital to the Mayor and Corporation of London, and this covenant included the grant of 'the house or hospital of Bethlem'. So the refounding of these two hospitals took place simultaneously. The latter was entirely for the insane, but there seem to have been no doctors or nurses of any kind, although there were 'keepers', of whose duties the records are silent. An old woman who was in charge of the dispensary is the only person mentioned as having given the poor inmates any medical or nursing attention. A record dated 21st June, 1578, states, 'It is granted that the old woman, the wife of David Thomson, who hath given medicine to the poor at Bethlem, shall have eight pence a week to keep two frantic persons in rooms there provided; she shall find them their diet and medicine. She reported she hath cured one William Horne, a rich man from North Cray, and also many others.'

In 1557 Bethlem had been handed over to the governors of Christ's Hospital, who were, of course, aldermen and commoners of the corporation, but they placed it under the management of Bridewell.

Treatment of the Insane.

Many of the demented seemed to have preferred the king's highway, although they were in all probability 'whipped from tithing to tithing', to the iron collar and chain that awaited them, not only in castle or court-house, but also in the 'asylums' for the insane; and in that they showed themselves not entirely bereft of their wits.

About 1630 a pamphlet licenced at Stationers' Hall and called 'The Petition of the Poor Distracted People in the House of Bedlam' set forth the deplorable conditions existing at that time; and Lupton, a writer of 'literary miniatures' at that period, says, 'It seems strange that anyone should recover here; the cryings, screechings, roarings, howlings, shaking of chains, swearing, fretting and chafing are so many, and so hideous.' It was this sort of pandemonium that gave rise to such phrases as 'Bedlam let loose'. One of the favourite pastimes of society, especially of the younger generation, was the Sabbath morning visit to Bedlam, where they spent an amusing hour or two provoking the more voluble patients, or plying them with drink, and making sport of their miseries.

They went to Bethlem in much the same spirit as the uncouth rustic goes to a menagerie or a travelling circus—to poke up the animals with an ash-stick—until, in 1766, a rule was made that the doors of the hospital were to be locked against all visitors on public holidays. Before that date there had actually

P   209

been a charge of a penny admission fee, and that appeared to give visitors the right to tease the poor unfortunate inmates. Until 1662 no attempt had been made to separate the distracted and demented women from the men, and then, in an effort to cope with an ever-recurring scandal, the following rule was made, 'The distracted women are to be continually kept from the distracted men, and a discreet, careful, and able single woman to be provided to take care of the women. She may call to her help any one or more of the men servants when she cannot rule any of the distracted women herself.' Unfortunately the first two women appointed were decidedly not discreet or of good behaviour, and so the experiment was, for a time, abandoned.

St Fillan was the heavenly specialist in lunacy, and in Scotland the practice of immersing the demented in the healing waters of St Fillan's Pool was followed as late as 1793. As Sir Walter Scott has sung in *Marmion*

> 'Then to St. Fillan's blessed well,
> Whose spring can frenzied dreams dispel
> And the crazed brain restore.'

The afflicted person was then bound hand and foot and laid on the floor of the church, or in a stone coffin, for the night; the bronze bell of St Fillan being placed beside him, or at his head. If in the morning he was found free of his bonds recovery from the madness was likely to take place. Those who recovered sometimes related marvellous visions that had appeared to them during the night. Often, however, the water cure took place at the nearest river, where the unfortunate victim, without any pretence at a religious rite, was ducked until his exhaustion was mistaken for restored sanity.

This martyrdom of the insane did not cease until well into the nineteenth century. In 1807 Sir G. O. Peele wrote to the Home Secretary of scenes which he had actually witnessed, 'There is hardly a parish in which there may not be found some unfortunate creature, chained in a cellar or garret of a workhouse, fastened to a leg of a table, tied to a post in an outhouse, or perhaps shut up in an uninhabited ruin; or sometimes left to ramble half naked, or starving, through the streets or highways; teased by the scoff and jest of all that is vulgar, ignorant and unfeeling.' There seemed to be a strange theory that lunatics could feel neither heat, cold, nor pain.

Pepys became a governor of the Hospital in 1662, and there are many allusions to Bethlem in his diary—to other governors, to patients and to physicians.

In 1676 the second hospital was built on the city moat at the edge of Moorfields, and the new Bedlam was as magnificent as a palace, a 'structure fair, royally raised'. The grandeur of its design and the spaciousness of its galleries and cells was reminiscent of thirteenth-century building and appeared to augur a much better future for the patients. But within a very few years visitors remarked chiefly upon the stench of some of the departments.

In 1752 Dr John Munro, who succeeded his father as physician at Bethlem, published the first edition of a remarkable little book which ran into three editions during the next twelve years, entitled *Low Life—or One Half of the World does not Know how the Other Half Lives*. In it he says, 'The nurses of Bethlehem Hospital are carrying the appointed messes in wooden bowls to the people under their charge, but putting by the best part of it for their own relations and more intimate friends who are to come and visit them in the afternoon.'

(*N.B.* This hospital has now been removed to Monks' Orchard, Beckenham, Kent; and it is one of the foremost of the modern Mental Hospitals of England.)

Refounding of St Thomas's Hospital.

It is said that Henry VIII. intended to refound St Thomas's Hospital under the name of the 'Hospital of the Holy Trinity' for lame, wounded and diseased soldiers, but that he was prevented from carrying out this plan by death. There was a good deal of money available for the project, which had accrued from the dissolution of the Savoy Palace Hospital. This had once been the residence of John of Gaunt. It was turned into a hospital and almshouse by the first Tudor king, Henry VII., but by 1538 it was full of 'common rogues and idle pilfering knaves'. Its revenues had been granted to St Thomas's, Bridewell and Christ's Hospitals, but we hear very little of any of these until about 1552. By that time the social problem had become most acute, and Ridley, Bishop of London, appealed to Edward VI. The boy-king directed that a letter be sent to the Mayor of London, authorising the election of a Committee of six aldermen and twenty-four commoners to draw up a report on the disgraceful condition of the streets and the most effective way of dealing with the scandal. In its report the Committee was careful to distinguish between the poor who ought to be assisted without delay, and the worthless and destitute vagabonds who ought to be punished with imprisonment and whippings before being trained to honest work. The suggestions made were:

(1) That those who were suffering from contagious diseases should be segregated, with adequate maintenance and proper discipline, in the Lazar or 'Lock' houses outside the city, at Knightsbridge, Hammersmith, Highgate, Kingsland, and Kent Street—the last named being the main thoroughfare, although little more than a lane in the sixteenth century, through which all who journeyed between London and the Continent had to ride. The present Great Dover Road was made close to, and parallel with, it.

(2) Fatherless and pauper children should be housed and educated in the dissolved convent of the Grey Friars, or Franciscans, which at that time was largely a collection of partly ruined buildings into which rogues and dissolute women crept at night for shelter.

(3) St Thomas's Hospital should be reorganised to receive the sick, the lame, and homeless old people.

(4) Lastly this committee grappled with the most difficult and

212

unpromising problem of their time—and, in fact, of all other times—the reformation and employment of the tramp, the rogue and the drunken or prostitute woman. They needed a prison which should also be a house of work with possibilities for amendment of character. The only building sufficiently large and conveniently situated for this was Bridewell Palace, and therefore they supplicated the King that he should, without delay, hand over the Palace, which was then falling into disrepair and was in the market for sale.

Of course such a comprehensive scheme would involve a large expenditure of money, much of which would have to be collected, but the citizens had already accomplished similar aims in connection with St Bartholomew's and Bethlehem Hospitals. Being men of business, the aldermen decided, in the first instance, to take a census of those whom it was supposed to benefit, and then to ascertain how much money might be collected. The result of the official investigation showed that some 2,100 persons came under the terms of the precept issued to each alderman. The total was made up as follows:

> Fatherless and other children, 300
> Sore and sick people, 200
> Poor people overburdened with children, 350
> Aged people, 400
> Decayed citizens, 650
> Idle vagabonds, 200

The methods adopted to obtain the necessary money followed the lines of all such efforts which, in the next two and a half centuries, resulted in the founding of our great voluntary hospitals and charities, and therefore it might be well to indicate the avenues by which the citizens were approached.

The committee first assessed themselves, then they divided the city up into parishes and appointed collectors to call upon the ministers and churchwardens of each parish, and ask that they should urge the parishioners to subscribe a sum each week to-

213

wards the expenses of the scheme. Each minister was supplied with a sermon, which included the figures and findings of the committee and was suffused with the spirit of evangelical philanthropy. Also, each householder was given a bill to exhibit, in his window or elsewhere, with a space for his name and the amount of his weekly contribution and collection.

The Work at St Thomas's Hospital.

In 1555 two hundred sick and aged were installed in St Thomas's Hospital, but the unaccustomed confinement and discipline proved too much for them and many ran away, so that guards had to be posted at the gates to prevent further exodus. The staff consisted of (a) two women, or sisters, to attend to the poor and wash their clothes when necessary or convenient, (b) one porter to open the gate to let the poor in or out, (c) one surgeon to cure the diseased who may be received therein, and (d) one honest, sober and pious man to survey the hospital and poorhouse, and to manage the revenues.

The first mention of a matron occurs in the minutes of 4th January, 1557, in the nature of a complaint that the husband of the said matron, whose name was Waymond, would meddle with her duties. A fortnight later one Amye Creade was appointed to the office during the matron's temporary absence, and provision was made for her permanent appointment in the event of the goodwife Waymond's further misdemeanours.

There is very meagre information regarding the kind of nursing given at this time. Sometimes the patients who had recovered were given work as porters or sisters at the hospital. The implements and utensils, which apparently included the surgeon's instruments, were under the care of the matron. The sick and needy seem to have been treated fairly well. An almoner attended at mealtimes every day to see that the rations were ample and were properly cooked. Meat was contracted for at 13d. a stone, and had to be of the 'best flesche except the neck and bluddie meate'; which probably meant liver and other viscera.

At the beginning of Elizabeth's reign there were three surgeons, no physicians, an apothecary, the matron and her staff, numbering twenty-five, although they decreased to fifteen in the next century. The prevalence of chronic ulcers at that period, due in part, probably, to the appalling hygiene of the age, was commented upon by a great Elizabethan surgeon, Thomas Gale, writing in 1562, 'I did see in the two hospitals of London called St Thomas's Hospital and St Bartholomew's Hospital, to the number of three hundred and odd poor people that were diseased of sore legs, sore arms and feet and hands, with other parts of the body so sore affected that a hundred and twenty of them could never be recovered without loss of a leg or an arm, a foot or a hand, fingers or toes, or else their limbs so crooked so that they were either maimed or else undone for ever.'

Early in the seventeenth century a physician was added to the staff. The matron and sisters were, according to the minutes, a frequent source of trouble to the governors, and were evidently drawn from a low class. Often they were before the governors on charges of drunkenness and brawling as well as more serious complaints, but one must remember that only their failings and shortcomings were recorded in the minutes. There are no statements about those who conscientiously carried out their duties in what must then have been a very insanitary and dangerous calling.

During the seventeenth century the hospital had fourteen wards each of twenty beds, but its only nursing staff was fourteen sisters and a matron. In February two more wards were added, but only one sister. In 1684 the number of patients was reduced to 160, except for six weeks in the Spring and the Fall, when extra patients might be admitted. In the Orders for the year 1700 the sisters are instructed to clean their wards by 6 a.m., to keep the yards clean and allow no hens to be kept therein. They are not to use the patients' fuel, nor to eat their victuals. Every tenth bed is to be left open for airing, and not more than one patient is to be put into each bed.

215

In 1752 the designation of 'sister' was changed to 'nurse', and that of 'nurse' to 'helper', and a new 'charge' was drawn up for the matron; but this consisted chiefly of details regarding the care of linen and the supervision of nurses and helpers.

Bridewell Hospital.

The essential problem with which it was proposed that Bridewell should deal was that of begging and thieving. Statutes of law had hitherto failed to cope with these evils and it was thought that the only permanent cure was labour. And at Bridewell it was proposed to train up poor children, and those who shewed no aptitude for learning, to various trades. Occupation should also be found for the sick and crippled when they were discharged from St Thomas's Hospital. Such a place of labour should serve to rid the streets of 'sturdy beggars'. The 'stubborn and foul' should be set to make nails and do the work of blacksmiths, whilst the weaker persons might 'make bedticks and bedding'.

The dissolute women, after being whipped, should be set to 'card wool and to spin'. Whipping was almost a universal punishment and panacea for mischievous conduct or offensive speeches, and chastisement was often administered as medicine—the dose to be repeated as often as necessary.

In the *Annals of Stow*, we read under the year 1553, 'The tenth of April, the lord mayor was sent for to the court at Whitehall, and there at that time the King's Majesty gave to him and the commonalty, and citizens, for to be a workhouse for the poor and idle persons of the city of London, his place of Bridewell and seven hundred marks, lands and rents of the Savoy, with all the beds, bedding and other furniture of the hospital of the Savoy, towards the maintenance of the said workhouse in his house of Bridewell, and the Hospital of St Thomas's in Southwark.'

The governors of Bridewell were empowered to appoint 'beadles' having the right to search all suspicious houses—ale-

216

houses, skittle-alleys, cockpits, dancing saloons, and gambling dens, and to convey to Bridewell the keepers of such places, together with 'ruffians and masterless men' arrested therein. Beadles were also attached to the hospitals. They attended the governors; but in their spare time they assisted in the work of 'cleansing the streets', and these men became the terror, not only of wrong-doers, but of many poor defenceless people.

By the end of Queen Mary's reign Bridewell had become a prison for the punishment of rogues and dissolute women. No attempt was made to introduce any system of apprenticeship; it had become a sort of sanctuary and exchange of vice where some 500 of the worst characters in England were housed at a cost of £2,000 a year, in fact, it had become such a sink of iniquity that the City authorities endeavoured to suppress it altogether, but without success for there was no substitute for it until the nineteenth century.

Christ's Hospital.

In 1555 the Convent of the Grey Friars was opened as Christ's Hospital to receive 380 children, but the mortality amongst them proved extremely heavy, due probably to their removal from their mothers and the free life of the streets and fields. However, the hospital has continued to receive and educate boy children ever since, and it ranks among the public schools of England, being known colloquially as the 'Bluecoat' school. It is now at Horsham, in Sussex, its London property having been taken over by St Bartholomew's Hospital. Christ's Hospital, St Thomas's Hospital and Bridewell were incorporated by the Charter of Edward VI. and they were allowed armorial bearings, which they share to this day.

CHAPTER XII

POST-REFORMATION NURSING ORDERS

*The Ursulines of France and Austria—The Order of St John of God—
The Orders of Camillus de Lellis—The Brignolines, or Daughters of
Our Lady of Mount Calvary—The Sisters of Charity of Vincent de Paul
—Founding of La Salpêtrière, or Hôpital Genéral—The foundlings of
Paris—Vincent's training of his Sisters—The Order of Vincent de Paul
in modern times—Administration—Nursing training—The Order of St
Charles de Nancy*

The Ursulines of France and Austria.

THIS Order was founded in 1537 by Angela of Brescia, who insisted that all the girls of her congregation should remain each in her parents' house, from whence she should assist the poor, visit the hospitals, tend the sick and carry out any work of charity that might be required. Later, the Order gave instruction to girls in reading, writing and the catechism. This led to a learned Council of Doctors of Law debating whether the teaching of females was not a work of the devil; but in spite of this the Ursulines of the seventeenth and later centuries became definitely a teaching Order of uncloistered nuns. Only in Canada did they continue to nurse the sick.

In 1639, the Duchesse d'Aiguillon, a niece of Cardinal Richelieu and one of Vincent de Paul's Ladies of Charity, who was left a widow whilst still a young woman, resolved to start some nursing work in Quebec. She possessed some of her uncle's practical genius for organisation, and through his influence she obtained a grant of land from the 'Company of New France', which had been given charge of the colonisation and development of

218

Canada by the French Government. With three Augustinian sisters and a small band of Ursulines she sailed from Dieppe on 4th May, 1639, and, after the many hardships of a stormy crossing which lasted for three months, they reached Quebec on 1st August. The Ursuline sisters had intended to teach Indian women—but on their arrival numbers of sick people were brought to them, including sufferers from small-pox. In a very short time they were overwhelmed with patients whom they tended in temporary quarters until they built a hospital at Sillery—the ruins of which may still be seen. After a few years it was deemed advisable, for protection against the inroads of the Iroquois, who were furiously attacking the settlement, to transfer the institution to the larger and better fortified town of Quebec. Accordingly, in 1658, they moved into the new and substantial building of the Hôtel Dieu in Quebec, which was for both natives and colonists. The Sisters organised an out-patients' department in connection with the hospital to which numbers of Indians came every day for treatment. War with the Iroquois was almost continuous, with the result that there were always wounded to be cared for in the hospital, and also a great deal of typhus fever.

The Hôtel Dieu of Quebec is still in existence, and it is now a recognised training school for nurses. It has been rebuilt several times; but, with the exception of the Hôtel Dieu of Montreal which was founded by Jeanne Mance in 1644, it is the oldest hospital foundation in Canada.

The Grey Sisters of Montreal are daughters of the Ursulines of Quebec, and both Orders, besides working in hospitals, nursed the sick in their own homes and taught the Indian women how to nurse.

The Order of St John of God.

The founder of this Order, John Ciudad, was born on 5th March, 1495. He was of humble birth and his early youth was spent in farming. Later, he became a soldier in the army of

Charles V. of Spain, and took part in that monarch's wars against France. He also fought with the Spanish against the Turks in Austria, but after the wars he again became a shepherd.

Hearing whilst at Seville of the cruel treatment meted out by the Moors to their Christian prisoners, he set out in an endeavour to aid and rescue them, but fell ill at Gibraltar. When 44 years of age, as a result of a vision of the Virgin and her Infant Child at Guadalupe, he went to Granada and rented a house where he might shelter the sick and infirm poor, and he went through the streets and squares of Granada searching for those who needed his ministrations, carrying on his shoulders those who were unable to walk. He issued forth every evening with a wallet and a hamper to beg for provisions for his patients. In this work he was joined by Antony Martin and Peter Velasco, and later, by Simon of Avila. Like Vincent de Paul a century later, he sought out abandoned infants and fallen women, finding help and shelter for them.

He died on his birthday, 5th March, 1550; but his work was then well established and was continued by his followers. Some years later it was duly recognised by the Popes. In 1571 Pope Pius V. gave them a Rule—under St Augustine—and authorised the wearing of a scapular and badge. The brothers took the usual three vows, but added a fourth—hospitality and life-long devotion to the poor and infirm. Their privileges were confirmed in 1576 by Pope Gregory XIII., who was so impressed by their far-reaching charity that he built for them the Hospital of St John Calybite in Rome, which is, at present, the central house of the entire Order.

The Order had its greatest development in France. It was first introduced into that country by Marie de Medici, wife of Henry V., in 1601. She established them in the Rue des Saints Pères, where a splendid hospital was built for their use. The Queen herself and the ladies of the court visited and helped at the hospital. This hospital is still in existence, but it is now a secular organisation.

In France the Order was known as the 'Brothers of Charity'. At the time of the Revolution in 1789 France possessed thirty-nine hospitals of the Order, in which no less than 4,125 patients were being cared for; but the Brothers of Charity shared the fate of all other religious Orders, and their houses and property were confiscated. The Order was reformed at Marseilles in 1819, and the Brothers took over all the nursing in the men's wards at the Hôtel Dieu of that city. Later, they did hospital nursing in many other towns in the south of France, and in 1826 they founded a branch near Lille—in the north of France—and a third at Dinan in Brittany in 1833.

At the present time the Order possesses two houses in Marseilles, one for aged poor and the other to supply nightly shelter for those who require it. At Paris, they have an establishment in Rue Lecourbe for the care and treatment of incurable children —the maimed, the blind, the deaf and dumb, etc. This has a seaside branch at Croisic, Loire Inferieure.

The English branch is at Scorton, in Yorkshire, founded in 1880 as a home for aged, disabled and incurable men and boys. The hospital stands in its own grounds of five acres, and all the brothers undergo a course of instruction in order to fit them for their nursing duties.

In 1882 a branch was founded in Ireland, at Stillorgan, near Dublin. This is a private home for mentally afflicted gentlemen, and it provides accommodation for 140 patients. There is a resident doctor, and the community consists of 24 brothers including a resident chaplain. It is recognised by the General Nursing Council of Ireland as a Training School for Mental Nurses, but all the brothers still live under the Augustinian Rule.

The Orders of Camillus de Lellis.

The founder of these two Orders lived from 1550 till 1614. He was a soldier, and in his youth a great gambler. In his twenty-fifth year he became a Franciscan friar and founded an Order of nursing priests that exists to this day. They were called the

221

'Ministers of the Sick', and they nursed sick persons, without consideration of creed or nationality, in their homes, in public or private hospitals and on the battlefields. The Second Order was of women who assisted in this work, and were known as the Daughters of Camillus.

In 1585 Camillus permanently founded his congregation in Rome. The Brothers and Sisters attended at the hospital of Santo Spirito every day, where they served the sick with most fervent charity—gave them food, made their beds, *cleansed their tongues* and exhorted them to patience. Cicatelli gives a most extraordinary account of these Camillines. He says, 'I myself have seen many a one of them, although he had been brought up with great delicacy, presenting food to sick men so covered with sores and so filthy that simply standing near them, not to say touching them, was enough to make any man sick. . . . The charity of the ladies in no way yielded to that of the brethren. Seeing them about the sick you would say that they could not be noble ladies whom all honour and respect, but slaves purchased to serve the hospital. Neither the dirt of the place nor the stench of the corrupting sores deters them, the most deplorable cases are the best served. They comfort them, they feed them, they warm them, they fan them, they smooth their beds, they comb and tie up their hair. There is no work of charity too difficult or too disgusting for their Christian fervour.'

One wonders why, with all this self-effacing piety, it never seemed to occur to them to *wash* their patients, or to *cleanse* their 'festering sores'. Surely that would have been more commendable than their stoic endurance of their patients' wretched condition.

Camillus obtained permission from Pope Sixtus V. for all the members of his Orders to wear a cross of red cloth on their cassocks and mantles. This badge had always been associated with Christian arms. Constantine adopted it for his legion in A.D. 312, and the Knights Templars had worn it on a white ground and carried it on their banners. The Camillines were bound to live

222

together in poverty, chastity and obedience, for the service of the sick and the plague-stricken. They were not bound by solemn vows, but stayed with the Order freely and voluntarily.

The Camilline Orders spread over Europe and into South America, and they have branches to-day in Italy, Belgium, Ireland, Germany and Holland. There is a branch of the Brotherhood in Spain. The Daughters of Camillus nursed during the last great plague of Barcelona, but none returned alive from the pest-houses and streets, and the Spanish branch of the Sisterhood then became extinct. England has never had branches, and France abolished its Camillines with the other religious Orders before the World War.

The Brignolines, or Daughters of Our Lady of Mount Calvary.

This Order was founded by Virginia Bracelli, who was born in 1587 at Genoa, and lived until 1651. During a great plague in Genoa in 1631 Virginia took orphans and rescued girls into her house and, later, she hired the deserted convent of the Friars of Bregara—known as Mount Calvary, and her followers took the robe of the Franciscan Tertiaries.

Ten years later the Government nominated three 'protectors' who were to provide for the necessities of the institution, and in 1650 Cardinal Brignole became the fourth 'protector'. Arrangements were made for the girls to serve in philanthropic institutions after the manner of the Daughters of St Vincent de Paul. The Order performed almost miracles of heroism during the plague epidemic of 1656, and its fame became so widespread that many Italian cities invited the Brignoline Sisters to form colonies in their midst.

Their Rule was almost identical with that of the Sisters of Charity of Vincent de Paul; but until 1840 the Brignolines nursed only women. Now they nurse men also.

Sisters of Charity of Vincent de Paul.

The Sisters of Charity are a French Nursing Sisterhood founded in the first half of the seventeenth century by Vincent de Paul, the third child of Jean de Paul, a small farmer of Pouy in Gascogne, near the Pyrenees. He was born on 24th April, 1576, and he had lived for nearly half a century before embarking upon the charitable and philanthropic works with which his name has ever afterwards been associated. He was educated at a Franciscan monastery, being destined for the priesthood. In 1605, during a short sea voyage from Marseilles to Narbonne he was captured by Turkish pirates and sold into slavery. He passed successively into the hands of three masters, a fishermen, an aged alchemist, and a wealthy farmer in the mountainous districts of Savoy. His third master released him in 1607 and he went to Rome, returning to France two years later. In 1613 he became tutor to the sons of M. de Gondi, a General of the Galleys. He was also confessor and spiritual advisor to Madame de Gondi, whom he assisted in the carrying out of various philanthropic schemes. After her death in 1625 he went to Paris, where, as in all other great cities of Europe, the social problems were acute. So long as the religious Orders had remained wealthy and generous the problems of poverty had been more or less in abeyance, but the civil wars of the sixteenth century had reduced all revenues, and the wide flow of charity had dwindled to a mere trickle that seldom reached those who most needed it. France had no Poor Law system such as had been introduced into England, there were no benevolent societies, no organisation of charity, and very few priests who recognised that they had any duties towards the poor; and yet poverty and ignorance, with all the evils that breed from their alliance, prevailed alike in the cities and country districts.

In the first year of his work in Paris Vincent founded the Company of Mission Priests. These were men who had renounced all ambitions regarding ecclesiastical preferment and devoted their lives to preaching in the villages and amongst the poor, pledged to a complete detachment from self-interest and to the service of Christ in the person of the poor, the sick, and the infirm. Eight years after their formation they made their headquarters in a monastery at St Lazare, with Vincent as their Superior; and therefore they became known as 'Lazarites'.

(*N.B.* This name had also been given to the chivalric Order of Knights of St Lazarus, but the two organisations must not be confused.)

The first movement in connection with the inauguration of the famous Order of Nursing Sisters was the outcome of visits paid to the Hôtel Dieu of Paris by Madame Goussault, the wife of a magistrate. She was appalled by the conditions she found there; the evils were so flagrant and, in her estimation, so harmful to the souls and bodies of all concerned that she went to the Superior of St Lazare feeling assured that he would intervene. The answer attributed to him was 'I have neither position nor authority to check abuses that exist there as they exist everywhere else. One must hope that those who undertake the management of this great institution will make the alterations that are needed.' Madame Goussault then appealed to the Archbishop of Paris, and he wrote to Vincent de Paul giving him the necessary authority and urging that he should make an effort to ameliorate the lot of the patients in the Hôtel Dieu. This was in 1634, and Vincent then set himself to study the conditions and the need for reform, and to organise a scheme to meet that need. He appealed for help to the great ladies of Paris, arranging a meeting at the house of Madame Goussault. The outcome of this meeting was the formation of a guild, known later as the Dames de Charité, with three officers—a Superior, a Treasurer, and a Keeper of the Wardrobe who was to have charge of stores other than money. About 120 ladies of quality joined this association, and they went in parties of four to cheer the sick, taking them soup, jellies, and other luxuries. Some 800 invalids were given comfort of this sort, although there were the inevitable difficulties, for the work of the Hôtel Dieu had been carried out for many years by the Augustinian Sisters assisted by the Grey Sisters, and, naturally, the introduction of 'lay' help was not altogether welcomed. Any woman, provided she was a Catholic, might become a Lady of Charity, if she had the consent of a male relation who claimed authority over her movements. Her first duty to the Order was the care of the sick, the second the relief of poverty.

After the first flush of enthusiasm had died down a little, the ladies ceased to be regular in the fulfilment of the duties they had undertaken. Health reasons, interference of husbands, and the claims of social and court duties intervened against the carrying out of their tasks, and many of them turned to the obvious recourse of the wealthy, and sent a paid substitute. It was so much easier to send a servant than to go in person; but that which had been a voluntary work of piety to the mistress was often only a disagreeable duty to the maid, and was carried out as a dull and uninspired routine. However, for four years these Ladies of Charity carried on their good work, but by 1638 the whole scheme needed reorganisation; and it was at that point that we have our first knowledge of the Sisters of Charity, or Servants of the Poor.

Some years earlier, in a quiet house in the parish of St Nicholas Chardonnet, Madame, or as she is more often called, Mademoiselle, le Gras had gathered around her a small company of young country-women, mainly of the peasant class, to aid her own efforts in the service of the poor. They were working under the guidance of Vincent de Paul, their tasks were laborious and homely, but they were showing greater stability in the doing of them than did their more favoured sisters among the society ladies; and when Mlle le Gras undertook the reorganisation of Madame Goussault's scheme, eager interest and liberal funds were forthcoming. The Company of the Sisters of the Poor developed rapidly both in numbers and in the sphere of usefulness of their work. There was no excitement or applause attendant upon the beginnings of this company, and the degrees by which

Mlle le Gras formed them into a Sisterhood are hardly perceptible. It was about eleven years after she first took helpers into her house that they were given a permanent Rule, although Vincent de Paul had permitted Mlle le Gras herself to take a vow eight years earlier, dedicating herself to the work of the Servants of the Poor. As Louise de Marillac she had married M. le Gras, Secretary to Marie de Medici—a man considerably older than herself—when she was twenty-two, and it was after his death in 1626 that she moved to the small house in Rue St Victor that was to be the birthplace of the Sisters of Charity.

Founding of La Salpêtrière, or Hôpital Genéral.

The problem that made the sharpest appeal to the hearts and minds of seventeenth-century philanthropists in Paris was that of dealing with habitual vagrants. There was hardly a semblance of protection for the public in a great city, and as soon as the daylight hours were over the streets could not be traversed by a peaceful citizen without grave danger to property, and even to life. No doubt many robberies were committed by the soldiery, or by lawless servants attached to the households of the nobility, but the difficulty of dealing with this evil was greatly increased by the hosts of homeless and destitute persons who crowded the streets, living on alms which were often extorted by force; and an individual malefactor became impossible to trace amongst such a crowd. There were places of refuge scattered about Paris where the beggars might congregate unmolested, and these came to be a sort of nursery, or forcing house, for crime.

In 1657, in order to deal with the menace, these beggars' sanctuaries were raided by the police, and for the first time street-lighting was introduced. These measures undoubtedly curbed the evil to some extent, but they did not provide a solution.

The enterprises of Vincent de Paul, especially with regard to the Mission Priests and the Dames and Sisters of Charity, had met with such amazing success that those who were striving to contend with the dangerous and degraded condition of the streets turned to him for direction. He laid the matter before the Queen Regent, Anne of Austria, and obtained a grant of the buildings and grounds known as La Salpêtrière, on the banks of the river opposite the Arsenal. The intention was that the Ladies of Charity should care for the homeless in that retreat, and that the needy should come to it voluntarily; but the magistrates took the matter in hand, and within a week of its opening, in May, 1657, the City Archers collected all the beggars who were still in the streets of Paris and compelled them to enter the Salpêtrière. The numbers increased rapidly until four establishments were required, and these became known as the Hôpital Genéral. In the main building young children, women and 250 aged married couples were housed. Of the other three buildings, Bicêtre was for men of all ages, Notre Dame de la Pitié was for boys under twelve and S Marthe de Scipion was used as the offices of the commissariat. The regulations provided that children should be educated and taught to work, and that all able-bodied men and women should be obliged to carry out their alloted share of labour. Vincent de Paul and his Mission Priests were the spiritual guardians of the vast colony, and the Sisters of Charity were the recognised servants of the poor thus congregated.

But the element of compulsion was not in accordance with Vincent's principles, and the indiscriminate treatment of vast numbers was quite incompatible with that respect for the individual which, according to Vincent's theory, was the right of every Christian. That may be the reason why we find so little mention either of Vincent or his Mission Priests in connection with the work at the Hôpital Genéral.

The Foundlings of Paris.

Another great problem of the Paris of that day was the number of deserted children in its streets, and the most familiar and picturesque representation of Vincent de Paul is in connection with his efforts regarding these waifs. About 1649 he hired a house outside the Porte St Victor in which he established twelve babies under the care of the Sisters of Charity, and very soon after this the Ladies and Sisters of Charity undertook the charge of all the foundlings in Paris. The Queen's interest was aroused, and subscriptions poured in. The work grew tremendously, and it was not until 1670, nearly ten years after Vincent's death, that the responsibility for it was taken over by the State.

Vincent's Training of his Sisters.

As has been stated, Vincent did not allow the Sisters of Charity to take any vows until 1642, and then one which bound them only for one year at a time. This vow was, and still is, renewed annually on 26th March. Vincent's training of his Sisters took the form of weekly 'Conferences', at which he both questioned and addressed them. In the streets and the poor houses of Paris they had no shelter or protection from insult save that which they erected and maintained for themselves. According to Vincent's oft-quoted dictum, they were 'a Community who have no monastery save the houses of the sick, who have for cells only a lodging or the poorest room, whose chapel is the Parish Church and who have the streets for cloisters. They are enclosed only by obedience; they make the fear of God their grille, and they have no veil but their own modesty'.

The life of a member of this company was a very hard one. A Sister must rise at four o'clock in summer and winter alike, she must eat sparingly and of the plainest food, and she must drink no wine. Her duties as a sick nurse were arduous and trying, she spent her whole life under a rigid Rule, in the daily toil of parish nursing and in the struggle to maintain order in the provincial hospital. Methods of alleviating pain were not yet known to medical science, and the Sister of Charity was often forced to witness the most horrible suffering. Moreover, she was constantly exposed to infection of all kinds, and many of her company contracted infections from which they died.

As time went on and their work became better known, the services of the Sisters of Charity were demanded more and more insistently, and they seem constantly to have been very overworked. After nearly thirty years' knowledge of them Vincent wrote, 'that while for the religious the one aim is the attainment of perfection for herself, the object of the Sister of Charity is the comfort and salvation of her neighbour.' (*Lettres*, Vol. ii, No. 550.)

It was Louise le Gras' constant and earnest wish that the work of the Sisters should not be separated from that of the Mission Priests, and, although at first Vincent had asked that they might be under special authority, he at length came to share the view that their hope of stability depended upon their direction by the Mission Priests; but it was ten years after their foundation that Letters Patent were issued to the Sisters of Charity, sanctioned by both the Church and the Crown, which placed them, in perpetuity, under the authority of the Mission Priests. Their numbers grew, but not in accord with the demands for their services. They travelled far and wide throughout their country, and worked in the army hospitals during the war with Spain in 1658, and among the sick and wounded soldiers in the hospitals at Calais. Within twenty years of their foundation the Sisters had about seventy mother-houses in France and Poland, and nearly four hundred members. As their leader and Superior, Louise le Gras was continually helped and encouraged by Vincent de Paul, and it was his training that made her great achievements possible; but she is a somewhat pathetic figure nevertheless, for obedience to duty taxed her powers almost to their limit, and ill-health during her last arduous years would have made her life a burden had her enthusiasm for her work ever flagged, or had the constant counsel and support of Vincent been withdrawn.

She died in 1660, six months before Vincent, but with the comfort of the knowledge that the affairs of the Sisters of Charity would be well ordered when her guidance was removed. And so it proved, for even during the Revolution when all other religious bodies were suppressed, their power and usefulness was such that the Government recognised their Order and permitted them to carry on their work. The height of their fame was reached early in the nineteenth century, and by 1850 it was estimated that there were twelve thousand women working as Sisters of Charity in various parts of the world.

The Order in Modern Times.

By no means the least astonishing part of the history of the Order of St Vincent de Paul is the tremendous advances it has made in the twentieth century. In this fourth decade it has branches in every European country with the exception of Norway, Sweden and Russia, and in many countries of the other continents. Although predominantly French until the nineteenth century it has now only 789 houses in France out of its total of 3,552, and of this total 432 are in America. The Order has some of the most up-to-date hospitals both in America and in Europe. In this country perhaps its most striking foundation is the St Vincent Orthopædic Hospital at Eastcote, near Pinner, Middlesex. As with so many of the organisations of the Order it is much more than a hospital, for, side by side with the strengthening of the misshapen or diseased body, the intellect is trained and developed, the character and outlook is moulded and everything possible is done to make the child forget its discomfort and suffering. In many cases the treatment is spread over a number of years. It may begin in the very early days of childhood and often it has not finished until adult age is reached. It may even continue in a modified form long after the cripple has become a wage earner.

In the special schools which are part of the hospital such subjects as dressmaking, stitchcraft, weaving on hand or foot-power looms, and many kinds of handicrafts are taught; whilst in the clerical section the patients work for certificates in shorthand and typewriting, and in the industrial classes boys are trained as bootmakers, carpenters, splint-makers, tailors and gardeners. They constitute the 4th Northwood Group of Scouts and Cubs, the 1st

Eastcote Extension of Guides and Brownies, and they have an Old Boys' Social and Cricket Club.

Administration.

Like most of the organisations of the Religious Orders for the relief of suffering in any form, the Orthopædic Hospital is most economically managed. The lives of the Sisters are dedicated to their work, and although bound only for a year at a time, their worldly needs are not great, for their permanent aim and ambition seems to be the practice of unlimited charity. There are no highly paid and luxuriously housed heads of departments, and there is no waste of stores or equipment.

Nursing Training.

The hospital accepts girls of 17 for a course of training lasting $2\frac{1}{2}$ years. This includes lectures and demonstrations not only in orthopædic nursing, but also in theatre and plaster work, ward management, and the treatment of all kinds of crippling and disabling diseases, including electrical and light treatments. The hospital gives its own certificate to those who successfully complete the course and pass their examinations, but it is not yet recognised as a training school by the General Nursing Council.

Other hospitals entirely nursed by the Sisters of Charity of St Vincent de Paul are the Italian Hospital in Queen Square, London, St Mary's Hospital, Lanark, the North Infirmary, Cork, and St Joseph's Orthopædic Hospital, Coole, Westmeath. These are all training schools or affiliated schools recognised by The General Nursing Council.

One of the most charming and beautifully organised of their smaller foundations is St David's Home, Castlebar Hill, Ealing. This is registered as a War Charity, and it provides a permanent home for totally disabled sailors and soldiers of all denominations, wherein they can find peace and comfort for the remainder of their days. Many of these War victims are quite helpless, requiring skilled nursing and frequent dressings. The degree of disablement makes the undertaking of such handicrafts as basket work and embroideries, which are so often a feature of such homes and which help so tremendously in filling otherwise empty hours, quite an impossibility at St David's; but a certain amount of leather work is done by the men, some of which is shown each year at the Exhibition of Work by Disabled ex-Service men held every November at the Imperial Institute, South Kensington.

Order of St Charles de Nancy.

This was an Order of women that was inaugurated in 1652. The Sisters were at first secular, and remained so for ten years; then they became monastic, taking life vows under Augustinian Rule with modifications to meet their needs as a nursing service. They nursed both men and women in homes and in hospitals; and they extended into Belgium, Prussia, Bohemia, and Italy. They are one of the few French Orders which survived the Revolution.

233

CHAPTER XIII

PROGRESS DURING THE EIGHTEENTH AND EARLY NINETEENTH CENTURIES

Guy's Hospital—The London Hospital—Two famous Irish Sisterhoods —Sisters of Charity and Sisters of Mercy—Pastor Fliedner and the Kaiserwerth Deaconesses

AT the beginning of the eighteenth century London, and in fact England, had only two general hospitals, St Bartholomew's and St Thomas's. As a substitute for the system prevailing before the Reformation every parish had been made nominally responsible for its sick poor by the passing of the Poor Law in 1601, and its various amendments. But this law was often harshly administered, without charitable feelings, and the provisions made to deal with the problems were quite inadequate to the needs.

Macaulay wrote that, in his day, there were no purely voluntary hospitals in England, for, although the two aforementioned had received back part of their pre-Reformation properties, which afterwards appreciated in value, they were dependent for a great deal of their support upon the citizens of London.

The eighteenth was a great hospital-building century in England, and the nineteenth and twentieth centuries have carried on this work very extensively. It will be impossible, and probably rather boring to the reader, to give the histories of many of these hospitals, so two have been selected as being typical of the various types of growth. One—Guy's Hospital—being founded, as a comparatively large building, by the philanthropy of one man, and the other—the London Hospital—starting in a small house, moving into larger premises, and then growing until it has become one of the largest in the world.

234

Guy's Hospital, and its Association with St Thomas's.

Thomas Guy was born about 1644 in the southern outskirts of London less than a mile from the site on which he was destined to build a hospital that should become world-famous. He was a publishing bookseller by trade, and in the opening years of the eighteenth century he became a governor, and a very great benefactor, of St Thomas's Hospital, then situated at Southwark, very near to his place of business. He erected three new wards on the north wing of this hospital about the year 1707, at a cost of more than £1,000—a very magnificent sum in those days. In 1724 he gave the hospital a new entrance, 'with piers and a pediment of stone', the latter being embellished with the arms of George I. The great gates of this entrance were of iron.

At this time St Thomas's was very concerned about the problem of treating incurables. Time and time again rules were made that they should not be admitted, and that no patient should be received a second time with the same disease; but there was no other provision made for these poor sufferers, and it was to meet this need that Thomas Guy founded a new hospital.

In the Minutes of St Thomas's Hospital, early in 1721, there is entered the first formal arrangement regarding this venture. 'Our worthy governor and benefactor, Thomas Guy, intending to found and erect a hospital for incurables in the close of this hospital, in the parish of St Thomas, we have agreed to grant him a lease, or to such persons as he may appoint, of several parcels of ground within the close of the hospital, and in the parish, upon several leases and under several ground rents, amounting to £17, 14s. 0d. per annum, purchased by the said Thomas Guy, or in trust for him, for 1,000 years at £30 per annum, tax free.'

He lived to see that hospital completed, and it was opened on 6th January, 1725—a little more than a week after its founder's death—sixty patients being admitted on the opening day.

The list of staff and salaries fixed during the early months after the opening of the hospital is interesting, particularly from the point of view of comparison between the various workers. The Treasurer's appointment was an honorary one.

	£	s.	d.
Treasurer	0	0	0
Clerk	40	0	0
Steward	80	0	0
Chaplain	80	0	0
Apothecary	80	0	0
Porter	35	0	0
Beadle	30	0	0
Matron	50	0	0
Eight Nurses, £16 each	128	0	0
Two Surgeons, £40 each	80	0	0
Two Physicians, £40 each	80	0	0
Butler, with his horse	67	2	0
Cook, with her Servant	32	0	0
Apothecary's Two Servants	78	0	0
Surgery Man	30	0	0
Eleven Sisters, £25 each	275	0	0
Twelve Watchwomen, £10, 8s. each	124	16	0
One Sister	25	0	0
One Brother (belonging to the lunatics)	35	0	0

The nurses and the servants were paid at a considerably higher rate than in any other hospital at the time, and this was an attempt to prevent them from extorting money from their patients —a practice strictly forbidden upon pain of losing their situations—but out of these stipends they had to provide their rations. The cure of souls was assessed at twice the value of the cure of the body, but the apothecary was as important as the chaplain. The employment of permanent watchwomen was not the customary practice at the time. The general rule seemed to be to summon these 'watchers' only when their services were required. They usually acted as night nurses, and did not live in the hospital buildings.

The London Hospital.

This began its career by the opening, on 3rd November, 1740, of a small house in Featherstone Street which became known as the 'London Infirmary'. The 'staff' consisted of a physician, a surgeon and an apothecary, who were to attend for two hours each morning. Nurses were not considered necessary, a man and his wife being engaged to carry out all the attentions required by the patients between the visits of the staff, and also to do all the domestic work that was necessary. There appears to be no record of the number of beds provided, but within three months of the opening of the house in Featherstone Street the work had so increased that a larger house had to be taken, the move being made in May, 1741, five months after the opening of the first house; and then a 'nurse' was appointed. Probably she was characteristic of the type of woman thought suitable for such work at that period, but it seems as though the patients might have been just as well off without her ministrations. The records state that she was called by her surname only, 'Squire', and that she was paid 5s. a week and lived out. Shortly after her appointment she was reported to the committee for having taken money from patients; but, as there was no rule which forbade this sort of thing, she was allowed to continue her work at the hospital. A night nurse was also appointed, and was paid 3s. 6d. a week. As the number of patients increased so did the number of nurses; and then a matron was appointed at a salary of £15 a year—a Mrs Elizabeth Gilbert—she was also paid 6d. a day for each patient, and with this sum she was to provide food. She ran up accounts with tradesmen for the very little food she was obliged to give the patients, and then decamped without paying the bills! No more experiments with regard to catering by the Matron were allowed, for the committee decided to keep the housekeeping in their own hands. The London Hospital appears to have been singularly unfortunate in the character and personality of its nurses during the eighteenth century—even at a time when nurses were renowned for drunkenness and dishonesty—if one may judge from the records of the committee meetings at which their misdemeanours were dealt with.

In 1743 it was decided that the nurses should be resident in the hospital at a salary of £6 a year for a nurse, and £4 for a watch, or night nurse. These were often elderly and rather decrepit women, and even as late as the early nineteenth century Sir William Blizzard, the great surgeon, complained that two persons upon whom he had operated for stone, and who required attention both night and day, had been left in the sole charge of an infirm old woman of seventy.

By 1745 the work had grown so that it had become necessary to take five more adjoining houses. One of these was known as 'The Jews' House', but there is no record of any special accommodation or diet being provided. At the present time one of the chief features of the hospital is its large department for those of the Jewish faith, comprising five wards in which all the religious rites of these people are carefully observed. A separate kitchen is provided which is under the charge of a Jewish cook, a special contract is entered into for the supply of Kosher meat, and the Jewish Sabbath—Saturday—is the weekly visiting day. There is also a Jewish mortuary for the dead.

In 1756 the nurse was honoured by having 'standing orders'. She was expected to come on duty at 6 a.m., and to continue at her post until 10 p.m. Days 'off' and holidays were, of course, unknown. Her duties were, amongst other things, to make the beds of the officers and servants, to clean the rooms, passages and stairs, and the Court- and Committee-rooms. In the face of such 'orders' we are not surprised to find that, when referred to in the minutes, she is classed with 'beadles, porters and other superior servants'. With regard to education and training no standards were required. In fact, as late as 1830 women who could neither read nor write were employed as nurses in most of the hospitals throughout Europe.

In 1847 a number of cases of serious illness is recorded among

238

the nursing staff of the London Hospital. A committee appointed to investigate the cause reports that—'The general disorder of the health of the nurses is brought on from excessive fatigue, induced by having to perform both Day and Night Duty, with but a short and hurried interval of rest between these periods of attendance in the wards'. It recommended that the staff should be increased, and consequently fourteen women were engaged as night nurses. They were non-resident, and were paid weekly at the rate of 1s. 6d. per night.

In 1874 definite practical training of nurses was introduced, but not until 1880 were lectures and demonstrations given to the nursing staff by Miss Lückes, the Matron, and by members of the Medical Staff.

In 1895 a preliminary training school was opened at Tredegar House, where probationers attended for a period of seven weeks before entering the hospital wards.

Two Famous Irish Sisterhoods: the Irish Sisters of Charity.

This Sisterhood was founded about 1815 by Sister Mary Augustine (Mother Mary Aikenhead, 1787–1858), and it was possibly one of the first moves towards the reorganisation of hospital nursing in English-speaking countries. The conditions in Ireland were, if anything, worse than in England, and in the wretched slums of Dublin they were indescribable; dirt, starvation and epidemics, particularly of typhus fever and cholera, brought in their wake an almost unequalled desolation. It was under these circumstances that the Sisters of Charity had their origin, with Miss Aikenhead as their first Superior, and Bishop Murray of Dublin as their Director. They took no vows of enclosure, for their work was to visit the poor in their own homes and nurse them in times of sickness. They also taught in the poor schools, and later they undertook the visiting of prisoners in the Kilmainham jail. During the cholera epidemics that occurred about 1820 they extended their activities to Cork, and they worked in the hospitals both in that city and in Dublin. In the next few

239

years the Order grew tremendously, and it extended into Waterford, Clonmel, Kilkenny and Merrion. But Miss Aikenhead realised that the ignorance of her Sisters frequently nullified their efforts to deal with cholera, typhus, tuberculosis and other diseases that were all too common in the noisome slums. She sought to harness science and sound practical training to the service of the sick, and she saw that, in order to do this, the establishment of a hospital was imperative. Hitherto, no woman had accomplished such a task as she visualised; but the means of realising her dream materialised when the money for a building was forthcoming as a gift of £3,000 from a Sister on her profession. However, before a hospital could be established it was necessary that suitable staff should be trained to conduct it. Accordingly, in the spring of 1833 Mother Aikenhead sent three of her sisters to the Hospital of Notre Dame de la Pitié in Paris, which was under the control of the Sisters of St Thomas of Villanova. It held, at that time, the reputation of being the best conducted hospital in Europe. Meanwhile, she purchased the Earl of Meath's Georgian mansion in St Stephen's Green, Dublin, and early in 1834, on the return of the Sisters from Paris, this was opened as a hospital for the sick poor and was dedicated to St Vincent.

It was the first hospital in these islands to be founded, organised and staffed by women. It was conducted on the principle that charity, to be effective, must be exercised on scientific lines and, in the century that has since elapsed, it has never lost sight of that principle.

> 'A mission born in a woman's mind,
> Simple and grand,
> To house the sick, their wounds to bind,
> Make suffering clean, the Cross more kind,
> Labour with love close intertwined
> This Mary planned.'

(John Mowbray. Written on the occasion of
St Vincent's Hospital Centenary in 1934.)

In their work and in the organisation of their community, Mother Mary's Sisters followed the lines laid down by Vincent de Paul, and they called many of their subsequent hospitals after him. At one time there was a question whether they should affiliate with the French Sisters of Charity, but it was decided that such an international alliance might bring undesirable consequences.

St Vincent's, Dublin, was undoubtedly the leading hospital of these islands at the time when Florence Nightingale was endeavouring to find some means of acquiring some sound training and experience in the nursing of the sick, and she made a great effort to find acceptance within its walls. But the point our great English pioneer failed to appreciate at that time was that neither her anxious keenness nor her influence and prestige could enable her, a Protestant woman, to enter a Sisterhood of Catholic nuns for a short period of a few months.

The following excerpts from her published correspondence with Cardinal Manning shews how very keen was her desire to be received at St Vincent's.

'(June 1852). For what training is there compared with that of a Catholic nun? . . . There is nothing like the training (in these days) which the Sacred Heart of the Order of St Vincent gives to women.'

'(July 1852). The question you were kind enough to say you would ask for me is whether they would take me in at the Hospital at St Stephen's on the Green in Dublin . . . for three months, as I am. I could not go for more at present and therefore it would not do for me to go into the Noviceship. Novices are seldom, and Protestants never, I believe, employed in the Hospital. I want to be employed there at once, for it is not for purposes of retreat that I go, which I could do elsewhere with less anxiety to my people, but to learn their trade. I have a particular reason for wishing to be under St Vincent. I have obligations to him. I do not wish to trouble you for information which I could get for myself. But I do not think they would take me on, on these terms, without a recommendation, which you alone could do for me.'

Later she wrote,

'I really don't know what I am going to do; but if I do not see you again, St Vincent's Hospital, St Stephen's Green, is the place, and the Reverend Mother's name is (or was) McCarthy. Eight years ago I tried to do this and failed.'

(N.B. Mother Francis Magdalen McCarthy succeeded Mother Mary as 'Superior General'.)

Present Work of the Irish Sisters of Charity.

This Sisterhood has grown until its numbers now extend into many thousands. They have hospitals, orphanages, convalescent homes and schools in Ireland, St Joseph's Home for the Dying, Hackney, and St Margaret's Home, Rockferry, Cheshire, in England, and they have branches in the United States; but their greatest development outside of Ireland is in Australasia, where they have a series of hospitals and schools. The first of their foundations in that continent was St Vincent's Hospital at Sydney.

All the nursing at St Vincent's Dublin, was done by the Sisters themselves until 1892 when a few lay nurses were accepted. The systematic training of secular nurses was introduced in 1894, and although many of the older religious Sisters viewed the development with some dismay, the standard of the Nursing School has continued to be in complete harmony with the traditions of the hospital. The nuns of this Order have always been specially noted for the beautifully finished technique of their nursing duties, for the order and completeness of their ward equipment, and for attention to detail in their ward and general management.

The Irish Sisters of Mercy.

This Sisterhood owes its origin to Catherine McAuley (Mother McAuley, 1787–1841). She was a wealthy woman, and her idea was to establish a society of ladies who, between the period of leaving school and settling in life, might spend a few hours daily in the instruction of poor girls in all kinds of needlework and knitting; and this developed into a religious Order. Mother McAuley founded a house of shelter for destitute girls in Baggot Street, Dublin; but the first actual nursing work done by the Sisters was during a cholera epidemic in 1832, when they helped in the Dublin hospitals. In the next few years they nursed in several hospitals in Dublin and Cork, founding their own hospital—the great Mater Misericordiæ Hospital of Dublin—about 1860. This is still the chief hospital of the Order, which has now hospitals in all parts of the English-speaking world, particularly in the United States; but the visitation of the sick in their own homes remains as one of the special duties of these Sisters of Mercy. It was Mother Warde, one of the original group of Sisters, who, with a small band of helpers, went to America in 1843. Their chief foundations in that country are the Mercy Hospitals of Pittsburg and Chicago, and the Misericordiæ Hospital of Philadelphia.

These two Irish Orders were very instrumental in bringing about the great reaction against the abuses that existed in American hospitals and other institutions in the second half of the nineteenth century.

Pastor Fliedner and the Kaiserswerth Deaconesses Institution.

One of the most epoch-making experiments of the first half of the nineteenth century was commenced in a small parish near Düsseldorf on the Rhine by a young Lutheran clergyman named Theodor Fliedner. In his work amongst his congregation he saw so much of the misery to which the very poor were doomed when sickness came upon them. The harshly administered laws sent men and women into prisons for very minor offences, and at that time, the conditions in the prisons were so deplorable that, when discharged, the prisoners were in no fit state to earn an honest living; and meanwhile there was no aid forthcoming for their wives or children.

In 1822 Pastor Fliedner went on a tour through Holland and England in order to collect funds for the needs of his parish. In the former country he saw the work of deaconesses and realised what an asset such an organisation would be in the work that he was trying to accomplish. In England he met Mrs Elizabeth Fry and was very greatly impressed by the work that she was starting among the women prisoners in Newgate. Four years later, in 1826, he founded a 'Prison Association' for the purpose of arousing public interest in the reforms that were so long overdue, and for the assistance of discharged prisoners. In 1828 he married Frederike Munster, a woman who possessed remarkable initiation and organising power, and she gave him invaluable assistance in the work of his parish. In 1836 he bought a house to be used as a hospital for discharged prisoners and orphans, intending to train women of good character as deaconesses to assist in the work involved. His first deaconess was Gertrude Reichardt, a woman of forty-eight who was the daughter of a doctor. Before the year was ended the number of deaconesses had increased to six. In 1839 he purchased two adjoining houses in order that the work might have room to expand. The institution was then known as Kaiserswerth, and it became very famous, not only for the work it was doing among the sick, but also as a training school for deaconesses. The training given included nursing tuition and practice, kitchen, laundry and garden work, and a considerable amount of Bible study. Nearly all the nursing instruction was given by Frederike Fliedner, who compiled notes in her journal, which became the standard of teaching at Kaiserswerth, and which, although never published, may be regarded as the first 'nursing textbook'. The deaconesses took no vows and received no salaries, but were maintained for life if they became unable to support themselves.

The starting of Kaiserswerth aroused considerable interest in England, although this interest had no immediate results. Many visitors from other countries came to study its methods or to undergo training, and numbers of experienced deaconesses were sent from Kaiserswerth to commence work in other localities. Mrs Elizabeth Fry spent some time there in 1840 and, inspired by the work that was being done, she returned to form her own 'Institute of Nursing Sisters' as an attempt to raise the standard of nursing in this country.

In 1842 Kaiserswerth was rebuilt on more suitable lines, as the capacity of the original building was far too small and cramped for the amount of work that was being done, for it had over two hundred beds; but in that year deep sorrow came to its founder, with the death of Frederike Fliedner. A year later, however, Pastor Fliedner married again, his second wife being Caroline Bertheau, who for three years had been in charge of the women's surgical department of the Hamburg Hospital. In 1846 he visited London with four deaconesses, and commenced the work of the German Hospital.

In 1850, Florence Nightingale spent a fortnight on a visit to Kaiserswerth, and in the following year she returned for four months' training, working as a deaconess.

At the time of the Crimean War Kaiserswerth had a hundred and twenty-eight sisters and deaconesses, and sixty-two probationers. Eighty of the sisters were stationed in different parts of Germany, five in London, three in Constantinople and two in Smyrna. A branch of the Deaconesses Institution had been established in Pittsburg, United States, by Pastor Passavant, and was carrying on a much needed work in that country.

When Fliedner died, in 1864, there were thirty-two deaconess houses and sixteen hundred deaconesses. Their sphere of work included hospitals, almshouses, orphanages, schools, and the homes of their patients. They also worked amongst prisoners and prostitutes.

The establishment of Kaiserswerth was a great landmark in the development of nursing because it was the first attempt to initiate a hospital that should also be a training school for nurses. As such, it marks an important turning point; and, when we consider the influence it had upon Mrs Elizabeth Fry, Florence Nightingale and Agnes Jones, we realise the very great debt that England, alone, owes to its founder. In addition to this, at least one well-known London training school traces its inception to Kaiserswerth—the Prince of Wales's General Hospital, Tottenham.

A Dr Michael Laseron, from Germany, started a Ragged School in Dawson's Buildings, Edmonton, in 1856. It does not appear that definite records were kept during the subsequent decade, but, in 1867, a Kaiserswerth sister from the German Motherhouse took a small villa in Snell's Park, Edmonton, and commenced to train six of the elder girls from the school to assist in nursing the sick in the district. She wore the Kaiserswerth uniform; consisting of a black dress and shawl, and a black bonnet without a veil. From that time an important Deaconesses Institution developed which utterly outgrew its accommodation; and then, in 1883, the foundation stone was laid of the present hospital on The Green, Tottenham. When this building was completed the deaconesses moved into it; and by almost imperceptible changes it became the Tottenham Hospital under the Superintendency of Lady Christian Dundas, a deaconess who had given £7,000 towards its establishment. She continued to wear the Kaiserswerth uniform, and as 'Sister Christian' she was greatly beloved, not only in the hospital but also amongst the poor of Tottenham. Many sisters who trained under her held administrative and ward sisters posts long after the erstwhile 'Tottenham Evangelical Deaconesses Hospital' had become the Prince of Wales's General Hospital, and had been recognised as a Training School by the General Nursing Council for England and Wales; and well into this century these sisters wore the Kaiserswerth cap, of white muslin with the characteristic double ruche, as part of their indoor uniform.

Following the Kaiserswerth tradition, some of the early sisters, when trained, were sent to work in other parts of the country, but remained under the Central authority. Nine sisters were sent to the Perth Infirmary in 1872, and 'this was the only hospital in Scotland where the nursing was done by a religious body',[1] and

[1]*History of Nursing*, Lavinia L. Dock, vol. iii, p. 68.

the work of the deaconesses is said to have been excellent. However, most of them were withdrawn by Dr Laseron in 1877, when he was organising a party of nurses to go out to the Russo-Turkish war.

At the present time there are, at least, two of the old deaconesses still living who receive a small pension from the Prince of Wales's Hospital; but the Kaiserswerth rule that sisters should be maintained in old age or infirmity has recently become an anachronism with the death of the last of the resident deaconesses. These ladies, when their working days were over, were each provided with a private room attached to a ward. As far as their health and strength permitted, they kept their own rooms clean and tidy. They walked in the grounds and sat in the sunshine, or under the shade of a tree they had known since girlhood. When in poor health they were tended by the nursing staff of the associated ward. Their presence lent something of an old-world atmosphere to the busy twentieth-century hospital, and served to remind the modern student nurse, training in accordance with the curriculum of the General Nursing Council and preparing for State Examinations, of the pioneer work of two generations ago.

247

CHAPTER XIV

NURSING DEVELOPMENT IN AMERICA

Early American-Indian medicine and hospitals—First European hospitals in America—General nursing conditions—Jeanne Mance and the Hôtel Dieu of Montreal—Dorothea Lynde Dix and the care of the insane—The American Sisters of Charity

Early American-Indian Medicine and Hospitals.

THE ancient American-Indians had a knowledge of medicinal plants and of how to prepare them for administration. During the sixteenth century the earliest white travellers and explorers observed this, and they brought back to Europe some very valuable drugs, such as cascara sagrada, balsam of Peru, quinine, guaicum, sarsaparilla, sassafras, jalap, balsam of Tolu and ipecacuanha.

Mexico is said to have had well-endowed hospitals, complete with men and women physicians, surgeons and nurses, long before the Spanish invasion; but there appears to be no authentic accounts of these. The earliest hospital in America of which we have any definite knowledge is the Hospital of the Immaculate Conception in Mexico, founded by Cortez, who, five years previously, had led an expedition over the mountains from Peru into the Mexican valley and destroyed the existing Aztec civilisation. The hospital was staffed by members of a Nursing Brotherhood; and it is said that Sir Francis Drake spent some months as a patient in one of its wards whilst suffering from an illness consequent upon his shipwreck.

First European Hospitals in America.

Several hospitals in the United States claim, on different grounds, to have the oldest foundation. In point of time, that honour seems to belong to the present Bellevue Hospital in New York City, for it descended from a hospital built, in the town then known as New Amsterdam, by the West India Company, in 1650. It was intended for sick soldiers and the negroes of the Company. Later, the hospital combined with the city poorhouse, the joint institution taking the name of Bellevue Hospital; but even in 1736 it had only one ward for the sick, and in 1816 it was a poorhouse, a penitentiary and an asylum for the insane.

Another claimant is a hospital started at New Orleans about 1720; being placed under the care of the Sisters of Charity and becoming a city poorhouse in 1811.

Then Blockley Hospital, now known as the Philadelphia General Hospital, which began as an almshouse in 1720, claims to be the 'oldest hospital in continuous service'.

Yet another to claim priority is the Pennsylvania Hospital which received its Charter in 1751. The ground for its claim lies in the fact that it has always been devoted entirely to the care of the sick, whilst older foundations included the care of orphans, the aged and the insane, and also the relief of poverty.

General Nursing Conditions.

Blockley Hospital was a poorhouse and a mental asylum as well as a hospital, and visitors were admitted, upon payment of a small fee, to be amused by the antics of the lunatics—just as they were at Bethlem Hospital in this country—and in spite of several investigations that took place towards the end of the eighteenth and the early nineteenth centuries there was very little improvement in the general conditions.

During a severe cholera epidemic Bishop Kindred of Emmitsburg sent a group of Sisters of Charity to undertake the nursing —which they did most effectually—but after they left it relapsed into its former inefficiency.

From all the evidence it appears that the two large hospitals of Bellevue and Blockley were epitomes of everything that such institutions should not be.

It seems that conditions in American secular hospitals until about 1875 were even worse than in England. In the city hospitals most of the work was done by the pauper inmates and the prisoners; or else by old, or otherwise undesirable, women who could obtain no other employment, and one is not surprised to learn that serious epidemics were of frequent occurrence.

Almost the only real nursing was carried out by the religious orders, especially the Sisters of Charity, the two Irish Sisterhoods, and the Ursuline nuns. The Sisters of Charity had founded, in 1828, the first permanent hospital west of the Mississippi River at St Louis. This was started in a log hut of three rooms, but the Sisters also did visiting nursing. A branch of the Lutheran Deaconesses Order began its work in America by opening a hospital at Pittsburg in 1850, under the direction of Pastor Passavant who had visited Kaiserswerth and influenced some of the deaconesses to return with him. This work spread into Milwaukee and Chicago, establishing hospitals in many cities.

Jeanne Mance, and the Hôtel Dieu of Montreal.

The oldest Canadian hospital which is still in existence is the Hôtel Dieu of Montreal which was founded by Jeanne Mance in 1644. Mlle Mance was a Frenchwoman born in 1606. She spent her early life with her father at Saint Sulpice in Paris. She wished to go to Canada as a missionary, and a very wealthy lady, Madame de Bullion, offered to furnish her with funds to build a hospital providing that she directed the institution herself. Accordingly, in 1641 she went to Rochelle to embark and there learned that a woman was required to accompany a contingent of soldiers, who were proceeding to Montreal, in order to nurse any who might fall sick during the voyage, and she offered her services. These were accepted on the condition that she should become an associate of the Society of Montreal. Thereupon, she sailed with the soldiers, but was obliged to pass the entire winter with the troops in Quebec, where they were building wooden barracks for transportation to Montreal. She took charge of their provisions, and even of their military stores; and on account of this work with the soldiers and her subsequent hospital work she is known as the 'Florence Nightingale of America', although she preceded that lady by over two hundred years.

She left Quebec on 8th May, 1642, reaching Montreal a few days later, and then she proceeded to build the hospital at Villemarie, of which she became the head. She had to take charge of numerous wounded soldiers from the almost daily combats with the Iroquois, and her labours increased as the town and the population grew. The available funds became exhausted and she received no answer to her appeals from the headquarters of the Society of Montreal in France, and so, in 1649, she herself returned to France in order to collect the necessary money. She found that the Society was thinking of abandoning the colonisation of Canada, but she prevailed upon them to continue their efforts, and she returned to Villemarie the following year. Shortly after her arrival the town was attacked by the Iroquois, and after enduring great dangers she was obliged to evacuate the hospital and retire with her patients into the fort. Seeing that the colonists must eventually succumb if they received no reinforcements, she persuaded the Governor, de Maisonneuve, to return to France for soldiers, giving him part of the money that still remained in her hands for the expenses of the hospital, on condition that when peace was restored lands should be given in exchange, from which the future revenue of the hospital might be obtained. During the absence of the Governor she did her utmost to keep up the courage of the colonists, only 17 of whom were able to bear arms. The return of de Maisonneuve restored security to the colony, the hospital buildings were repaired and enlarged, and Mlle Mance was able to leave the fort with the sick and reenter the hospital. The resolution of this courageous woman and the money she gave at a critical time to arm and pay soldiers not only saved Montreal but the whole of Canada to France, a fact that was recognised by the Government.

The hospital continued to grow until she was no longer able

to manage it alone, so de Maisonneuve arranged to visit France and collect a band of nuns to help with the nursing and to succeed her in the management. During his absence a fall of ice injured her right arm, and as funds were again badly needed for the support of the hospital she decided to go to France herself. On her way home plague broke out on the vessel, and her attendance on the sick in addition to her injured arm resulted in her own prostration; but she recovered and returned to Canada in 1659 accompanied by three Hospital Sisters of St Joseph from the Convent of La Fléche at Anjou. One of these, Judith de Bresoles, opened a dispensary in connection with the hospital.

Jeanne Mance took yet another journey to France in 1662 in order to defend the interests of the colony, and upon arrival she found the Association of Montreal thoroughly disorganised. She thereupon persuaded its members to dissolve it and to cede the rights over Montreal to the Sulpitians.

She died at Montreal in June, 1673, but she will never be forgotten in Canada. Her statue stands on the Maisonneuve monument at Montreal, and a very beautiful portrait of her hangs in the Hôtel Dieu to this day. The hospital became a School of Nursing in 1901, and it was affiliated with the University of Montreal in 1920, but nuns from the Sisterhood of St Joseph are still working there, and it has over three hundred beds.

Dorothea Lynde Dix and the Care of the Insane.

Dorothea Lynde Dix was born on 4th April, 1802, in the town of Hampden, Maine. Her childhood was very unhappy on account of her tyrannical and fanatical father, and at the age of twelve she ran away to her grandmother's home at Boston. This lady brought the child up under very strict discipline and educated her to be self-supporting. At the age of 19 she became a school teacher; but after some years she completely broke down in health, developing tuberculosis. She then spent a year of rest in England, and whilst in this country she became very interested in the reforms that were being carried out with regard to the poorhouses, the prisons and the insane.

At the age of thirty-nine, after her return to America, she undertook to give religious instruction to the inmates of the East Cambridge House of Correction, where, for the first time, she was brought into contact with the deplorable conditions then existing in penal institutions. Twenty women were crowded into one filthy room with no beds or facilities for heating, and several of them were insane—and then she started her campaign for a drastic improvement in these conditions.

She enlisted the support of Dr Howe of Boston and he attacked the situation through the medium of a daily paper—the *Boston Advertiser*. His articles met with protests and denials, and no improvements followed. Then Miss Dix set out to visit jails and almshouses throughout Massachusetts in order to collect her own statistics. In two years she had accumulated accounts of misery and outrages sufficiently appalling to stir any but the most heartless out of their indifference, and she sent her report to the Legislative Council of Massachusetts.

The ultimate result of this was that State funds were voted for the building of an asylum for the insane who were then in jails and almshouses. Miss Dix next extended her activities to Rhode Island where she collected facts and published her report in the papers in order to arouse public sympathies. Here, again, her efforts met with success, and during the ten years that followed she travelled through thousands of miles of America, from Nova Scotia to Louisiana, mainly in the discomfort of stage coaches and waggons plodding their way through mud and over the roughest of roads. In addition to her tuberculosis, which persisted throughout her life, she contracted malaria, so that her activities were often held back by her physical disabilities; but in each State she remained long enough to arouse the sympathy of the public and the activity of the Legislative Councils. One by one these States erected buildings for the shelter, care and kindly treatment of the insane, and many of them wished to name institutions after the intrepid Miss Dix; but with one exception she refused this recognition of her work. The Dixmont Hospital of Pennsylvania is the only institution bearing her name, and even that is in a modified form.

In 1856 she again visited the British Isles. She travelled through parts of Scotland collecting information with regard to abuses in the institutions for the insane in this country. Her disclosures led to the appointment of a Royal Commission empowered to correct these scandals wherever they existed.

Then followed a year of similar work on the Continent, after which she returned to America, and, although still working for the building of new asylums and the betterment of conditions in those already existing, another sphere of activity opened up for her. In 1861, at the age of 59, she was invited to organise the nursing staff of the Union army, and she became the Superintendent of Nursing during the Civil War of 1861-1865. The country honoured her at the close of hostilities, the following Order being issued by the War Department and signed by Edwin M. Stanton, the Secretary for War.

'Washington City, 3rd December, 1866,

'In token and acknowledgement of the inestimable service rendered by Miss Dorothea Dix for the care, succour and relief of the sick and wounded soldiers of the United States on the battlefield, in camps and in hospitals during the recent War, and of her benevolent and diligent labours and devoted efforts to whatever might contribute to their comfort and welfare, it is ordered that a Stand of Arms of the United States National Colours be presented to Miss Dix.'

The flags thus officially presented to her she bequeathed to Harvard College where they now hang in the Memorial Hall. But the work for which her name will for ever be remembered is the reformation in the care and treatment of the insane. The material result of her work was the founding, during her lifetime, of thirty-two asylums in the States, and the raising of the greatest sums of money ever subscribed for a strictly benevolent object; but with all that effort, the use of iron manacles for the insane was not abolished until 1886.

Miss Dix died in 1887, and was buried in Mount Auburn cemetery, near Boston. Perhaps the finest commentary on her life and work might be found in the letter written to Dr Tuke of England by the Rev. Dr Nicholas after the brief memorial service—'Thus has died and been laid to rest in the most quiet and unostentatious way, the most useful and distinguished woman America has yet produced.'

The American Sisters of Charity.

These Sisters constitute an Order formed early in the nineteenth century by Mrs Eliza Seton, their Mother-house being at Emmitsburg in Maryland. At first these sisters cared chiefly for unmarried mothers, foundlings and orphans, but quite early in their history they organised hospitals for the sick, the injured and the insane. The first of these was the Baltimore Infirmary, opened in 1823, and for more than fifty years they carried out all the nursing therein. The earliest American hospitals that were built exclusively for consumptives belonged to this Order. They founded St Vincent's Hospital in 1840, and out of this grew 'Mount Hope'—a refuge for the insane which was one of the earliest asylums in America, wherein the victims of insanity were treated under humane conditions. The American Sisters of Charity are now affiliated with the Order of Vincent de Paul.

The nursing and general administration in the secular hospital of Blockley in Philadelphia had, by the middle of last century, reached the limit of their deterioration, and then as a climax came a severe cholera epidemic with which the nurses completely failed to cope. The nearest Order of Sisters was Mother Seton's community at Emmitsburg, ninety miles away. There was no railroad and no telegraphic communication, so a messenger was sent on horseback with a request that some of the Sisters should come and help. Accordingly, with the consent of

Bishop Kindred, their director, six Sisters set out on horseback, that being the only available mode of conveyance, and it took them three days to make the journey. They did not, however, remain at Blockley after the epidemic had subsided; but the incident gives some indication of their readiness to undergo hardship and danger in the carrying out of their work for the sick.

At the present time they have homes for the old and incurable, general hospitals, tuberculosis sanatoria, foundling homes, and asylums for the insane; in fact, for every phase of human need they have a response, and there are now over ten thousand Sisters of this Order working in America alone. One of their most important foundations is the New York Foundling Asylum. It was here that Dr Joseph O'Dwyer worked out his system of intubation for obstructive laryngeal diphtheria. The blocking of the small opening into the larynx by the diphtheritic exudate was the cause of a high mortality amongst these foundling children whenever there was an epidemic of diphtheria—which happened nearly every year. Dr O'Dwyer's idea was not entirely a new one. The practice of inserting a tube into the larynx from the mouth had been tried by the Greeks two thousand years earlier, it was also tried by the French in the Medical School at Montpelier; but the methods used had failed in their purpose of affording relief. It was only after many years of experimentation that Dr O'Dwyer succeeded in perfecting his apparatus. Now, as all nurses know, O'Dwyer's method of intubation has saved countless lives and has proved even more valuable for adults than for children, although at the present day it has been greatly superseded by the operation of tracheotomy; and the general use of antitoxic serum has diminished the necessity for either of these measures.

256

CHAPTER XV

EARLY NINETEENTH-CENTURY CONDITIONS IN ENGLAND

Social conditions—English Nursing Sisterhoods—Institute of Nursing Sisters—Park Village Community—The Sisters of Mercy—St John's House Sisterhood—The All Saints' Sisterhood—General progress

Social Conditions.

AT the dawn of the nineteenth century in this country nursing was looked upon as an inferior, disagreeable and repellent form of domestic service. Women were employed without any preliminary enquiries as to character, and without previous experience, in order to induce them to serve for very low wages. Most of them were middle-aged or elderly, and all the hospital records of that time teem with instances of nurses being reported for drunkenness, fighting, bad language, pilfering and extracting money from patients. But it should be realised that only those who gave trouble were brought to the notice of the Committee and had their misdemeanours reported in the minutes. A great many of the others may have been quite respectable and conscientious in the carrying out of their duties, but they did not make history as did their undesirable sisters. And however one may be appalled by a study of the conditions existing in hospitals, Poor Law institutions and asylums for the insane in the early half of the nineteenth century, when these are viewed in their true perspective—as part of the general social system prevailing at that time—they are seen to be comparatively humane in an age that tolerated such terrible evils as the slavery of women and little children in mines, collieries, brickfields, mills and factories, the revolting cruelties meted out to poor unfortunate

s   257

children in cheap boarding schools, and the unspeakably filthy conditions in lodging houses. Even when the Ten Hour Factory Act was passed in 1844 its conditions were not applicable to children, who could therefore be made to work much longer hours.

But, as in all other ages and countries, the cry of the oppressed did eventually reach the ears of those who were willing to sacrifice time, money, and social or political advancement in order to champion their cause.

John Howard and Elizabeth Fry had awakened the public conscience with regard to prison conditions. Lord Ashley, afterwards the seventh Earl of Shaftesbury, had flung all the weight of his rank and influence into his fight for humane legislative control of the conditions under which the very poor lived and worked, and he was, undoubtedly, the master figure in nineteenth-century social and industrial reforms. Charles Dickens, Thomas Hood and Charles Kingsley were using their literary gifts in an attempt to bring home to the minds of the more educated classes some conception of the unnecessary hardships and sufferings endured by those whose lot had been cast in less favourable circumstances, and to arouse in them a sense of their individual and collective responsibility towards these blots upon civilisation.

English Nursing Sisterhoods.

In the English hospitals of the middle nineteenth century the conditions were so bad as to be almost unbelievable. Many of the buildings were dirty and most unhygienic, there was practically no vocational spirit amongst nurses, and the medical and surgical treatments, in the absence of anæsthetics and antiseptics, were subject to many limitations and were fraught with dangers such as the present generation can hardly understand. When reading medical articles contributed to the various journals, and the textbooks of medicine published at that time, one is struck by the dependence placed upon whisky as a remedy for all continued fevers and exhausted conditions; and it was prescribed in very large doses, often as much as a quart a day for one patient. It must have been rather easy for nurses to obtain it, and in their overworked and underpaid employment one can, perhaps, begin to understand why so many of them became noted 'tipplers'. They certainly seemed to have reached the limit of their inefficiency just before the Crimean War. Without religious inspiration to refine drudgery, without education to appreciate the aims of medical science, without sufficient wages or leisure to maintain a decent existence, these nurses were a pitiable and unrespected class of women.

The great need of the country was not only for a rebuilding of hospitals with a thorough reorganisation of hygienic conditions, but also the substitution of respectable and intelligent women upon whom some reliance could be placed for the nurses who were proving so utterly unsuited to their responsibilities. And that seemed rather hopeless of attainment because respectable women, with the exception of such reformers as Elizabeth Fry and, later, Florence Nightingale, tended to avoid every possible contact with hospitals and nurses, and there was no such thing as friendly visiting of the hospitals by women of the better classes.

Naturally, the sick shewed great reluctance to enter the hospitals as patients except as a very last resource. In Roman Catholic countries many religious Orders, as we have seen, were nursing the sick in their own homes, but in Protestant England there was no such organisation until well into the nineteenth century; and then a whole crop of Sisterhoods arose. These not only gave immediate help to the sick and injured, but they prepared the way for the great reorganisation that was to come in the later part of the century.

Institute of Nursing Sisters.

This was the first organisation of women to act as district or private nurses. It was founded in 1840 by Mrs Elizabeth Fry, who, in spite of her home duties and her many children, found time to work amongst the sick poor who lived in the neighbourhood of her country home. Very early in her married life she had become interested in the terrible conditions, both physical and moral, that existed in the prisons. In 1813 she commenced her visits to women prisoners in Newgate, and in 1817 she instituted sewing and teaching classes for these women, and she was instrumental in forming the 'Association for the Improvement of Female Prisoners in Newgate'. This aimed at the entire separation of the sexes, the classification of criminals, female supervision for the women, adequate provision for religious and secular instruction and for their useful employment. The movement rapidly extended to other prisons not only throughout the United Kingdom, but also into Italy, Denmark and Russia.

In 1840, whilst visiting prisons in European countries, Mrs Fry came into contact with Pastor Fliedner of Kaiserswerth. She then realised the great necessity for something analogous to his deaconesses in England, and on her return she founded the 'Institute of Nursing Sisters' at Raven Row, Whitechapel. It moved twice during the next two years, finally becoming established at 4, Devonshire Square, Bishopsgate. The Sisters were women of good character who were at least able to read and write, and they were selected principally from the higher domestic or small farming and trading classes. The regulations with regard to their dress and conduct were somewhat rigid. They were required to wear a neat and becoming uniform. They were maintained and paid by the Institute, and they visited and nursed the poor in their own homes; but they also nursed many patients who paid definite fees to the Institute for their services. They visited Guy's Hospital daily for a few months in order to learn what they could from the nurses there, but that was probably not very much considering the type of women then engaged in the wards. However, the Sisters must have become familiar with the aspect of patients suffering with various diseases, and have learnt much from their observations. Guy's was an institution likely to commend itself to Mrs Fry, because it had been founded especially for the care of the sick in chronic illness.

Some of the Sisters were sent to the London Hospital for similar training and experience, but in 1842 it was reported that 'such was the uncleanly state of that establishment that the Secretary is desired by his Committee to inform the Committee of the London Hospital that unless an improvement can be made the nursing sisters cannot be allowed to continue on duty there'. This communication obviously received attention, for the Sisters did continue to work at the London Hospital.

This organisation still survives although the need it was formed to meet has long since become non-existent. However, it does meet a very definite need of modern times, for, to quote from its own prospectus, its purpose is 'to supply *fully trained* nurses to those who require skilled nursing, but who, owing to limited means, are unable to afford the standard fee that is rightly charged for such Nurses by other Private Nursing Institutions. It is with this object that the Nursing Sisters Institution still exists, and the Committee asks for the kind co-operation of the Medical Profession and of other Private Nursing Institutions to ensure that the services of the Staff may reach those for whom they are intended.'

The Nursing Sisters' Institution, as it is now designated, has removed from Devonshire Square to 10, Collingham Road, S.W.5; and it was under the patronage of her Royal Highness, the Duchess of York, until her accession as Queen Elizabeth.

The Park Village Community.

This was founded near Regent's Park, London, in March, 1845, by the Rev. E. B. Pusey for the service of the poor in the district of St Pancras. Dr Pusey had visited Mother Aikenhead's foundation in Dublin, and was greatly impressed by the work that was being done. The Sisters of the Park Village Community spent about five hours each day in ministering to the needs of the poor, and especially those that were sick, but they had no hospital training.

The Sisters of Mercy.

Inaugurated by Miss Sellon at Devonport, the Sisters of Mercy were very similar in their aims and activities to Dr Pusey's community. They worked during a cholera epidemic in Plymouth, acquiring knowledge and practical skill for which some of them found a wider outlet a few years later among Miss Nightingale's unit in Scutari. This sisterhood later amalgamated with the Park Village Community, forming what is known as the Ascot Priory.

St John's House Sisterhood.

This was definitely under clerical control and was the first purely nursing Order in the Church of England. It was started at 36, Fitzroy Square in 1848, three hundred years after the establishment of the Protestant Church, a tardiness that must surely be a cause of consternation and wonder to all students of the history of the Churches' work in the care of the sick. Instruction and practical training was given to the women who joined this Order in one of the following hospitals—the Middlesex, Westminster, or King's College. They paid £15 for two years' training, but were bound to work for St John's House for five years, receiving board, lodging and a small salary. The inhabitants of other houses in Fitzroy Square were aghast at having a community of nurses in their midst, and also there was a general terror of contagion. Mainly owing to their antagonism, the St John's House Sisterhood moved to 5, Queen Square, Westminster, in 1853, from thence to Norfolk Street, Strand, and at the very end of the century to Queen Square, Bloomsbury, which is still their headquarters.

This Order helped tremendously in the reform of nursing that came after the Crimean War by taking over the whole of the work at King's College Hospital from 1856 onward, until nurses

262

of the new order, as established by Miss Nightingale, could assume the responsibility. They did not sever their connection with 'King's' until 1885. They rendered the same service to Charing Cross Hospital from 1866 to 1889, and to other London hospitals for shorter periods.

Six St John's Sisters accompanied Miss Nightingale in 1854 to Scutari, and twenty more followed during the next year. Training in midwifery, for which they went to King's College Hospital, was introduced into the St John's House curriculum in 1861, and for many years towards the end of the nineteenth century the sisters worked under the direction of the All Saints' Sisterhood. The Sisters of St John the Divine, who still work in Deptford and Poplar, are a branch of St John's House, being founded by Miss Caroline Lloyd in 1883. She had been Sister Superior at St John's House from 1870 until she left to found the daughter Sisterhood.

The organisation in Queen Square is no longer under clerical control. It was taken over by St Thomas's Hospital in 1919, and is now known as St John's and St Thomas's House. It is an institution for fully trained private nurses working on a co-operative basis.

The All Saints' Sisterhood.

This was founded by Miss Brownlow Bryon in 1851 and in many respects it worked on very similar lines to St John's House. It established a home for incurable women in Fitzroy Square, and from 1857 to 1899 the sisters undertook a great deal of the nursing at University College Hospital. In 1883 the two sisterhoods—that of St John's and All Saints'—were amalgamated. The greatest work, historically speaking, of these two sisterhoods was the part they played in carrying on with the nursing in London hospitals during the gap between the ousting of the old uneducated and unreliable 'Sairey Gamp' type of nurse and the establishment of the new order of trained nurses drawn from the better educated classes, and holding ideals of conduct and ser-

263

vice consistent with the real spirit of their work for humanity. Neither Mrs Fry's nor the Anglican Sisterhoods took any part in drawing up the great schemes for the reform of hospital nursing, but the help that they gave for many years with the actual work in the hospitals enabled the reorganisation to be accomplished in a much shorter time than could otherwise have been possible.

General Progress.

About the time that these Sisterhoods were initiated many scientific medical advances, for example, the control of smallpox by vaccination, the invention of the microscope, the campaign against puerperal sepsis and the introduction of anæsthesia, were all tending to mitigate human suffering, and were opening up almost illimitable fields of future progress in the fight against disease. It is doubtful whether nursing could ever have developed as a profession for refined and tenderhearted women but for the introduction of anæsthesia, for few women have such nerves of iron that they could have endured the shambles that was then an operating theatre, with its great wooden table and strong straps for securing the hapless patient. Neither could surgery have developed, for surgeons were as unable to inflict unlimited pain as patients were to endure it. Other momentous discoveries hovering on the horizon of that age were those of Louis Pasteur and Joseph Lister, with the consequent development of aseptic surgery and of a new curative science—bacteriology—having, as its practical offshoot, all the possibilities of sero-vaccine therapy. And then, just at the psychological moment, came the Crimean War, which made possible, and threw a floodlight of publicity, upon the work of a woman—Florence Nightingale—with a vision that brought to a sick world a great dream of healing, and the genius and the power to accomplish that dream.

264

Part III : A Profession

CHAPTER I

FLORENCE NIGHTINGALE

Parentage and early life—Continental travel—Desire to become a nurse —Visits to London and to Rome—Interest in Kaiserswerth—Visit to the Near East, and then to Kaiserwerth—Efforts to obtain training again frustrated—In Upper Harley Street—The Crimean War—Want of hospital organisation—'The Times' Fund, and the appeal for nurses— Mr Sidney Herbert's Letter—Miss Nightingale's acceptance, and departure for Scutari—The hospitals on the Bosphorus—Appalling conditions at Scutari—Reorganisation—Visit to the Crimea—Fall of Sebastopol, and after—Return to England

PROBABLY no other figure of the nineteenth century has been surrounded by so much glamour and public adoration, both during her active career and since her retirement and subsequent death at the great age of ninety years, as has Florence Nightingale. As her biographer, Sir Edward Cook, says, 'she became a legend in her lifetime'. But legends arc apt to be augmented by the imaginations of the people to whom they belong, and they grow so persistently rooted amid the verbiage of popular and sentimental ideas that it becomes increasingly difficult to tell the story afresh in its truc perspective.

Immortalised by Longfellow's 'Santa Filomena' and Miss Yonge's *Golden Deeds*—to say nothing of the less enduring hosts of soldiers' ballads, prize poems at the universities and sentimental verses set to music for the Victorian drawing-room and concert platform—the prevalent idea of Miss Nightingale was of a lovely girl of noble birth who forsook the pleasures of high society for the horrors of war on the bleak and inhospitable shores of the Sea of Marmora, and who went about the wards of

267

the Barrack Hospital at Scutari at night with a lamp in her hand, ministering to the sick and wounded, and shedding an angelic peace upon all the suffering and dying victims of the Crimean War.

Such a figure is apt to become a little intangible, and there was nothing intangible about the clear-headed organiser who was the Lady-in-Chief at the Eastern front, facing gigantic practical problems of sanitation in the filthy, vermin-ridden hospitals, with dysentery, cholera, enteric and typhus fever accounting for a greater mortality than all the shells and bullets that came from the guns of the enemy. Those two years, however, filled as they were with such stupendous and self-sacrificing labour in the cause of human suffering, held but a small part of the work she was to accomplish, not only for her contemporaries but also for posterity. Even she, with all her clear-sighted vision of possible future developments, could hardly have visualised the far-reaching results of the movements she started for the reconstructing of hospitals, the founding of the modern profession of nursing and the reforming of the sanitary administration of the British Army and of India.

A life such as hers cannot be justly dealt with in one brief chapter of a book. Only the merest outline can be given, with the hope that the interest of the reader will be stimulated to pursue the subject further in other literature.

Parentage and Early Life.

Although born into a wealthy and cultured family there was nothing remarkable in Miss Nightingale's parentage. Her father was William Edward Shore, but he changed his surname to Nightingale in 1815 on succeeding to the property of his maternal great uncle, Peter Nightingale. Her mother was the last of the eleven children of William Smith of Parndon Hall, Essex. Their first child was a daughter born at Naples in 1819, and named Parthenope after an old Greek settlement on the site of her birthplace. Florence was also born in Italy, on 12th May, 1820, and she, too, was named after the city of her birth.

The following year her parents returned to England, and eventually settled at Lea Hurst, in Derbyshire. But as this was rather bleak in the winter months, Mr. Nightingale purchased another property on the edge of the New Forest. This was Embley Park, in the parish of West Wellow, near Romsey, and it became the winter home of the Nightingale family.

Florence and her sister spent most of their childhood and early girlhood between Lea Hurst and Embley Park. They were educated at home under the supervision of their father, and Florence proved singularly apt in Latin, Greek, modern languages, music and abstract sciences. As she grew up she took her place in accompanying her mother on visits to poor and sick neighbours, and in arranging village entertainments and school treats; but she does not appear to have been more interested than the average daughter of kind-hearted country gentry, who accepted responsibility for the physical welfare of their dependents. Stories are told of the way in which she tended wounded birds and animals, nursed sick dolls and tried to mend their broken limbs or heads, but she was not extraordinary in that, for all normal girl-children do such things.

Continental Travel.

At seventeen she accompanied her parents and sister on a continental tour, chiefly through France and Italy, which lasted for eighteen months. Throughout this time she studied music, art, French, German and Italian, and joined in picnics, concerts, soirées and balls, meeting thereat some of the most famous, aristocratic and cultured people in Europe. During the second winter abroad she was introduced into the brilliant circle of one of the last of the Paris *salons*, where she met Mary Clarke, afterwards Madame Mohl, who became one of her most intimate friends, and remained so until she died in 1882, more than forty years later.

Desire to become a Nurse.

Although Florence Nightingale always accepted the wealth and social position into which she was born without questioning, she became dissatisfied with the desultoriness of the social life she was forced to live. She needed some definite aim in life, and, having found it, she was thrown into revolt against the environment of her own home. All her letters of this period show that she longed for a wider sphere of usefulness in the world, in which she could be of service to less fortunate humanity; and it was then that her thoughts turned definitely to nursing. But this was not work that might seriously be undertaken, at that time, by a young woman of good social standing. A hospital ward was considered to be no fit place for any modest woman of sound character and family.

It is recorded, by Mrs Julia Ward Howe, that when she and her husband were staying at Embley Park in 1844 Florence took Dr Howe aside and asked him, 'If I should determine to study nursing, and to devote my life to that profession, do you think it would be a dreadful thing?', and he replied, 'Not a dreadful thing at all, I think it would be a very good thing'. But Dr Howe was a very great philanthropist, and although Florence valued his opinion highly, that opinion was not likely to be shared by her own family. She evidently tried to enter a hospital soon after that. Among her friends were Dr Fowler, physician to the Salisbury Infirmary, and his wife; and in December, 1845, Florence wrote to her cousin, Hilary Bonham Carter, of a frustrated plan. She says:

'It was to go to Salisbury Hospital for these few months to learn the "prax", and then to make such wondrous intimacies at West Wellow under the shelter of a rhubarb powder and a dressed leg; let alone that no-one could ever say to me again, your health will not stand this or that. I saw a poor woman die before my eyes this summer because there was no-one but fools to sit up with her, who poisoned her as much as if they had given her arsenic. And then I had such a fine

270

plan for those dreaded latter years, if I should outlive my immediate ties, of taking a small house in West Wellow.—Well, I do not like talking about it, but I thought something like a Protestant Sisterhood without vows, for women of educated feelings, might be established. But there have been difficulties about my very first step, which terrified Mama. I do not mean the physically revolting parts of a hospital, but things about the surgeons and nurses which you may guess. Even Mrs Fowler threw cold water upon it; and nothing will be done this year at all events, and I do not believe, ever; and no advantage, that I see, comes of my living on, except that one becomes less and less of a young lady every year, which is only a negative one. . . . I shall never do anything, and am worse than dust and nothing.'

It is rather hard for the nurse of to-day to realise the difficulties that stood in the way of a woman who wished to devote herself to secular nursing work a century ago. The objections were deeply rooted in the conventions of the age, which did not countenance the exposure of gentlewomen to dangers and temptations in such unrefined and unpleasant surroundings as those of a hospital ward. One can understand that the idea of allowing their carefully nurtured daughter to work with the coarse, intemperate, and sometimes immoral nurse of the time was repugnant to Miss Nightingale's parents, and they tried very hard to find some outlet that should divert her energies into more acceptable channels.

Visits to London and to Rome.

Miss Nightingale paid a long visit to London in the spring of 1847, 'doing the exhibitions and hearing Jenny Lind'; and then in the autumn of that year she went with two great friends of hers, Mr and Mrs Bracebridge, to spend the winter in Rome. Her mental unrest was beginning to play upon her health, and her parents hoped that foreign travel would provide a new and satisfying interest. It proved, however, to be a big step towards the fulfilling of her vocation, although that was not apparent at the time; for among other English people wintering in Rome she met Mr and Mrs Sidney Herbert, who became her lifelong friends; and also Archdeacon Manning, who later became a Cardinal.

Interest in Kaiserswerth.

Florence had heard of the work of Pastor Fliedner at Kaiserswerth through a pamphlet given her by a German friend, and her interest in it was immediately aroused. It was a kind of 'school of nursing' which a Protestant mother might allow her daughter to enter. Her sister wrote in 1848, 'Flo is exceedingly full of the Hospital Institutions of Germany, which she thinks so much better than ours. Do you know anything of the great establishment at Kaiserswerth, where the schools, the reform places for the wicked, and a great hospital are all under the guidance of the Deaconesses?'

In the autumn of that year Mrs Nightingale and her elder daughter were arranging to go to Carlsbad for treatment, and Florence hoped that they should all meet Madame Mohl and her husband at Frankfurt, and that from there she should visit Kaiserswerth. But, owing to disturbances at Frankfurt, the whole plan was abandoned. In a letter to Madame Mohl Florence expressed her bitter disappointment. She wrote:

'I am not going to consign to paper for your benefit all the cursings and swearings that relieved my disappointed feelings, but oh! what a plan of plans I had made out for myself! All that I most wanted to do at Kaiserswerth, Brussels and Co. lay for the first time within reach of my mouth, and the ripe plum has dropped.'

During the next year she found a new interest in inspecting hospitals in London, and in working in the Ragged Schools; and very dearly she loved her 'little thieves at Westminster' as she called them.

Visit to the Near East, and then to Kaiserswerth.

In the autumn of 1849 she again accompanied Mr and Mrs Bracebridge on a foreign tour, this time to Athens and Egypt.

All that winter they travelled, and not until the end of the following June did they return to Europe. Then, after visiting Dresden and Berlin, they came to Kaiserswerth on 31st July. Florence stayed for a fortnight with Pastor Fliedner and his wife, after which she rejoined her friends at Dusseldorf, and the next day they crossed to England. She wrote a pamphlet entitled 'The Institution of Kaiserswerth on the Rhine'. In it she described the work of the Deaconesses and appealed to Englishwomen to start similar institutions. This was printed by the Ragged Schools Press, and was published anonymously.

It was not until July, 1851, that she achieved her ambition to return to Kaiserswerth, and this time she stayed for three months, working with the Deaconesses, and finding great joy and satisfaction in the experience.

Efforts to Obtain Training again Frustrated.

After this her life at home proved still more irksome to her. She realised, however, that she could never nurse as she wished to do unless she obtained some definite training, but how or where such instruction could be had was indeed a problem. It was at this time that she begged Cardinal Manning to use his influence to get her accepted for three months training at the Hospital of the Irish Sisters of Charity at St Stephen's Green, Dublin. He could not do this, but he did obtain permission for her to study under the Sisters of St Vincent de Paul in Paris. With that intention she went to stay with M. and Madame Mohl, and having obtained permission from the '*Assistance Publique*', she spent some time in visiting and inspecting hospitals and other institutions, and had the privilege of watching some of the most famous Paris surgeons at work. But just as she was about to enter the Sisters' hospital, the Maison de la Providence, she was recalled to England by the illness of her grandmother, whom she nursed until her death.

T

273

In Upper Harley Street.

The next event of nursing interest in her life was her appointment as Superintendent of a small hospital in London for sick ladies in reduced circumstances. Her friend, Mrs Herbert, was a member of the committee, and it was decided that the hospital should be moved to new premises in Upper Harley Street, that the Lady Superintendent should be resident, and that she should enter upon her duties as soon as the move was accomplished.

Whilst waiting for this, Miss Nightingale returned to Paris, and again endeavoured to gain experience by working with the Sisters of Charity. This time she did actually enter their hospital, but almost immediately developed measles and had to be nursed herself. However, she made a rapid convalescence and returned to London a month later.

On 21th August, 1853, she took up her duties at 1, Upper Harley Street, where, except for a short holiday at Lea Hurst and a few weeks spent in volunteer nursing at the Middlesex Hospital during a cholera epidemic, she remained until the following year when she embarked upon her great work in the Crimean War, for which all her previous life had been an unconscious preparation.

The Crimean War.

An outbreak of hostilities between Great Britain and Russia had been impending for some months, and at length, on 28th March, 1854, the formal declaration of war was read from the steps of the Royal Exchange. England and France were allied for the protection of Turkey.

The first great battle was fought at Alma on 20th September, and England's brilliant victory was acclaimed with a burst of exultation that inspired Archdeacon Trench's famous verses:

'Thou on England's banner blazoned with the famous fields of old,
Shalt, when other fields are winning, wave above the brave and bold,

274

And our sons unborn shall nerve them for some great deed to be done
By that twentieth of September, when the Alma's heights were won.
O ! thou river ! dear for ever to the gallant and the free,
Alma, roll thy waters proudly, proudly roll them to the sea.'

In the guarded words of the official bulletin, such a victory
'could not be achieved without a considerable sacrifice', and
although many homes were plunged into mourning, the country
did not, as a whole, grudge the sacrifice. But hot upon the mood
of national rejoicing came consternation and bitter resentment,
for news of another kind began to arrive. This was the first war
in which the 'Special Correspondent' attached to a newspaper
played a conspicuous part. Hitherto, news from a battle zone
had been carried by runners and horsemen; but with the introduction of postal services and telegraph wires, these gave place
to war correspondents, who furnished much fuller accounts of
victory or defeat, the numbers slain or wounded, and the attention given in dressing stations or hospitals, than could possibly
have been carried by hand. Mr William Howard Russell, the
'Special Correspondent' attached to *The Times*, sent a dispatch
dated 'Constantinople, 30th September', which was published
in *The Times* of 12th October, 1854. In it he said:

'No sufficient preparations have been made for the proper care of
the wounded. Not only are there not sufficient surgeons—that, it
might be urged, was unavoidable; not only were there no dressers or
nurses—that might be a defect of system for which no-one was to
blame; but what will be said when it is known that there is not even
linen to make bandages for the wounded. The greatest commiseration
prevails for the sufferings of the unhappy inmates of Scutari, and
every family is giving sheets and old garments to supply their wants.
But why could not this clearly foreseen want have been supplied? Has
not the expedition to the Crimea been the talk of the last four months?
And when the Turks gave up to our use the vast barracks to form a
hospital and depot, was it not on the ground that the loss of the
English troops was sure to be considerable when engaged in so
dangerous an enterprise? And yet, after the troops have been six

275

months in the country, there is no preparation for the commonest surgical operations. Not only are the men kept, in some cases, for a week without the hand of a medical man coming near their wounds; not only are they left to expire in agony . . . though catching desperately at the surgeon whenever he makes his round of the fetid ship; but now, when they are placed in the spacious building, where we were led to believe that everything was ready that could ease their pain or facilitate their recovery, it is found that the commonest appliances of a workhouse sick-ward are wanting, and that the men must die through the Medical Staff of the British Army having forgotten that old rags are necessary for the dressing of wounds.'

On the following day another letter was published in which Mr Russell wrote:

'The worn-out pensioners who were brought as an ambulance corps are totally useless, and not only are surgeons not to be had, but there are no dressers or nurses to carry out the surgeons' directions, and to attend on the sick during the intervals between the visits. Here the French are greatly our superiors. Their medical arrangements are extremely good, their surgeons more numerous, and they have also the help of the Sisters of Charity, who have accompanied the expedition in incredible numbers. These devoted women are excellent nurses.'

Want of Hospital Organisation.

The truth was that in the British forces there had been a general breakdown of surgical and hospital organisation. Food and clothing were stowed in holds of vessels beneath cargoes of ammunition, and were therefore inaccessible. Lint, bandages, and other requisites for hospital and ambulance work were rotting in storehouses on the shores of the Bosphorus because no orders had been issued through the correct channels for their delivery. No women nurses were attached to British military hospitals at that time. The question of including them had been considered before the army left England, but, on account of the general character of hospital nurses, the military authorities had

276

decided to employ only male orderlies working under the direction of the Medical Staff.

'The Times' Fund, and the Appeal for Nurses.

The Times accompanied the letter published on 13th October by a leading article appealing for help, and a Fund was started by Sir Robert Peel with a donation of £200 to provide comforts and necessities for the sick and wounded. Two days later, in a letter published in *The Times*, a correspondent asks:

'Why have *we* no Sisters of Charity? There are numbers of able-bodied and tender-hearted English women who would joyfully and with alacrity go out to devote themselves to the nursing of the sick and wounded, if they could be associated for that purpose, and be placed under proper protection.'

Quite a number of English ladies had evidently been thinking along similar lines, including Lady Maria Forrester, a daughter of Lord Roden, who offered to contribute a considerable sum of money towards sending out some nurses. To Lady Verney, the sister of Florence Nightingale, she said, 'I am so anxious that something should be done that I would have gone myself, only that I knew that I should not have been the slightest use.' Undoubtedly, the one woman who *could* successfully have taken out a party of nurses to work in a barrack hospital was Miss Nightingale, and the one statesman who could inaugurate such a scheme was the Secretary *at* War, Mr Sidney Herbert; and by a very fortuitous circumstance these two were close friends. Both their minds were busy with the same project, and Miss Nightingale wrote to Mrs Herbert offering to bear the expense of taking herself and one nurse out, whilst Lady Forrester had given money for three more. She asked if it would be of any use applying to the Duke of Newcastle for his authority (he was the Secretary *for* War).

277

Mr. Sidney Herbert's Letter.

Meanwhile Mr Herbert was writing a long letter to Miss Nightingale on the same subject, in which he carefully explained the position, and led up to the request that Miss Nightingale should undertake to superintend the whole scheme. He pointed out that hitherto none but male nurses had ever been employed in military hospitals, giving the reasons, and continued:

'But at Scutari, having now a fixed hospital, no military reason exists against their introduction, and I am confident that they might be introduced with great benefit, for hospital orderlies must be very rough hands, and most of them, on such an occasion as this, very inexperienced ones. I receive numbers of offers from ladies to go out, but they are ladies who have no conception of what a hospital is, nor of the nature of its duties.'

He then mentioned two offers which seemed to him to be worth considering, but adds:

'There is but one person in England that I know of who would be capable of organising and superintending such a scheme; and I have been several times on the point of asking you, hypothetically, if, supposing the attempt were made, you would undertake to direct it'. He continues, 'The selection of the rank and file of nurses will be very difficult, no one knows it better than yourself. The difficulty of finding women equal to a task, after all, full of horrors, and requiring, besides knowledge and goodwill, great energy and great courage, will be great. The task of ruling them, and introducing system among them, great; and not the least will be the difficulty of making the whole work smoothly with the medical and military authorities out there. This it is which makes it so important that the experiment should be carried out by one with a capacity for administration, and experience. A number of sentimental ladies turned loose into the hospital at Scutari would probably, after a few days, be "mises à la porte" by those whose business they would interrupt, and whose authority they would dispute'. . . .'If this succeeds, an enormous amount of good will be done now, and to persons deserving everything at our hands, and a prejudice will have been broken through and a precedent established which will multiply the good for all time. I hardly like to be sanguine as to your answer. If it were "yes" I am sure the Bracebridges would go out with you and give you all the comfort you would require, and which their society and sympathy alone could give you.'

Miss Nightingale's Acceptance, and Departure for Scutari.

Mr. Herbert saw Miss Nightingale on the following day, 16th October, the matter was arranged between them; and five days later Miss Nightingale, accompanied by Mr and Mrs Bracebridge and thirty-eight nurses left London. Her uncle, Mr Samuel Smith, went with the party as far as Marseilles, and many details of the journey, and of the departure from that port, on board the *Vectis*, on 27th October, are obtained from his letters. He was the husband of 'Aunt Mai', of whom more will be told later.

Whilst the expedition was being fitted out, its headquarters were established at Mr Herbert's house in Belgrave Square, where Mrs Bracebridge and Miss Mary Stanley, sister of Dean Stanley, interviewed applicants; but the material offered was anything but promising. Miss Stanley wrote:

'Here we sit all day. I wish the people who may hereafter complain of the women selected could have seen the set we had to choose from. All London was scoured for them. We sent emissaries in every direction to every likely place. We felt ashamed to have in the house such women as came. One alone expressed a wish to go from a good motive. Money was the only inducement.'

Eventually, by recruiting from the various Sisterhoods, the number was obtained as follows: ten Roman Catholic Sisters—five from Mother McAuley's Sisters at Bermondsey and five from Norwood—eight Anglican Sisters from Miss Sellon's Home at Devonport, six nurses from St John's House, and fourteen from various English Hospitals. Mr Herbert had pointed out to Miss Nightingale the very great necessity to avoid any kind of criti-

279

cism regarding religious partisanship, for this was an age of heated and rather bitter sectarian controversy. She was anxious, therefore, to include all schools of Christian thought, so that it might be found that, however her helpers differed with regard to theological opinion, they might still work together in a common cause for the brotherhood of man.

By 4th November, the party reached Constantinople, and on the afternoon of the same day they arrived at the hospital at Scutari.

The Hospitals on the Bosphorus.

Actually, there were four hospitals at that base. The first to be established was the General Hospital, to which reference was made in Mr. Russell's dispatch. It had been designed, originally, as the Turkish Military Hospital, and was handed over to the British in May, 1854, partially equipped. North of this was the Selimiyeh Barracks, a great building with square towers at each angle which had been made over for use as a British Hospital after the Battle of the Alma. This was known as the Barrack Hospital, and was Miss Nightingale's headquarters throughout her stay at Scutari.

South of the General Hospital were various buildings belonging to the Sultan's summer palace. These were pressed into service in January, 1855, as the Palace Hospital. This was not under Miss Nightingale's jurisdiction. It was principally for sick officers and was under the direction of Mrs Willoughby Moore, the widow of a very gallant officer who had died earlier in the war. She was assisted by four nurses sent out to her from England.

There were also hospitals at Koulali, about five miles farther north on the Asiatic shore of the Bosphorus, which were opened about a month after Miss Nightingale's arrival. At first they, too, were under her supervision, but when, in January, 1855, Miss Mary Stanley arrived with a party of forty-seven nurses, the Koulali hospitals were given over to her. The administration was not very successful and therefore they were broken up in November, 1855.

In addition to these hospitals there were five in the Crimean Peninsula itself, on the opposite side of the Black Sea, but Miss Nightingale did not visit these until late in the Spring of 1855.

Appalling Conditions at Scutari.

The conditions in the Barrack Hospital upon her arrival were even worse than Miss Nightingale had been led to expect from the reports that had reached England. The absence of proper sanitation, the general filth and the prevalence of vermin were evils that needed drastic reforms before ever the nursing work could be organised; and with her characteristic thoroughness and practical ability she tackled these difficulties.

To give Miss Nightingale's own words, in her report to the Royal Commission of 1857:

'It is impossible to describe the state of the atmosphere of the Barrack Hospital at night. I have been well acquainted with the dwellings of the worst parts of most of the great cities of Europe, but have never been in any atmosphere which I could compare with it. . . . The sheets were of canvas, and so coarse that the wounded men begged to be left in their blankets. It was indeed impossible to put men in such a state of emaciation into those sheets. There was no bedroom furniture of any kind, and only empty beer or wine bottles for candlesticks.'

The Battle of Balaclava had been fought on 25th October— whilst Miss Nightingale was on her journey to the East—and the Battle of Inkerman took place on the day after her arrival. The ships that brought the wounded across the Black Sea from the Crimea were terribly ill-equipped, and the journey from Balaclava to Scutari took eight and a half days. Needless to say, a number of the men died during the voyage, and many of those who survived were in an extreme state of emaciation and weakness, from wounds, frostbite and dysentery. All arrived still in their uniforms which were stiff with blood and discharge, covered with filth and thoroughly verminous; even their beards were full of vermin. The hospital possessed but the scantiest of water supplies, and no vessels in which to wash the patients, no soap, towels or hospital clothing.

It indeed required a woman of experience, bold initiative and great practical ability to cope with such a situation. Miss Nightingale set the orderlies to scrub the filthy wards and corridors. Her nurses assisted in the making of clean chopped-straw pallets, and of shirts, pillows and slings, and by the 8th of November, four days after their arrival, the hospital had over 2,000 patients. Miss Nightingale, in a letter to her friend of Harley Street, Dr Bowman, the ophthalmic surgeon, says:

'On Thursday last (November 8th), we had 1,715 sick and wounded in the Hospital (among whom 120 cholera patients), and 650 severely wounded in the other building called the General Hospital, of which we also have charge, when a message came to me to prepare for 510 wounded on our side of the Hospital, who were arriving from Balaclava. . . . I always expected to end my days as a Hospital Matron, but I never expected to be a Barrack Mistress. We had but half an hour's notice before they began landing the wounded. Between 1 and 9 o'clock we had mattresses stuffed, sown up, laid down, alas! only upon matting on the floor. . . . We have had such a sea in the Bosphorus, and the Turks, the very men for whom we are fighting, carry in our wounded so cruelly, that they arrive in a state of agony. . . . Twenty-four cases died on the day of landing. . . . We have now four miles of beds, and not eighteen inches apart. . . . The wounded are now lying up to our very doors, and we are landing 540 more from the Andes. . . . In all our corridor I think we have not an average of three limbs per man. And there are two more ships "loading" at the Crimea with wounded. . . . I am getting a screen now for the amputations, for when one poor fellow, who is to be amputated to-morrow, sees his comrade to-day die under the knife, it makes impression and diminishes his chance. . . . We have erysipelas, fever and gangrene, and the Russian wounded are the worst. . . . If ever you see Mr Whitfield, the House Apothecary of St Thomas's, will you tell him that the nurse he sent me, Mrs Roberts, is worth her weight in gold, . . . Mrs

Drake is a treasure. . . . The other four are not fit to take care of themselves, but they may do better bye and bye if I can convince them of the absolute necessity for discipline.'

Another difficulty Miss Nightingale had to tackle almost immediately upon her arrival was the provision of suitable laundry facilities. There was a contract for the washing of the hospital bedding, and of the linen of the patients. Miss Nightingale found that the bedding was washed in cold water, that many of the articles sent back as clean had to be destroyed owing to their verminous condition, and that the number of shirts washed during the past month was six.

Reorganisation.

As has already been stated, *The Times* was organising a Fund to supply the soldiers with necessities and comforts. Mr Macdonald was sent out to administer that fund in co-operation with Miss Nightingale, and she found his assistance invaluable. Her first request to him was for 200 hard scrubbing brushes, and sacking for washing the floors. Next, he assisted her to provide a laundry. She took a Turkish house, had boilers fixed, and employed soldiers' wives to do the washing. Then she arranged extra Diet Kitchens in different parts of the hospital. Hitherto, all the cooking had been done in thirteen large coppers situated at one end of the vast building, and as there were four miles of beds, it was found that it took three to four hours to serve the patients' ordinary dinner; and there were no facilities for preparing food between the stated mealtimes. Miss Nightingale had three supplementary boilers fixed on one of the staircases for the preparation of arrowroot and other articles of light diet. Early in 1855 a most invaluable volunteer arrived in the person of M. Alexis Soyer, a famous chef of the Reform Club. To him was handed over the culinary department, and he rearranged and extended Miss Nightingale's kitchens.

Mr Macdonald and Miss Nightingale established a store, independent of Government supplies, for clothing as well as food, and, to give but one figure, 50,000 shirts were issued to the patients from this store. It was not because the Government had failed to send the necessary clothing that these supplies were required, for on one occasion Miss Nightingale knew that 27,000 shirts had already been landed and were in the Purveyor's store, but he could not unpack them without a 'Board'—and three weeks elapsed before the Board of Survey released those shirts'. War Office regulations assumed that every soldier brought an adequate kit into hospital with him. However, three out of the four generals had so confidently expected Sebastopol to fall after a few days siege that they decided not to disembark the men's knapsacks, but to march light. In Miss Nightingale's report of 8th January, 1855, she gives the reasons for the want of hospital equipment as follows:

'The extraordinary circumstance of a whole army having been ordered to abandon its kits, as was done when we landed our men before Alma, has been overlooked entirely in all our system. The fact is that I am now clothing the British Army. The sick were re-embarked at Balaclava for these hospitals without resuming their kits, also half-naked besides. And when discharged from here they carry off, small blame to them, even my knives and forks—shirts, of course, and hospital clothing also. The men who were sent to Abydos as convalescents were sent *in their hospital dresses*, or they must have gone naked. The consequence is that not one single hospital dress is left in store, and I have substituted Turkish dressing gowns from Stamboul. (Three bales in the passage are marked Hospital Gowns, but these have not yet been "sat upon"). To purvey this hospital is like pouring water into a sieve, and will be till regimental stores have been sent out from England enough to clothe the naked and refill the kit.'

To a woman with less resource, initiative and decision, or of less administrative energy, the task of bringing order out of such chaos would have been fraught with insuperable difficulties; but by the Spring of 1855 everything was working comparatively smoothly in the hospitals at Scutari. The mortality had fallen from 42 per cent to 22 per *thousand*.

284

Visit to the Crimea.

Sebastopol was still not relieved, and as the siege was likely soon to be accompanied by assaults it was decided to develop the hospitals at Balaclava so that the wounded might be spared the sufferings of the sea voyage to Scutari. Instructions from the War Office, dated 27th April, 1855, invested Miss Nightingale with full authority to inspect the regimental hospital and the five general hospitals established there; and on 2nd May, leaving Mrs Bracebridge in charge, she set forth from Scutari accompanied by Mr Bracebridge, M. Soyer and another cook, four nurses including Mrs Roberts and Mrs Drake, and a boy, Thomas. In the comparative rest of the voyage she wrote several letters, in one of which she said:

'What the horrors of war are no one can imagine. They are not wounds and blood and fever, spotted and low, and dysentery, chronic and acute, and cold and heat and famine. They are intoxication, drunken brutality, demoralisation and disorder on the part of the inferior; jealousies, meanness, indifference and selfish brutality on the part of the superior.'

And then she proceeds to propound schemes for the recreation and better employment of the convalescent which, later, materialised as reading-rooms and class-rooms, with books, writing materials and games.

The sea voyage was accomplished in three and a half days, and with characteristic energy Miss Nightingale set to work investigating the hospital accommodation, planning new huts, and, in conjunction with M. Soyer, the erection of kitchens for extra diets; but after a very few days she went down with a serious attack of Crimean fever. For a time her life was despaired of, and the anxiety felt, not only at the Crimea but also in England, proved how sincerely she had gained the love and admiration of the English people. Throughout her illness she was most capably and devotedly nursed by Mrs Roberts. The months of

285

both physical and mental overstrain that she had endured at Scutari doubtless rendered the subsequent exhaustion much more severe than it might otherwise have been. She was strongly urged to return to England for at least two months' rest, but she refused to do so, and after a short convalescence at Therapia, she resumed her work at Scutari in August. Mrs Drake, whom she left at Balaclava, contracted low fever, and died on 9th August; and although this was not the first death among her nurses, Miss Nightingale felt the loss most keenly. In that month the Bracebridges returned to England, but their place was taken by Mrs Samuel Smith—Miss Nightingale's 'Aunt Mai'.

Fall of Sebastopol, and After.

Sebastopol fell on 8th September, after assaults which resulted in tremendous casualty lists, and from then until she finally returned to England Miss Nightingale divided her time between Scutari and Balaclava. During those months she was wrestling not only with disease and death, but also with jealousies, intrigues and other difficulties. At Balaclava she met with more annoyance and obstruction than she did at Scutari. Her official designation was 'Superintendent of the female nurses *in Turkey*', and this gave an opening to her opponents on the other side of the Black Sea to show that they regarded her as an interloper. However, when the attention of the War Office was called to this technical 'irregularity' Miss Nightingale was immediately given the official status necessary for carrying out her work on that front also.

Peace was signed in Paris on 30th March, 1856, but there was still much to be done in the Crimean hospitals, and Miss Nightingale did not leave until July.

Return to England.

The Government offered a British man-of-war to bring the national heroine home, but she declined this. All England was now alert to discover her plans and the hour of her arrival in this country, but, apart from her habitual shrinking from public plaudits, she was so weary from the long strain on both mind and body that she dreaded the reception that the people were prepared to give her. Instead, she travelled with her aunt, stayed at a quiet hotel in Paris for one night, and then travelled as 'Miss Smith', her aunt's daughter; and thus she arrived quite unobserved at Dover, and proceeded by train to London, where she spent the night. The next day she visited the Sisters at Bermondsey, in accordance with a promise she had made earlier in the war; and after having rested for a few hours in the peace of their convent, she completed her journey to Lea Hurst, still unrecognised, and just walked up from the station to her home, after nearly two years of absence.

287

CHAPTER II

THE NIGHTINGALE FUND, AND THE ESTABLISH-
MENT OF NURSING SCHOOLS

*Raising of the Fund—Suggested uses in establishing 'schools of nursing'
—Administration of the Fund—A nursing textbook—Difficulty in ob-
taining probationers—Miss Nightingale's letters to her nurses—The
Nightingale Scheme in other hospitals*

DURING the summer of 1855 public opinion ran high in appreciation of the work Miss Nightingale was accomplishing in the
Crimea, and it was resolved that it should be given some tangible
expression. She was consulted as to the form this should take, it
being suggested that an establishment resembling 'Kaiserswerth'
might be founded in this country under her direction. A public
meeting was held on 29th November, 1855, at Willis's Rooms,
but they proved too small for the enthusiastic gathering which
assembled there. The Duke of Cambridge presided, and Mr
Sidney Herbert, Lord Stanley and Lord Lansdowne were
among the speakers. The meeting arrived at the decision that the
memorial should take the form of a 'Nightingale Fund', which
should enable Miss Nightingale to establish and control an institution for the training, sustenance and protection of nurses. A
copy of the resolution was sent to her, and in her reply, dated
'Scutari, 6th January, 1856' she says:

'Dear Mr Herbert, In answer to your letter (which followed me to
the Crimea and back to Scutari), proposing to me the undertaking of
a Training School for Nurses, I will first to say that it is impossible
for me to express what I have felt in regard to the sympathy and the
confidence shown to me by the originators and supporters of this

288

scheme. . . . I must add, however, that my present work is such as I would never desert for any other, so long as I see room to believe that what I may do here is unfinished. May I, then, beg you to express to the Committee that I accept their proposal, provided that I may do so on their understanding of this great uncertainty as to when it will be possible for me to carry it out.' (Report of the Nightingale Fund. Addenda, pp. 1-2.)

Contributions from all ranks flowed into this Fund, although in some high quarters the whole scheme was thought to be just a futile fad. In one of Lord Granville's letters he says:

'Lady Pam thinks the Nightingale Fund great humbug. "The nurses are very good now. Perhaps they do drink a little, but so do the ladies' monthly nurses, and nothing can be better than them; poor people, it must be tiresome sitting up all night".' (*Life of the Second Earl Granville*, Fitzmaurice, Vol. I, p. 136.)

But in spite of such criticism the Fund reached the sum of £44,000 by the time Miss Nightingale returned to England.

When first she arrived from the East she was on the edge of a nervous breakdown, and she needed a period of rest and seclusion; but within three months she was working again. She realised that this was the psychological moment to urge the necessity for carrying out reforms in the conditions of barracks and military hospitals, before public enthusiasm and interest had time to cool, and therefore this was the task that claimed her immediate attention. To give her own words, in answer to an address from the parishioners of West Wellow in December, 1856:

'We can do no more for those who have suffered and died in their country's service. . . . It remains for us to strive that those sufferings may not have been endured in vain—to endeavour so to learn from experience as to lessen such sufferings in future by forethought and wise management.'

And in her 'Private Notes' occurs the following, 'I stand at the altar of the murdered men, and while I live I fight their cause.'

Mainly owing to her endeavours a 'Royal Commission' on the

u · 289

'Health of the Army' was appointed in 1857, and for the next three years she was almost entirely engaged in writing reports for it. This Commission enquired into the glaring and terrible blunders in the organising work of the Army Medical Service, and it initiated reforms in the Sanitary organisation of the Army. Miss Nightingale was not, herself, appointed on the Commission, for it was contrary to the conventions of the age that a woman should take so public a part in War Office affairs. Nevertheless, she was the moving spirit of its activities, and not until after its Reports were published did she feel at liberty to organise reforms in Hospital Nursing.

The experiments at Scutari had conclusively demonstrated two things: that there was room, and great need, for women nurses in the British Military Hospitals, and that it was imperative that a new order of nurses should be created, organised on a secular basis. These nurses should not only be devoted to their calling, as were the Sisters of the Religious Orders, but be educated women specially instructed in all the branches of science that enter into the work of a nurse, as well as in the practical procedures carried out in the ward or sickroom.

Medical and surgical sciences were making great progress during this age. The anæsthetic properties of chloroform and ether had been demonstrated, and these substances were being used extensively both in surgery and in midwifery. Louis Pasteur was working in his laboratory in Paris, elaborating his theories of fermentation and putrefaction. Joseph Lister was already a qualified surgeon and was almost on the eve of his great discoveries which resulted in the introduction of antiseptics. Cohn, the founder of bacteriology, and Parkes and Chadwick, the founders of modern hygiene, were all young men engaged in the investigations that led to the development of the sciences with which their names are associated. Sanitary science was making rapid advances, and such social and industrial reformers as Lord Shaftesbury, William Tuke and Josephine Butler were arousing the general public to a realisation of its responsibilities towards its dependents, its fellow workers and its less fortunate neighbours.

At no other period in modern history was the stage so perfectly set for the introduction of the professional nurse of good character and mental ability, trained, not only in ward and sickroom management, but also in the theoretical part of her work, so that she could be an intelligent colleague of the physician or surgeon under whom she was working, with a clear understanding of the patients' symptoms, and of the aims and objects of the remedies and treatments used.

That such a reorganisation was desirable was, however, by no means a unanimous opinion among those whose influence counted in the development of such a profession. Many medical men held the view that nursing was a menial occupation for which education and training were quite unnecessary, and might even prove a menace. A rather heated correspondence on the subject was published in *The Times*, near the end of 1857. One correspondent says:

'A poor woman is left a widow with two or three children. What is she to do? She would starve on needlework, she is unfit for domestic duties, she knows nobody to give her charring and she has no money to buy a mangle. So she gets a recommendation from a clergyman and is engaged as a Hospital Nurse.'

It is difficult in any country to set about doing something that has not been done before. Especially was this so in Victorian England; and the cause which Miss Nightingale sponsored involved the breaking through of custom and of precedent.

One of the staunchest defenders of the old system, before Miss Nightingale 'began to interfere', was Mr South, a famous surgeon of St Thomas's Hospital. He wrote:

'That this proposed hospital nurse-training scheme has *not* met with the approbation and support of the medical profession is beyond doubt. The very small number of medical men whose names appear in the enormous list of subscribers to the Fund cannot have passed unnoticed. Only three physicians and one surgeon from one (London) hospital, and one physician from a second are found among its supporters.'

He was, himself, perfectly satisfied with the existing type of nurse at that time. He says,

'As regards the nurses or wardmaids, these are in much the same position as housemaids and require little teaching beyond that of poultice making.' (*Observations on Training Establishments for Hospitals*, 1857, p. 16.)

Administration of the Nightingale Fund.

Meanwhile the Nightingale Fund, which with the accumulated interest now amounted to £48,000, was invested in the name of trustees; and a Council was nominated by Miss Nightingale for the administration of the Trusts. The net income from the Fund amounted to £1,426, and she intended to found or conduct an Institution on her own lines, and to become the Superintendent of it herself.

But her health did not improve sufficiently for such active work to be possible, and she realised that she must work through existing hospitals and be content with directing the activities of other persons. Her choice for the experiment fell upon St Thomas's Hospital, for Mr Whitfield, the Resident Medical Officer, was in sympathy with her project, the hospital, then on its ancient site in the Borough, was large and well managed, and the Matron, Mrs Wardroper, was a woman after Miss Nightingale's own heart. Perhaps the very fact that St Thomas's was on the eve of leaving the site that had been its home for over six hundred years influenced Miss Nightingale in her choice, for she had the foresight to realise that, in the better and more modern hospital that would be built, a fitter accommodation could be given to her probationers than in any existing hospital of her day.

The Committee of the Nightingale Trust accordingly met the

Governors of the hospital and an agreement was drawn up for the foundation of the 'Nightingale School', by the terms of which the hospital was to provide facilities for the training of nurses, and the Nightingale Fund was to bear the cost, including the payment of the nurses' salaries. On 24th June, 1860, fifteen probationers were accepted for one year's training, their board, lodging, washing and uniform being provided by the Fund, and also a salary of £10 per annum. An upper floor of the new wing of the hospital was adapted for their accommodation. It provided a separate bedroom for each, a common sitting-room and two rooms for the Sister in charge of them. This constituted the first 'Nurses' Home' in an English hospital. The probationers were under the direct authority of the Matron, who acted under the instruction of Miss Nightingale. They wore a uniform consisting of a brown dress with a white cap and apron, and they served as assistant nurses in the wards, receiving instruction from the Sister and from members of the Medical Staff. Their progress was reported in a 'Monthly Sheet of Personal Character and Acquirements of each Nurse', which Miss Nightingale had drawn up and Mrs Wardroper was required to fill in.

A Nursing Textbook.

In December, 1859, Miss Nightingale had published a little book entitled *Notes on Nursing*, in which she preached a new gospel of hygiene, applicable both to the home and the hospital. Although its published price was 5s.—a much larger sum then than now—15,000 copies were sold during the first month. A cheaper edition at 2s. quickly followed. Two years later a popular, abridged, sevenpenny edition appeared, with an additional chapter called 'Minding Baby', intended for the instruction of the bigger sister. This had a very large circulation and was reprinted in America, and also translated into German, French and Italian.

Naturally, Miss Nightingale's *Notes on Nursing* became a textbook for the school at St Thomas's. It was described as 'an incomparable treatise on nursing'. In it she combats the idea that 'it requires nothing but a disappointment in love, or an incapacity for other things, to turn a woman into a good nurse'. She taught that nursing was an art, and like any other art it needed in its votaries the sense of a calling and then a diligent apprenticeship.

Difficulty in Obtaining Probationers.

In spite of the example Miss Nightingale had set and the excellent arrangements at the Nightingale School, recruits were very slow to take advantage of the opportunity for training. Convention was still not approving of nursing as a profession, parents were afraid of infection, the fastidious thought that attendance upon the sick was not compatible with the delicacy of a lady's feelings, and it was considered derogatory for a gentlewoman to become a wage-earner.

Miss Nightingale wrote a kind of prospectus at that time, setting forth clearly the aims of the School and the conditions for training. She wrote:

'We hear so much of idle hands and unsatisfied hearts, and nowhere more than in England. All England is ringing with the cry of "Woman's Work", and "Woman's Mission". Why are there so few to do the work? . . . We require that a woman be sober, honest, truthful, without which there is no foundation on which to build. We train her in habits of punctuality, quietness, trustworthiness, personal neatness. We teach her how to manage the concerns of a large ward or establishment. We train her in dressing wounds and other injuries, and in performing all these minor operations which nurses are called upon both day and night to undertake.

'We teach her how to manage helpless patients in regard to moving, changing, feeding, temperature, and the prevention of bedsores.

'She has to make and apply bandages, line splints and the like. She must know how to make beds with as little disturbance as possible to their inmates. She is instructed how to wait at operations, and as to the kind of aid the surgeon requires at her hands. She is taught cooking for the sick; the principles on which wards ought to be cleansed, aired and warmed; the management of convalescents, and how to observe sick and maimed patients so as to give an intelligent account to the physician or surgeon in regard to the progress of cases in the intervals between visits—a much more difficult thing than is generally supposed. We do not seek to make medical women, but simply nurses acquainted with the principles which they are required constantly to apply at the bedside.

'For the future superintendent is added a course of instruction in the administration of a hospital, including, of course, the linen arrangements and whatever else is necessary for a matron to be conversant with.

'There are those who think that all this is intuitive in women, that they are born so, or at least that it comes to them without training. To such we say, send us as many geniuses as you can, for we are sorely in need of them.' (*Life of Florence Nightingale*, by Sarah Tooley, 1905, pp. 257–8.)

With the opening of the new St Thomas's Hospital—on the banks of the Thames opposite the Houses of Parliament and Westminster Abbey—all the available Nightingale probationers were taken on the staff; six as sisters and fourteen as nurses. The claims of the larger hospital, with its eight pavilions, made increasing demands upon the time of the Matron, Mrs Wardroper, and left her less able to supervise the training and general 'home' life of the probationers. A new post was, therefore, created, with the title of 'Home Sister', in 1874. This was held for twenty-one years by Miss Crossland and nearly six hundred nurses completed their training under her care.

Miss Nightingale's Letters to her Nurses.

Beginning in 1872, Miss Nightingale sent an 'Annual Letter' to the nurses in training, and those who had been trained, at St Thomas's. The letter was read aloud, often by Sir Harry Verney, Miss Nightingale's brother-in-law and Chairman of the Nightingale Fund. It was then printed and a copy was given to each nurse. These letters are not only full of practical and helpful advice, but they strike a marvellous note of encouragement and inspiration, applicable just as much to the nurse of to-day as to those early probationers. To give a few quotations:

'A woman who takes a sentimental view of nursing (which she calls "ministering" as if she were an angel), is, of course, worse than useless. A woman possessed with the idea that she is making a sacrifice will never do; and a woman who thinks that any kind of nursing work is "beneath a nurse" will simply be in the way.'

'For us who nurse, our nursing is a thing, which, unless in it we are making progress every year, every month, every week, take my word for it, we are going *back*. The more experience we gain the more progress we can make. The progress you make in your year's training with us is as nothing to what you must make each year *after* your training is over. A woman who thinks in herself, "Now I am a full nurse, a skilled nurse, I have learnt all there is to be learnt," take my word for it, she does not know *what a nurse is*, and she will never know; she is gone back already. Conceit and nursing cannot exist in the same person.'

'I have been in position of authority myself, and have always tried to remember that to use such an advantage inconsiderately is— cowardly. To be sharp upon them is worse in me than for them to be sharp upon me. No one can trample upon others and govern them. . . . We ought to *be* what we seem, or those under us will find out very soon that we only seem what we ought to be.'

'After all, all that our training can do for us is to teach us how to train ourselves. . . . Do we look enough into the importance of giving ourselves thoroughly to study in the hours of study, of keeping careful "Notes of Lectures", and of type cases—and of cases interesting from *not* being type cases—so as to improve our powers of observation, all so essential if we are *in future to have charge?* Do we keep in view the importance of helping ourselves to understand these cases by reading, at the time, books where we can find them described, and by listening to the remarks of physicians and surgeons in going round with the students? So shall we do everything in our power to become proficient, not only in knowing the symptoms and what is to be done, but in knowing the "Reason Why" of such symptoms and *why* such and such a thing is done; and so on, till we can some day train others to know the "reason why". Many will say, "We have no time, the ward work gives us no time." But it is so easy to develop into a mere drudgery about the wards when we have goodwill to do it and are fonder of practical work than of giving ourselves the trouble of learning the "reason why".'

In one of her later letters—the one written in 1888—she seems apprehensive with regard to the growing importance placed upon examinations, fearing that practical work might thereby suffer. This was the year after the formation of the first important 'Nurses' Association' for the purpose of establishing a General Register of professional nurses, an aim with which she was never in sympathy. She says:

'The Ambulance Classes, the Registration, the Certification of Nurses and of Nursing (and of Midwifery), especially any which demand the minimum of practice, or may substitute for personal progress in active proficiency, mere literary or word progress, instead of making it the material for growth in correct knowledge and practice, all such things may tend this way. It is not the *certificate* which makes the nurse or the midwife. It may *un-make* her. The danger is lest she let the certificate be *instead* of herself, *instead* of her never-ceasing going up higher as a woman and a nurse.' (From *Florence Nightingale to her Nurses*, Preface by Rosalind Nash, Macmillan, 1914.)

The Nightingale Scheme in Other Hospitals.

To return to those first probationers of 1860. When they finished their year of training they were expected to continue as hospital nurses, either at St Thomas's or in some other hospital, taking charge of wards or groups of wards and directing and controlling the work of the untrained nurses. Of those who finished that first year's training, six were given appointments at St Thomas's Hospital, two in Poor Law Infirmaries, and the rest in other hospitals. Each year this 'drafting out' increased until after ten to fifteen years nearly every hospital in England had at least one Nightingale nurse, and many of them had become training schools for nurses, adopting much the same principles as those of St Thomas's Hospital. These were, briefly, that the probationer nurses lived at the hospital under definite discipline which maintained a moral and social tone vastly superior to that previously found in lay hospitals, they were directly under the authority of the Matron and not of a male head, and they received theoretical teaching, including instruction in the basic sciences, from the Medical Staff; and practical teaching in the wards under the Sisters. And thus was born the modern conception of nursing, not only as an art and a vocation, but also as a profession based upon moral and educational requirements.

298

CHAPTER III

EXTENSION OF TRAINING TO OTHER FIELDS OF NURSING

Introduction of organised District Nursing and the Reform of Poor Law Nursing—Work of William Rathbone and Agnes Jones—Death of Agnes Jones, Miss Nightingale's tribute—Reforms in London—Hospitalisation of Poor Law Infirmaries—Development of District Nursing—The Metropolitan and National Nursing Association—The Queen Victoria Jubilee Nursing Institute

Introduction of Organised District Nursing, and the Reform of Poor Law Nursing.

Two great names—those of William Rathbone and Agnes Jones—stand out in connection with the introduction of district nursing in the great cities of England, and with the reform of nursing in Poor Law Infirmaries.

William Rathbone, of Liverpool, was born in 1819. He was the son of a Unitarian cotton merchant who had worked very hard and effectually in the movement for the abolition of slavery.

Early in 1859 his wife became ill, and she died on 27th May. During her illness she was attended by a very able nurse named Mary Robinson. Mr Rathbone then began to realise what illness must mean in the homes of the poor, where comforts, appliances and skill were lacking; and after the death of his wife he resolved to try an experiment. He engaged Nurse Robinson for a further period of three months to nurse poor patients in their own homes in a certain district of Liverpool, providing such nourishment, medical comforts and appliances as were required to render the nursing as effective as possible in a poor and often unhygienic home.

299

At the end of the first month she went to him and begged to be released from her engagement, for, accustomed though she was to many forms of illness and death, she was not able to endure the sight of the misery she encountered in the homes of the poor. Mr Rathbone persuaded her to persevere for a little longer, pointing out that her work was an experiment which, if successful, might prove to be the beginning of organised effort to reduce the evils which were so distressing to her, and that the satisfaction of abating these would be sure, in time, to reconcile her to the work. This prediction was entirely fulfilled by the end of the three months, for she found that many of the people were most responsive to the teaching she gave them in the tending of their sick; and the restoration of the breadwinner, or the mother, to health often restored the whole family to independence and tolerable comfort. Moreover, it helped to prevent the drunkenness and recklessness that lead to the moral ruin that so often follows upon hopeless misery in the home.

Obviously, she was marvellously fitted for such work, and she then asked to be allowed to devote herself entirely to nursing the poor instead of nursing in wealthy families as she had done hitherto. Mr Rathbone felt that it was his duty to extend the work that had had such a very successful beginning. There was no doubt that the necessary funds would be forthcoming, but the great difficulty was that skilled nurses could nowhere be found. He applied to the 'Nightingale School' at St Thomas's Hospital, and also to King's College Hospital where the St John's House Sisters were working; but neither could spare a single nurse, for all who had undergone training were needed for the work of introducing the new system into other hospitals. He consulted Miss Nightingale, and she suggested that Liverpool should train its own nurses. The principal Liverpool hospital, the Royal Infirmary, had, at that time, no facilities for training on the new lines. But Mr Rathbone undertook to build a suitable School with a Nurses' Home and present it to the Infirmary Committee if it, in turn, would undertake to carry out the training of nurses for a sufficiently long period to give it a fair trial. If the scheme failed, the building was to become the property of the infirmary, and to be turned to any suitable use.

In July, 1862, the completed building was handed over to the Committee of the Infirmary, and it was placed under the direction of Miss Merryweather, who had been trained in the Nightingale School. Its three main objects, as set forth in the prospectus were:

(1) To provide thoroughly educated professional nurses for the Infirmary.

(2) To provide district nurses for the poor.

(3) To provide sick nurses for private families.

By 1865 the whole of Liverpool had been divided into eighteen districts. Each district had been placed under the care of a nurse, and of a lady or group of ladies, who undertook to superintend the work of the nurse, pay for her lodging and provide nourishment and medical comforts for the patients who were too poor to obtain them for themselves.

Poor Law Nursing.

Very soon another problem presented itself for solution. It often happened that the district nurse was called upon to minister to patients who, for some reason or another, could not be nursed satisfactorily in their own homes, and yet were suffering from some prolonged or incurable malady which rendered them ineligible for admission into a general hospital. The only place for such patients was the Parish Infirmary at Brownlow Hill, and the respectable poor had such a horror of this institution that they were willing to endure almost any suffering rather than enter its portals. It housed twelve hundred sick and infirm persons, many of whom were very old or entirely helpless; and the only nursing was done by pauper women from the adult wards of the workhouse.

The conditions at Brownlow Hill were no worse than in most

301

other workhouse infirmaries in the kingdom, for none of them had trained nurses at that time; but most of the able-bodied women who were living in a workhouse were either mental or moral derelicts, and especially was that likely to be the case in a seaport town like Liverpool. The night conditions were, if anything, worse than those of the day, for where the inmates were too sick or infirm to create any disturbance, the wards were locked up at night, and were not visited until morning. Other wards were patrolled by policemen in order to maintain a certain amount of order and discipline.

The improvement of these conditions was the next task that claimed the benevolent interest of Mr Rathbone. He volunteered to bear the cost of introducing trained nurses for a period of three years, and he asked Miss Nightingale if she would choose twelve nurses trained at St Thomas's, and also a Lady Superintendent. To supplement these he proposed that the same number of probationers should be obtained from good class homes in Liverpool. The remaining nurses should be chosen from among the more able-bodied and respectable of the women in the workhouse; but these should be taken off the books as paupers, be paid a small salary and be given a more liberal diet than that issued to inmates.

The Committee had hesitated, at first, to agree to such a plan on account of the expense it would involve, and Mr Rathbone's offer did not meet with much approval, for if the scheme were to prove successful the ratepayers would, eventually, have to bear the cost. It was urged by the supporters of the plan that the cheapest way to treat the sick was to cure them. To quote one question asked by the Vestry Clerk of an honorary physician from St Thomas's, 'If you had to cure the sick at so much a head, and had to choose between unpaid pauper women allotted to you gratis, or paying yourself for skilled nurses, which would you choose?' Unhesitatingly, the answer came, 'To pay for skilled nurses, certainly.' (Quoted from *Workhouse Nursing, the Story of a Successful Experiment*, 1867.)

Eventually, it was agreed that the scheme should be given a trial, but in the male wards only; and for the superintendence of this important pioneer work Miss Nightingale's choice fell upon Miss Agnes Jones, an Irish girl, who was the daughter of Colonel Jones of Fahan, Londonderry, and the niece of Sir John Lawrence. In 1860 she had undergone a period of training at Kaiserswerth, and after that she had worked with Mrs Ranyard at a Bible Mission in the East End of London. In 1862 she entered St Thomas's Hospital as a Nightingale probationer for a year's training, and having completed this course she worked as a nurse in the Royal Northern Hospital, London, until she went to Liverpool on 16th May, 1865. In a letter to Madame Mohl, Miss Nightingale described her as 'ideal in her beauty, like a Louis XIV. shepherdess'.

When she took over the charge of Brownlow Hill Infirmary it was so crowded that some of the patients were sleeping two or three in a single bed. Hers was indeed almost as difficult a task as Miss Nightingale's had been at Scutari, for it was the age of 'Mr Bumble and Mrs Corney', and, although the officials were, doubtless, well-intentioned, their general attitude was not such as to make the work of a well-bred and sensitive Lady Superintendent a very easy one. Among the patients she was sent to nurse there were a number of malingerers—able-bodied men with sore arms or legs which they took care should not get well. The foul language, the drunkenness and vicious habits, and the mental and physical degradation at first appalled her. In her earliest letter from Liverpool, she herself described the wards as 'like Dante's Inferno'. She found that some of the men had worn the same shirts for seven weeks, and the bed clothes were sometimes not washed for months.

She tackled the problem of the overcrowding by persuading the new Governor, who was an extremely able man, to institute a labour test; and within a month two hundred men took their discharge, saying that if they had to work they might as well work outside. This brought the number of inmates somewhat nearer to the number of beds, and thus gave more scope for the skill of the nurses.

The project of training pauper women to help with the nursing was an utter failure. These women were quite untrustworthy in every way. Many of them spent their first salary in getting hopelessly drunk. Out of the fifty-six whom Miss Jones endeavoured to train, not one turned out even a tolerable nurse, and at the end of the first year this part of the experiment was abandoned. During the second year the scheme with regard to the nursing of the sick by trained women was extended to include the whole of the infirmary and it succeeded beyond all expectation. The Guardians then announced their intention of making the scheme permanent, and of charging the cost of it upon the rates.

Death of Agnes Jones.

Before the third year was ended Agnes Jones fell a victim to typhus fever. Her resistance had been lowered by overwork and all the anxiety attendant upon such pioneer work as she was carrying out in Liverpool, and she died on 19th February, 1868.

Whilst she was working at the Bible Mission in London before going to Liverpool she had discussed with Mrs Ranyard the possibility of forming a band of nurses to work amongst the poor. In 1868, partly with the idea of a memorial to her, Mrs Ranyard organised a nursing branch of the Mission, but these women were not trained except in the way that the members of the lay Sisterhoods were trained—by spending a few months in a hospital in order to gain what useful knowledge they could. The Ranyard Nurses still exist and do extremely useful work, but they are now all fully trained nurses with the same professional standards as the 'Queen's Nurses'.

Miss Nightingale's Tribute.

Miss Nightingale wrote a very beautiful tribute to the memory of Agnes Jones, entitled 'Una and the Lion'. This was published in *Good Words* for June, 1868, and in it she says:

'One woman has died, a woman attractive and rich, young and witty. . . . She died as she had lived, at her post in one of the largest workhouse infirmaries in the kingdom—the first in which trained nursing has been introduced. . . . Una and her paupers far more untamable than lions. In less than three years she had reduced one of the most disorderly hospital populations in the world to something like Christian discipline, and had converted a Vestry to the conviction of the economy, as well as the humanity, of nursing pauper sick by trained nurses.'

But ere she died the reforms had been consolidated, for the nurses trained under her were able to carry on the work she had so well started; and the name of Agnes Jones will for ever be associated with the great reform of Poor Law Nursing.

Reforms in London.

Liverpool had shewn the way, and London followed. The state of the Metropolitan workhouses, as reported upon by the Poor Law Board of 1866, showed that the sick wards were, for the most part, insanitary and overcrowded, that the beds were insufficiently and unevenly padded, and almost inevitably produced bedsores, and there was a deficiency of basins, towels, brushes, and combs. The eating and drinking vessels were unclean. The food of patients was cooked by paupers and was frequently served cold. There were insufficient medical officers, and the only nursing was done by pauper women, whose love of drink often drove them to rob the sick of stimulants and whose treatment of the sick was neither gentle nor intelligent. Very few of them could read or write, and sometimes a patient had no attention for several days because the pauper in charge of him was herself bedridden. Cases were reported in which the patient's bed had not been made for four or five days. A scheme was drawn up by Mr. H. B. Farnall, Poor Law Inspector from the Metropolitan area (in conjunction with Miss Nightingale and Dr Sutherland), insisting upon the separation of the sick, the insane, the incurable and the children, with the provision of suitable accommodation and treatment for each; but all were to be under a single Central administration.

The Bill that made this possible was Mr Gaythorne Hardy's Metropolitan Poor Act passed on 29th March, 1867, and when this came into operation the reforms started in real earnest. Under this Act it was proposed to build a new Infirmary at Highgate. The plans were submitted to Miss Nightingale by Mr (afterwards 'Sir') William Wyatt, the leader of the reform in the St Pancras area. The Infirmary was built and was opened in 1869; Miss Elizabeth Torrance being appointed Matron with nine trained nurses under her. Amongst other reforms which Miss Torrance introduced was the occupation of the inmates by useful work. Her own accounts of this are amusing. In 1871 she wrote, 'The achievement I am most proud of is getting the men's suits cut out and made. I found a tailor in No. 2 Ward who cut out some, and I sent them into No. 1 and 4 to be made; but there was a tailor in No. 1 who made difficulties. "You see, ma'am, it's such a very old-fashioned cut".'

Hospitalisation of Poor Law Infirmaries.

In June, 1871, the Local Government Board issued three Orders for the separate administration of Metropolitan Infirmaries—those of Wandsworth and Clapham, St George's in the East, and St Mary, Islington. Thus began a decisive movement in the 'hospitalisation' of Poor Law Infirmaries; but the progress was somewhat slow, and it was another eight years before the first provincial infirmary—Leeds—followed London's example.

In 1897—thirty years after the initiation of the reforms—the employment of pauper nurses was finally forbidden, and from that date the training of paid nurses in Poor Law Infirmaries continuously improved. The infirmaries were under the administration of a master and a matron, there being a visiting Medical Officer who undertook all the ordinary surgical procedures. For special cases a consultant from a voluntary hospital was called in.

At the beginning of this century all the larger infirmaries had a resident medical officer, a superintendent nurse, charge nurses and probationers; but an important change in their central control occurred in 1919, with the establishment of the Ministry of Health, which took over the duties of the Local Government Board.

The next epoch-making event was the passing of the Local Government Act in 1929, for under its provisions all the functions of the Boards of Guardians throughout the country, including the control of the Poor Law Infirmaries, passed to the County and County Borough Councils, who were empowered to convert the infirmaries into general public health hospitals. This Act came into operation on 1st April, 1930, and more than twenty former Poor Law Infirmaries, mainly in the large cities and towns of the midlands and the north, immediately became 'general hospitals'. The conditions upon which such a change could be made were that all aged and infirm inmates, apart from those who were definitely sick, were to be removed to other institutions, and the ordinary units of a general hospital for the nursing and treatment of acute medical and surgical cases were to be provided.

Nearly a hundred former Poor Law Infirmaries in London and the provinces have now become general hospitals under the control of the Ministry of Health. Unhampered by debts, financial difficulties and chronic shortage of beds, as are the large voluntary hospitals, they bid fair to become the leading hospitals of this country when they shall have succeeded in shaking themselves quite free of the clinging spirit of 'Bumbledom'. The great traditions of our voluntary hospitals may be an intangible asset, but it constitutes a very real power, based as they are upon a selfless spirit of service, and a considerate kindness and courtesy to all within their walls, whether patients, staff or visitors; and it is that that lends the charm and dignity which characterises so many of our voluntary hospitals. The municipal hospitals have yet to make their traditions, with the help of the mellowing influences that can come only with the years. Although many men and women working in, and for, them are striving to this end, they are still feeling the somewhat shattering effect of the double transition; and the danger of the municipal system, involving as it does, a central controlling authority, is that of becoming merely mechanical. It is difficult for each hospital to maintain the individuality which is due to the wholehearted interest and zeal of those who are working in it, and, to a certain extent, developing their own ideas; and the compilation of voluminous records may, unless the tendency is carefully watched, somewhat cramp the main function of the hospital, which is, of course, the care of the patient. However, there is no real danger of such a regrettable development whilst the spirit still lives which activated the reforms of the past century.

Development of District Nursing.

In a comparatively short time the system of Poor Law nursing inaugurated in Liverpool and London spread, as we have seen, over the whole country as a complete revolution in the nursing of the sick in workhouse infirmaries; but there still remained the almost destitute in their own homes.

The first organisation of trained nurses to deal with this problem, apart from the Liverpool nurses, was the East London Nursing Society, founded by the Hon. Mrs Stuart Wortley and Mr Robert Wigram in 1868. This conformed, in its main features, to the Liverpool scheme, and in a very short time it had extended its activities throughout the whole of the East End of London. Its object was, and is, to provide trained nursing for the sick poor in their own homes, without distinction of creed or nationality. It became affiliated with the Queen's Institute of District Nursing in January, 1891, but it is controlled by its own Committee and manages its own finance and general affairs. Its head office is now in Queen Victoria Street, E.C., its Northern Division Home is in Bow Road and its Southern Division Home is in Stainsby Road, Limehouse. During 1936 nearly twelve thousand patients were nursed by the staff of this Society, and an extension of the work which is now being carried on is the attendance of two nurses at the Medical Relief Stations established by the London County Council.

The Metropolitan and National Nursing Association.

In 1874, as a result of conferences between Mr William Rathbone—then a member of Parliament and resident in London for half the year—and Sir Edmund Lechmere and other philanthropists connected with the English Branch of the Order of St John of Jerusalem, the movement which created the Metropolitan and National Nursing Association was started. Its promoters invited the support of the Duke of Westminster, and began by appointing a sub-committee (of reference and enquiry) 'To enquire into the state and need of district nursing, the training schools already existing capable of training women for nursing the poor in their own homes, and the hospitals suitable for such institutions; the district nurses already at work, and the places where need of nurses is felt.'

The findings of this sub-committee proved to be the turning point in the history of district nursing. The need was shewn to be so great, and the facilities almost non-existent. There were, in fact, almost a hundred nurses working amongst the poor in London, but at least one-third of these were untrained, and the hospitals were unable to supply the number of trained nurses that were needed. The criticisms of the existing system were that there was too much indiscriminate charity and too little nursing. There was not sufficient control or direction, and inadequate instruction was given by the nurse to the patients' friends or relatives with regard to ventilation, cleanliness, disinfection, the toilet of the patient and all the other things that make for effective nursing; and there was far too little communication between the doctor and the nurse.

The recommendations made were that the nurses should receive more complete and systematic hospital training based upon the 'Nightingale Scheme'; that they should work under the supervision of inspectors or superintendents who should themselves be nurses of higher professional, social and general qualifications, that they should be in closer touch with the medical men and work as much as possible under their direction; and that the duty of granting relief should be separated, whenever possible, from the nurses' duties, being left to parish authorities, clergy, district visitors and charitable missions.

The objects of the Association, as stated in its own prospectus, were as follows:

(1) To train and provide a body of skilled nurses to nurse the sick poor in their own homes.

(2) To establish in the Metropolis, and to assist in establishing in the country, district organisations for this purpose.

(3) To establish a training school for district nursing in connection with one of the London hospitals.

(4) To raise, by all means in its power, the standard of nursing and the social position of nurses.

The Committee proposed to establish a Central Home and Training School for nurses in district work, and then to extend the work by opening other homes in suitable local centres. Each home was intended to lodge and board about six nurses working under a trained District Superintendent. This home was established in Bloomsbury Square, W.C.1., and was opened in December, 1875.

The first Superintendent of the Central Home was Miss Florence Lees, a Nightingale nurse; and much of the success of organised district nursing in London was due to her great practical skill and energy. She interviewed and selected the candidates, who had to be gentlewomen; for it was thought that district nurses would be placed in positions of greater responsibility in carrying out the doctors' orders than were nurses working in hospitals, and that women of education should be more capable of exercising such responsibility. Also, that the vocation would attract a large number of women of the better classes who were anxious to enter some employment that would give them independence, and that their higher social position would give them greater influence over their patients and tend to raise the status of the whole body of professional nurses in the consideration of the general public. All this has been fully justified by experience.

After selection the candidate remained in the Central Home for a month in order to learn something of the general nature of district nursing. She was then sent to a hospital for one year, and having satisfactorily completed this course she returned to the Central Home for a further six months in order to undergo specialised training.

Applications for the services of the nurses were received from doctors, clergy or other charitable workers. The patient was visited, if possible, by the Superintendent herself, and if, in her opinion, it was a suitable case for district nursing she assigned the patient to a nurse, to whom she gave directions as to management. The nurse visited daily and kept a record of each case, having communicated with the doctor and obtained his instructions in writing. The time spent with each patient depended entirely upon the nature of the individual case and the conditions under which he, or she, was being nursed. On the first visit the nurse might need to put the room into nursing order and to instruct some woman of the household in certain duties. What exactly was meant by 'putting the room into nursing order' is well explained by Miss Lees herself. She says:

'Upon entering a close, ill-ventilated room, too often in an indescribable state of filth and vermin, the nurse's first duty is to see that the bed of the patient is so arranged as to have the greatest amount of air, light and space possible, which, in most cases, necessitates a total rearrangement of the furniture in the room. That done, the nurse washes and arranges the patient, makes the bed, applies any dressings required, then dusts the room, ventilates it, empties and washes all utensils, dirty glasses, etc., and when necessary, disinfects utensils and drains, sweeps up the fireplace, fetches fresh water and fills the kettle. With helpless patients, she takes the necessary precautions against the formation of bedsores; and in serious cases, or when desired to do so by the doctor, takes a strict note of the variations in the disease which a nurse ought to know and observe. In fact, as far as possible, the patient's room is made to resemble a small ward in a well-arranged hospital.'

The Association maintained its high standard of nursing, but in a very few years it was seriously hampered by want of funds; and by extending its activities in the formation of new branch homes it had incurred considerable debts. It was then found advisable to reorganise the Association, making the branch homes independent of the Central Home, and requiring them to find their own means. This not only reduced the expenditure of the Central Home but it quickened local interest and liberality. Henceforth only when a new centre was formed did the Association provide funds.

The work of district nursing was now very successfully launched in London, and it quickly spread throughout the provinces and eventually into Scotland and Ireland.

In 1880 Miss Lees married the Rev. Dacre Craven. She then became an honorary inspector, and nine years later she published the first textbook dealing with this form of nursing, entitled *A Guide to District Nurses and Home Nursing* (1889); written at the request of the Trustees of the Queen Victoria Jubilee Fund. The details of this scheme have been given fairly fully because the principles involved are still accepted as the foundation of district work and of all the branches of Public Health nursing which have subsequently developed. As the scope of the work has extended, the teaching has broadened in order to keep pace with it; but ever since the commencement of such organised work it has been realised that hospital training forms but the basis of the tuition and experience required, and that specialised instruction and practical training must follow after the attainment of the hospital qualification. Moreover, the nurse engaged in any form of Public Health work must be a 'Missionary' of hygiene, and be forever teaching the laws of health to the patient and his household.

The Queen Victoria Jubilee Nursing Institute.

In 1887 an immense impetus was given to this work amongst the poor in their own homes. Queen Victoria herself became most interested in the organisation and she directed that the bulk of the 'Women's Jubilee Offering', which amounted to some £70,000, should be devoted to the extension and development of district nursing schemes, appointing the Duke of Westminster, Sir James Paget and Sir Rutherford Alcock as trustees, in consultation with Mr William Rathbone. The interest on this fund amounted to some £2,000, and this was applied to the founding of an Institute for the training and maintenance of district nurses.

In the following year the Queen Victoria Jubilee Institute for Nurses came into being with branch centres throughout the kingdom; and to it was affiliated the Metropolitan and National Association. By its Charter granted in 1889 it was connected with St Katherine's Royal Hospital, Regent's Park, which had been founded and endowed by Queen Matilda, the Consort of Stephen, in the twelfth century. It was handed down, with all its estates, by Queen Philippa, and the Queens of England became its patrons throughout all the intervening centuries. But this association of the Jubilee Institute with St Katherine's was terminated by a Supplemental Charter granted by King Edward VII in 1904, which gave permission for part of the income of the Institute to be applied to the training of midwives. Subsequently, its headquarters were removed to Victoria Street, S.W.1., but its Central Office is now in Lower Belgrave Street.

The first Queen's Nurse to be enrolled and the first General Superintendent of the Queen's Institute was Miss Rosalind Paget, who received the honour of Dame of the Order of the

British Empire in 1935. Dame Rosalind is now an invaluable member of the Council.

The regulations for the training of Queen's Nurses are on the same general lines as when the Institute was founded, although the qualifications have advanced with the scientific developments of the time. The candidate is required to have undergone at least three years training in a general hospital approved by the General Nursing Council and to have obtained her State Registration Certificate. Then, after a trial period of a month, she continues her special training for a further five months. In addition to the practical training, special courses of lectures are given on Maternity and Child Welfare, Social Economics, Tuberculosis, and on other subjects relative to district nursing. The object of this training is to teach the nurse to adapt her knowledge and skill to the conditions of her work in the homes of the people. If she accepts this training she is bound by an agreement to work for a further twelve months at least, wherever the Institute might require her services.

Under a revised Charter granted in 1928 the name of the Institute was changed to the 'Queen's Institute of District Nursing'. This was considered to be more suitable as the reigning, or existing, Queen will always be the Patroness of the Institute. It is now governed by a Council nominated by Her Majesty, Queen Mary, and a certain number of its members are appointed directly by her, including, at the present time, four of the Royal Princesses.

The scope of the Institute is national, it has a Scottish and an Irish branch, and over 7,000 nurses are working in connection with it. In scattered rural districts the Queen's Nurse often acts also as a Health Visitor and a School Nurse.

In many country districts there is neither work nor funds to justify the engagement of a Queen's Nurse, and yet there is a great need for someone to care for the ordinary ailments and chronic cases and, above all, for midwives and maternity nurses. A special class of nurses, who have not had full hospital training but have had training in district nursing and midwifery, is provided for these areas. They are called Village Nurse-Midwives. In addition to securing a high standard of training and work, the Queen's Institute acts as an advisory and executive centre for the Nursing Associations in the general organisation of their work, in negotiations with the Government Departments, and in connection with national schemes such as the agreements with the Approved Societies of payment for the nursing of their members.

315

CHAPTER IV

NINETEENTH-CENTURY REFORMS IN THE CARE OF THE INSANE

Historical note—St Dymphna, a patron saint of the mentally afflicted— The present work at Gheel—The insane in Britain—The work of Dr Philippe Pinel in Paris—William Tuke and the Retreat at York— Legislation—The padded room—Modern developments

Historical Note.

THE history of the treatment of lunacy seems to show that it was during the three centuries following the Reformation that there developed, in civilised countries, the system of appalling neglect and revolting cruelty towards the insane that called for the drastic reforms of the nineteenth century.

In the early middle ages the insane were received into general hospitals and were treated on very humane lines. Paul of Egina, writing in the seventh century, indicates the employment of general procedures which are quite closely followed in the mental hospitals of to-day. He says, 'Those who are subject to melancholy from a primary affection of the brain are to be treated with frequent baths and a wholesome and humid diet, together with suitable exhilaration of mind, and without any other remedy unless, from its long continuance, the offending humour is difficult to evacuate, in which case we must have recourse to more powerful and complicated lines of treatment. . . . The diet for melancholics shall be wholesome and moderately moistening, abstaining from beef, roe's flesh, dried lentils, cabbages, snails, thick or dark-coloured wines, and whatever things engender black bile.' Maniacs were to be treated on the same lines, with

316

the addition of mild restraining measures. 'But above all things they must be secured in bed, so that they may not be able to injure themselves or those who approach them; or be swung within a wicker basket in a small couch suspended from on high.'

St Dymphna, a Patron Saint of the Mentally Afflicted.

Contemporary with Paul of Egina lived St Dymphna, the beautiful daughter of an Irish prince, who as a result of persecution by her father, fled with her chaplain, Gerebern, to Gheel in Brabant. Thence they were followed and put to death by the father. A shrine to St Dymphna was erected on the site of their martyrdom, and here manaics are said to have recovered their sanity. The intercessions of St Dymphna were believed to be very valuable in helping children of a low grade mentality who were brought to the shrine, often from long distances. When the prayers of the relatives were not immediately answered the children were sometimes left near the shrine in the care of the villagers, so that they might continue to have the benefit of the saint's intercessions. As a consequence of this custom many of the houses in the village contained one or more of these defectives, who were cared for as members of the family. The feeling that they were under the strict patronage of the saint made them the objects of special care and solicitude. They were given simple tasks to perform, were shielded from the cares and irritations of everyday life as much as possible, and were kept out of the current of the busy life that existed in towns.

Other villages followed this example, as did many monastic houses in Belgium, and thus arose the first known 'mental defectives' colonies'. As the children grew up they were able to carry out many useful tasks, which not only gave them a definite interest in life but helped to defray the cost of their support. Gheel has remained a sanctuary for those who are 'troubled in mind' ever since. About A.D. 1200 a church, which is still in existence and to which an asylum was attached, was erected at the shrine. Visitors to 'l'Eglise Ste Dymphne' are still shown the 'maison des malades', although it is no longer used for the accommodation of patients; and in the crypt of the church are a number of small cells with strong bars and heavy doors which were used for the more acute or violent patients.

The Present Work at Gheel.

This 'village community' is so remarkable that some account of its organisation and work appears to be justified. It is situated in a flat agricultural part of Brabant about 50 kilometres along a fairly good motor road from Antwerp, or 80 kilometres from Brussels; it can also be reached by train. It covers an area of about 27,000 acres and has a population of 18,000. Of these, 3,000 are mental patients. Some of the houses are two-roomed thatched cottages many centuries old, whilst others are quite modern-looking red-bricked villas. The community is not entirely Catholic. There are about 400 Jews and a good proportion of Protestants, and their religious needs are ministered unto by a Rabbi and a Lutheran Pastor. The patients are not exclusively Belgian, for many come from other European countries, including England, and from America.

The State undertook the reorganisation of the Colony in 1925. There is now a Central Hospital with 50 beds for men and 50 for women. Each bed is daintily curtained, thus ensuring a degree of privacy for the patients not often found in a mental hospital ward. The Administrative Block contains a Convent wherein live ten Sisters, and also an observation ward. The Colony is under the charge of a Medical Superintendent assisted by six doctors and eighteen visiting nurses. The latter include both sexes and all are qualified in mental nursing. Each householder is allowed to board two patients of the same sex, but he must be able to show that he has a source of income apart from the money received for patients. The Province pays about 10s. 6d. a week for each patient. Of this, the foster parent is paid about 8s. and the balance is used for the hospital and administrative expenses. Private patients pay anything from £100 to £250 per annum, from which 15 per cent is deducted towards the overhead expenses of the Colony. As far as possible patients are boarded out with people of their own social class, so that mental strain and bewilderment consequent upon trying to adjust themselves to an unusual routine is avoided.

All new patients are received into the Observation Ward of the hospital until the character of his, or her, malady is ascertained and a suitable environment is chosen for boarding out. Not all patients can be treated on this system, and those for whom it is deemed impracticable are sent to an asylum apart from the Colony. Each doctor has 600 patients under his care and each nurse has 180 houses to visit.

A doctor must call on each of his patients at least once a month; but in addition to this the patients may visit at the Central Hospital on any day and at any time—there is always one doctor in attendance. The nurse visits each patient once a fortnight, or more often if it is deemed necessary, and keeps a written report of the patient's condition and progress.

The rules regarding general hygiene in the houses in which the patients are received are very strict. The patients are free to go about as they wish, but they must be in by 4 o'clock in the winter and 8 o'clock in the summer. The village has cafés but no public houses, indeed, alcohol is forbidden. There are no restrictions with regard to visitors even in the hospital itself. The men patients work in the fields or in the market gardens and they receive payment for the work they do. The women are employed in sewing and in laundry and domestic work, but there is no compulsion with regard to this.

Many patients improve greatly with the advantage of family rather than institutional life, and, for suitable cases, this certainly seems the ideal method of treatment. But, successful as it is at Gheel, one must remember that the villagers have had more than twelve hundred years' experience in making homes for the mentally afflicted. The young are born into that ministry, and as they grow up they seem to accept, as their own, a part of the

319

responsibility for the care and well-being of the boarders. About 300 patients improve sufficiently to be discharged each year; but some of them have found such peace in the community that they do not wish to leave. They are then allowed to live in the Colony, but they are not regarded as patients.

This system of 'boarding out' chronic lunatics was tried in Scotland towards the end of last century, at Kennoway in Fifeshire; but the effort was not very successful. In Finland and Sweden it has been definitely established with regard to a few of the larger asylums, and the results appear to be satisfactory.

The Insane in Britain.

Some account of the hardships and cruelties suffered by lunatics in England has already been given in Part II, Chapter XI, but it was not only in this country but throughout Europe and America that such conditions prevailed, and although the nineteenth century was well advanced before any radical reforms occurred, the cause of the insane had found many champions during the preceding centuries.

Most eloquently did Daniel Defoe protest against the abuses of asylums in his day, and in 1706 he published a 'Scheme for the Management of Madhouses'. He draws attention to the practice of men sending their wives to madhouses at every whim or dislike in order that they might be undisturbed in the pursuance of their own ways. He asserts that this custom had reached such lengths that the private madhouses were greatly on the increase in, and near, London. He characterises the procedure as 'the height of barbarity and injustice', and 'worse than a clandestine inquisition'. He says that even if not totally suppressed, these houses should be subject to examination. He asks, 'Is it not enough to make anyone mad to be suddenly clapped up, stripped, whipped, ill-fed and worse used?' And he continues, 'If this tyrannical inquisition, joined with the reasonable reflection a woman of any common understanding must necessarily make, be not sufficient to drive any soul stark staring mad, though before she were never so much in her senses, I have no more to say.' He urges that it should be considered no less than a felony to confine any person, under pretence of madness, without due authority, and he calls upon Queen Caroline to begin her auspicious reign by requesting that a Bill might be brought into the House to regulate these abuses.

But nothing of the kind was done for many years afterwards. True, there was an Act of Parliament passed in 1744, but this appears to be rather for the protection of society than for the care of the lunatic. It refers to those who are 'so far disordered in their senses that they may be too dangerous to be permitted to go abroad'. It authorises any two justices to apprehend them and have them securely locked up and, if necessary, chained; but there is no provision for a medical examination.

In 1763 a Committee of the House of Commons was appointed to enquire into the state of the madhouses in the kingdom. On this committee sat such eminent politicians as the elder Pitt, Fox, Lord North, Wilkes, Grenville and Townsend; and although their report was very cautiously worded it shewed that Defoe had not exaggerated the conditions. It emphasises the alarming facility with which the liberty of the subject could be taken away on the plea of insanity, and the frequency with which persons availed themselves of this means of getting rid of a troublesome relative or dependent.

The Committee passed the following resolution, 'That it is the opinion of the Committee that the present state of the private madhouses in this Kingdom requires the interposition of the legislature.' One might have expected that something really effective should have followed such a report, but all that happened was that, ten years later, a Bill for the 'Regulation of Private Madhouses' was passed by the Commons but was thrown out by the House of Lords, whilst another, which proved almost a dead letter in its operation, was passed in the following year. The Commissioners in Lunacy, appointed in 1845 under the Chairmanship of Lord Ashley (afterwards the 7th Earl of

Shaftesbury), characterised this Act of 1774 as 'utterly useless in regard to private patients, though in terms directing visitations to be made to lunatics', and stated that the provisions 'did not even apply to the lunatic poor, who were sent to asylums without any authority except that of their parish officers'.

The Work of Dr Philippe Pinel in Paris.

In spite of the frequent checks that were met with by reformers, the long martyrdom of the insane was nearing its end, both in Britain and on the Continent. In France the chief mover in the reforms was Dr Philippe Pinel, who had, on his appointment as Director in 1793, introduced some new methods of treatment at the Bicêtre Hospital in Paris. As a direct consequence not only of his compassion but of his medical researches he adopted the bold procedure of freeing the lunatics in the Bicêtre from their fetters, and he also revised their dietary, increased their comforts and arranged for employment suited to their powers. From the moment he instituted a more humane system of treatment he found that scenes of turbulence and excitement were much less frequent, and his patients were in a more favourable state for medical observation; therefore his opportunities for research into the causes and manifestations of psychiatric conditions were greatly augmented.

Ten years later the second great mental hospital of Paris, the Salpêtrière, came under his Directorship, and this gave him a wider field for his reforms. Like most other pioneers he met with a good deal of opprobrium at the time, but he lived for another thirty years during which he wrote a great many books on the pathology and treatment of insanity. His work was carried on by his son, Scipion, and his pupil, Jean Esquirol, who has justly been called the 'Hippocrates of Psychological Medicine'.

William Tuke, and the Retreat at York.

There was at York an asylum founded about 1777, no doubt with the best intentions on the part of its promoters, but by 1791 the treatment meted out to the poor inmates was the subject of many scandals, although the time had not yet come for its public exposure. Instead, it was proposed by a citizen of York, William Tuke, that an asylum should be erected wherein the patients should be treated with all the kindness their condition allowed. This proposition was made in the Spring of 1791 before an assembly of the Society of Friends. It was adopted, the funds provided and the necessary steps taken for the erection of a suitable building in a healthy locality in the neighbourhood of York. No bars or gratings were affixed to the windows and the building was supplied with neither manacles nor chains. It was surrounded by a large garden, and ample provision was made for work by the men patients in the open air, both in the garden and associated farm. The women patients were employed in sewing, knitting and in domestic duties, and all patients were given a plain but nourishing diet. The managers of the Retreat seemed to recognise, for the first time in these islands, that because a person is mad upon one particular subject it does not follow that he is insensible to feelings of kindness and gratitude, or that he is in a state of mental degradation.

Although Pinel's work in Paris had started before the establishment of the York Retreat, neither Pinel nor Tuke were aware of the other's efforts to bring about such drastic reforms in the treatment of lunacy. Each saw the wretchedness, misery and suffering of the insane and was moved by compassion to effect a complete reform; and each succeeded so well that never again, in their respective countries, could the previous conditions be accepted without protest. Their work demonstrated conclusively that any form of coercion was an evil and that gentleness should take the place of violence, the best form of restraint being self-restraint. Also, that self-restraint could be engendered by appealing to the instinct of self-regard rather than to the instinct of fear, and that the mind of melancholics could be diverted by bodily exercise in the performance of useful duties, or by walks, conversation, reading, or other recreations. The only type of physical restraint used was the wearing of a belt with light leather straps.

But the Retreat at York proved an isolated, if glorious, experiment in this country for very many years, although the question of the 'better regulation of madhouses' was the subject of serious debates in the Commons for the next thirty to forty years, led most strenuously by Lord Ashley (Earl of Shaftesbury) who was an indefatigable reformer of abuses connected not only with the treatment of lunatics but with every section of helpless and oppressed humanity.

In 1828 a Bill was passed and fifteen Commissioners in Lunacy were appointed, but little progress was seen until, following the Reports of the Commissioners, the first really effective Lunacy Act was passed in 1845. This received the Royal assent in the August of that year, and it has well been called the 'Magna Charta of the Liberties of the Insane'. Since that date other Acts have been passed as amendments, or as safeguards against possible evasion of certain clauses, especially with regard to certification of the insane.

No single legislator ever earned the gratitude both of the insane and their friends as did Lord Shaftesbury, who for more than fifty years devoted himself to the task of making proper provision for the care and treatment of the afflicted in mind. It was, to a great extent, due to his untiring efforts that the separation of criminal lunatics from those who had not seriously transgressed the law was made possible in 1863, by the establishment of Broadmoor in Berkshire, about four miles from Bracknell, on a site covering three hundred acres and commanding extensive views. It was built to carry out the provisions of the Insane Offenders' Act of 1860.

The Padded Room.

One of the greatest innovations of the nineteenth century was the invention, by a German professor, Dr Autenrieth, of the padded room, the walls and floor of which were covered with rubber stretched over layers of cork chips. On such a surface a maniac might expend his futile fury without any injury to himself or damage to property, and this rendered the use of any drastic means of restraint quite unnecessary. The padded room was introduced into Bethlem Hospital about 1844, and every mental asylum of to-day is equipped with such rooms. The bed is usually made up on a mattress on the floor and the room is specially heated. This is a great comfort in cold weather as the patients frequently toss off the bedclothes and may even discard their own clothing. In addition to this, the warmth itself may help to induce somnolence and thus quieten the patient.

Modern Developments.

A new era had now dawned in the history of the insane. With the abolition of mechanical restraint and the introduction of humane and scientific treatments involving hydrotherapy and rest in bed, accompanied by the necessary attention to the daily toilet of the patient and special dietetic and medicinal treatment, it became imperative that skilled and intelligent nursing should also develop; and the advance in psychiatric nursing has kept pace with the rapid progress in all other branches of medicine and nursing. At the present time most countries have two grades of mental nurses—the qualified mental nurse and the attendant nurse. These are of both sexes, for in no other branch are men nursed by their own sex to so great an extent as in mental hospitals and homes. Attendants are untrained in that they do not undergo a specialised course of instruction and study with a view to passing qualifying examinations, but among their ranks may be found many devoted and intelligent men and women who have gained, by clinical experience and observation, such an understanding of the special needs and the management of the insane that, at least under present conditions, their services are indispensable in the asylums of this and many other countries. In private work also, acting under the direction of a doctor, they find a large sphere of usefulness.

The trained mental nurse of to-day in England may have

qualified under one of two systems. She, or he, may have received training and passed examinations in psychiatric nursing only, or the mental training may have been taken as a postgraduate course after a general nursing qualification has been obtained. In Great Britain the Nurses' Registration Acts of 1919 provide for a supplementary register of mental nurses, the prescribed course of training being three years. The Royal Medico-Psychological Association also holds examinations of its own for nurses who have undergone the training and instruction included in its curriculum of mental nursing, but the certificate of this Association does not give admission to the State Register.

The modern tendency, and the ideal for the future, is to include psychiatric training in the basic curriculum of general nursing, and many general hospitals, especially those under the Ministry of Health, have now a special psychiatric department, where early or mild cases of 'mental sickness' are investigated and treated in an out-patient clinic, whilst more acute cases are nursed in special wards as are the sufferers from any other particular form of illness. The teaching of mental hygiene in schools and colleges and the promotion of mental health as a branch of Public Health work is recognised as being one of the greatest medical developments of this age; and the collaboration of nurses with a clear understanding of the ordinary psychiatric problems is of immense value both in the preventive and curative branches of this work.

The interaction of mind with bodily processes is now so widely recognised that all modern teachers of nursing are including in their curriculum some instruction in the elementary facts and problems of psychology, although, at present, it seldom constitutes a special course of lectures during general training. However, the time is undoubtedly not far distant when psychiatric nursing will be as much a part of general training as is the nursing of disorders of the endocrine system or the preparation of a patient for a surgical operation.

326

CHAPTER V

HENRI DUNANT AND THE RED CROSS

The battle of Solferino—Convention of Geneva—The second Geneva Convention—The Third Geneva Convention—Peace Conference of the Hague, 1907—The Joint War Committee—The work of the Red Cross Societies during peace—The Junior Red Cross—Nursing training given by Red Cross Societies—The Red Cross and the Florence Nightingale Foundation—Other recent developments of Red Cross work—The Red Cross Society's Blood Transfusion Service—The Aeroplane Hospital Service

ONE of the greatest and most effective of the nineteenth century humanitarians was surely Henri Dunant, who was born at Geneva on 8th May, 1828; for it was due to his keen realisation of the agony of mind and body endured by the wounded on the battlefield after fighting had finished, and his persistence in seeking the interest of kings, princes, churchmen and generals of armies, that a new and far-reaching movement was started for the alleviation of the sufferings of the wounded soldier.

It was not the first time that the idea underlying the Red Cross movement had been put into operation, for the care of *enemy* wounded was recorded during the Athenian war with Sparta, when the people of Lacedæmon took the wounded into their own houses irrespective of race. This was an advance upon ancient practice. Again, during the Crusades some work of the kind had been accomplished. Then, towards the end of the fifteenth century Queen Isabella of Castile had introduced field ambulances and mobile dressing stations; but these efforts were comparatively shortlived. During the next three centuries various conventions, agreements and treaties were entered upon which

327

regulated the status of captured hospitals and the freedom to be accorded to the medical personnel; but it remained for Henri Dunant to stir up the machinery for putting the ideas into an organised practice, capable of developing into an international compact that should be enduring in its operation.

In June, 1859, M. Dunant, a young man of thirty-one, was spending a holiday travelling in Lombardy. Austria and France were then at war, and the battle of Solferino was fought on 24th June.

Both armies were already tired by long marches when they met in the early dawn of what proved to be an intensely hot day. The battle front was fourteen miles long and covered a succession of hills and ridges with little villages and fruitful farms nestling in the hollows and valleys. All that day the battle raged, it developed into hand-to-hand fighting with infantry, cavalry and artillery inextricably mixed; and many were the miracles of valour and endurance performed by heroes whose names were never recorded for posterity. The farms, gardens, orchards and vineyards were laid waste, and the non-combatants to whom the battlefield had been home, found themselves plunged from peaceful thrift into homeless destitution.

The next morning Dunant's travels brought him to a hill overlooking the battlefield whereon lay fifteen thousand dead and wounded, with swarms of flies and carrion birds hovering around; and in the appalling anguish of that sight was born the determination to leave no stone unturned to bring about such an international covenant as should render a repetition of that scene forever an impossibility. But the immediate need was to obtain dressings, medical aid and temporary hospitals for the wounded lying on that sun-baked Lombardy plain, and Dunant gathered together the inhabitants of the neighbouring village of Castiglione and set them all to work. Even the children collected straw to spread in the churches, monasteries and public squares whereon to lay the stricken men. Dunant pressed other tourists and everyone he could find into service, and all day long they laboured under the broiling sun to dress wounds, and give food, water and medicines to the wounded. The few surgeons present could give attention to but a small proportion of the sufferers. The supplies of dressings and bandages gave out, and water became very scarce. The transport of the wounded was much delayed by the lack of vehicles and of men to load them. The sights, sounds and smells from that inferno of suffering caused many of the helpers to collapse, and Dunant realised most clearly that however willing a band of unorganised and untrained volunteers might be, it was utterly incapable of dealing effectively with the stupendous task in hand; and when the work of caring for the wounded at Solferino was ended he interviewed field marshals and generals, and laid before them the scheme that was taking shape in his own mind.

He wrote a little pamphlet entitled 'Un Souvenir de Solférino' in which he described the sufferings of the wounded with very vivid effect, and tried to show how much of that suffering might be avoided in the future. He pointed out that one must have volunteer nurses previously trained and officially recognised by the commanding officers of the armies, and that there was a precedent for such an organisation. In 'Un Souvenir de Solférino' he wrote, 'The picture of Miss Florence Nightingale going through the vast wards of the military hospitals during the night, with a small lamp in her hand, noting the condition of each sick man, will never be obliterated from the hearts of the men who were the objects or the witnesses of her admirable beneficience, and the memory of it will be engraven in history.' This pamphlet was translated into several languages and was eagerly read by all classes of people. Dunant travelled through Europe using all his powers of persuasion to make others see what was so clearly outlined in his own mind; but it was four years after the battle of Solferino, on 26th October, 1863, that the Geneva Society of Public Utility, of which Dunant was a member, held a meeting that was attended by thirty-six delegates from various countries. Meanwhile, two other authors, an Italian named Palasciano and a Frenchman named Arrault, had also used their pens to urge that international recognition should be accorded to the neutrality of the sick and wounded and to the inviolability of medical personnel and ambulances.

Convention of Geneva.

The discussion at Geneva lasted for four days, but as the delegates had no power to act for the nations they represented, they made plans for another meeting at the same place in the following year for the purpose of drawing up a treaty that should be binding upon all nations that signed it. The members of the commission nominated by the Geneva Society of Public Utility ultimately constituted The International Committee of the Red Cross, which continues to have its headquarters at Geneva. The second Conference, which lasted from 8th to the 26th August, 1864, resulted in the signing of 'The Treaty' or 'Convention of Geneva' by delegates from sixteen countries. This convention was an international agreement for improving the conditions of wounded soldiers on the field. Its chief provisions were the neutrality of ambulances and military hospitals as long as they contained any sick or wounded, the care of the sick or wounded irrespective of nationality, the wearing of a brassard by neutralised individuals, and the use of a distinctive and uniform flag for hospitals and ambulances, accompanied always by the national flag. The emblem for both the flag and the arm badge was to be a red cross on a white ground.

A curious omission which led to a good deal of confusion later was any decision as to the designation for the national organisations. Consequently a number of different titles were used. In England the unwieldy name of 'The National Society for Aid to the Sick and Wounded in War' was adopted. The Dutch Society was the first to use the title 'Red Cross', and other countries followed its lead.

The Second Geneva Convention.

In the Austro-Prussian War of 1866 it was realised that both the powers and the limitations of the Geneva Convention of 1864 were imperfectly understood, many questions being raised as to the interpretation of certain clauses, and so a Second Geneva Convention was called in 1868 to settle the various controversial points. This Convention paid special attention to problems connected with naval warfare and drafted ten articles on this subject. The decisions of this Convention were not, however, confirmed by the Powers until the Convention of 1906.

In England, during the years that followed the Second Convention, the Red Cross and the St John Ambulance Association both developed and combined their organisations, assisting the wounded in every war that occurred. Meanwhile, the Army Nursing Service Reserve, which owed its inception to H.R.H. Princess Christian, had come into being and was proving a very valuable adjunct to the Army Medical Service; but by the beginning of this century it was felt by the Central British Red Cross Council that there might, with advantage, be much more unification of effort in the British Empire, and that during peace times arrangements should be made to anticipate all the necessities likely to arise during war. The result of the enquiries and deliberations of the Council was that, in July, 1905, one comprehensive British Red Cross Society for the whole Empire was formed, with Queen Alexandra as its President. The members and associates were recruited from all classes throughout the Empire, and the Society was entirely voluntary. A notification of this reconstruction of the British Red Cross Society was sent to the International Committee at Geneva.

During the various wars that occurred during the latter part of the nineteenth century the armies of Europe had had opportunity to master the principles and practice of the Red Cross movement as laid down in the articles of the Geneva Conventions of 1864 and 1868. Some of the paragraphs in these articles were alleged to be vague, and the experience gained during the wars of the intervening forty years had emphasised the necessity for a certain amount of revision and clarification of the original statutes.

The Third Geneva Convention.

On the invitation of the Swiss Government a Conference met at Geneva in 1906 and was attended by forty-one delegates. This Conference formulated a new Convention consisting of thirty-three articles. These were arranged under the following headings: (1) The wounded and sick. (2) Medical units and establishments. (3) Personnel. (4) Material. (5) Convoys of evacuation. (6) The distinctive emblem, etc.

The plain red cross on a white ground was officially authorised because it was realised that it must be clearly distinguishable from a distance, and that any heraldic details might lead to errors of observation, but the Convention of 1906 also emphasised the fact that the emblem had no religious significance. This was necessary in order to preserve uniformity, for Turkey had already replaced the Cross by the Crescent.

Peace Conference of the Hague, 1907.

In the year following the Third Geneva Convention, the Second International Peace Conference met at the Hague 'for the purpose of giving a fresh development to the humanitarian principles which served as a basis for the work of the First Peace Conference in 1899'. Forty Powers were represented at the Conference by their official delegates, and thirteen Conventions were drawn up. Although these have very little to do with the work of the Red Cross, the Geneva and the Hague Conventions are so often confused that it may be well to draw a clear distinction. The topics of the Hague Convention were: Pacific Settlement of International Disputes, Opening of Hostilities. Laws and Customs of War on Land. Rights and Duties of Neutral Powers. Laying of Automatic Submarine Contact Mines. Bombardment by Naval Forces. Adaptation of the Principles of the Geneva Convention to Maritime War.

It will be seen that only in the last section is there any definite relation to the Articles of the Geneva Convention; but an article in this section gave authority to Turkey to use the Red Crescent, and to Persia to have a Red Lion and a Red Sun on its 'hospital' flag, thus breaking the uniformity agreed upon at Geneva.

The Joint War Committee.

During the early months of the World War the British Red Cross Society and the Order of St John of Jerusalem formed the 'Joint War Committee' in order the better to co-operate in the responsible duties they had undertaken, and this became the largest single organisation for the care of the sick and wounded in war that the world had ever known. It controlled field dressing stations and stretcher-bearing units, motor ambulances, hospital trains, sea transport, a stores department dealing with dressings, equipment, food supplies, garments and comforts, auxiliary and base hospitals, casualty clearing stations, rest stations, convalescent homes, hostels for the relatives of the wounded, and medical, surgical and trained nursing staffs.

The League of Red Cross Societies.

At the conclusion of the War the Red Cross Society had several thousands of workers under its control. Many of these had become most proficient in the work they had been doing, having acquired considerable experience and technical skill. It was felt that this power could still be utilised in some public service if only a suitable organisation could come into being to direct it. To this end a Medical Conference was convened at Cannes in April, 1919. A section was devoted to 'nursing', and was attended by representatives from Great Britain, the United States, France and Italy. An important outcome of the Conference was the formation of the League of Red Cross Societies in May, 1919. This is controlled and administered by a Board of

333

Governors which includes a representative from each of the sixty affiliated countries, although the authority is actually centred in an Executive Committee of eleven. The headquarters of the League are at 12, Rue Newton, Avenue d'léna, Paris, and the present head of the Nursing Department is Mrs. Maynard Carter, A.R.R.C., an English nurse who was appointed in 1927. Previous to that date the appointment had been held consecutively by two American nurses, Miss Fitzgerald and Miss Olmsted. The work of the nursing section of the League of Red Cross Societies is to help in establishing training schools for nurses and in developing Public Health work in those countries where such work is not yet established; and also to arrange a system of scholarships to enable trained nurses to receive the necessary supplementary education to qualify them as teachers or as Public Health nurses. In addition, it collects, analyses, publishes and distributes information on many subjects relating to nursing and to Public Health work in general.

It will be seen therefore, that the League of Red Cross Societies is a federated body in which the national aspect of Red Cross work assumes importance, whereas the International Red Cross Committee, with its headquarters at Geneva, has an independence that enables it to deal with difficulties, and with delicate situations in which opinion is divided, with a detachment that would not be possible with the League. However, the International Committee and the League work in close cooperation and they share joint responsibility; for example, representatives of the International Committee sit with the League delegates on the governing body of the Florence Nightingale Foundation, whose creation was due to the initiation of the League of Red Cross Societies, and the Committee has been entrusted with the awarding of the Florence Nightingale Medals to very distinguished nurses of all countries.

334

The Work of the Red Cross Societies during Peace.

In this brief sketch it is quite impossible even to outline the magnificent work that has been, and is still being, done by the Red Cross organisations throughout the world. These organisations are unique both in their magnitude and their efficiency, and they are carrying out, more thoroughly than ever before, the suggestion made by M. Dunant, in 'Un Souvenir de Solférino', that such societies could render great service in times of peace during epidemics, industrial strikes, earthquakes, fires, floods, or any other national disasters. The Supplemental Charter of the British Red Cross Society, dated 12th December, 1919, declares that although the primary object of the Society is the furnishing of aid to the sick and wounded in times of war, it should, in addition, 'include the improvement of health, the prevention of disease, and the mitigation of suffering throughout the world'. Thus there was opened up an almost illimitable field of activity in combating malaria, tuberculosis, typhus and yellow fever, dysentery and cholera, and in dealing with all kinds of public calamities.

The Junior Red Cross.

In 1920, at a General Council of the League of Red Cross Societies, a resolution (No. IV) was passed, 'That a national Red Cross Society should organise the youth of its country for Red Cross Service.' By May, 1926, thirty-seven countries had entered upon this work, with a total membership of over eight million junior members. Its numbers now exceed seventeen and a half million, with branches in fifty-one countries. In Britain, the Junior Branch is now an integral part of the Red Cross Society's organisation. It has its own Director and its own literature, in the form of textbooks and a magazine. It gives training in personal hygiene and in First Aid, it encourages an interest in sick and crippled children, arranges correspondence with Juniors in

335

other lands, and is steadily increasing in numbers, efficiency, and in the scope of its activities.

Nursing Training Given by Red Cross Societies.

Ever since the inception of the Red Cross idea it has been realised that instruction and training must be given in times of peace so that the necessary nurses are prepared to undertake the work required during war. In some countries elementary instruction only is given, whilst in many others a full three-years' course is arranged in the Red Cross Hospitals, for example, in Japan and Bulgaria, Sweden and Latvia.

The Red Cross and the Florence Nightingale International Foundation.

It has already been mentioned that at the Conference held at Cannes in 1919 it was resolved, amongst other things, that a system of scholarships for trained nurses should be established that should enable their holders to undergo an educational course which would qualify them as Public Health nurses or as Tutors. In 1920, the British Red Cross Society officially appointed the College of Nursing, 1a, Henrietta Street, Cavendish Square, London, W.1., to make the necessary arrangements, in conjunction with King's College of Household and Social Science (University of London), and a course of instruction in Public Health Nursing was initiated. This was transferred to Bedford College for Women, London, in the following year. Nurses from nearly every country affiliated with the League were selected by their respective Red Cross Societies to enter Bedford College for the scholastic year, that is, from September to July, in order to undergo training in Preventive Medicine. In 1924 an additional course for nurse-administrators and teachers in schools of nursing was arranged, and a hostel for these international students was opened at 15, Manchester Square, London, W.1. The League was responsible for the upkeep and management of this establishment, which contained 21 bedrooms and very well-arranged sitting rooms; but when, in 1933, the Florence Nightingale International Foundation was formed by the joint action of the League of Red Cross Societies, and the International Council of Nurses, the League gave the Foundation the leasehold of the house, which is a fine example of the Adam period, dating from about 1783. The original lease is a very large and imposing document signed by one of the Adam brothers himself. The house is now known as the Florence Nightingale International House, and is the headquarters of the Foundation.

On 26th June, 1936, the certificates gained by the International students during the preceding year were presented by H.R.H. the Duchess of Kent. Nurses from New Zealand, Australia, Sweden, Finland, Switzerland, Lithuania, India, Canada and Great Britain gained certificates as nurse-administrators and teachers, and students from the Philippine Islands, New Zealand, United States and Great Britain for Public Health work.

Other Recent Developments of Red Cross Work.

The British Red Cross Society has now extended its peace-time activities in many directions. Nearly every municipality has a local branch of the Red Cross and many of these branches organise a series of lectures by lady doctors or trained nurses, giving instruction to women on the conservation of health in the home, the care of infants and the principles of home-nursing. London branches have Treatment Centres in connection with the elementary schools of the London County Council at which dental and eye troubles and many minor ailments receive attention, the County Council making a capitation grant for each child and paying the salary of the doctor and nurse attached to the Centre; the Branch of the Red Cross Society being responsible for all other expenses and also for the administrative arrangements.

In 1922 a Physical Treatment Centre for Civilians was opened at Kensington, where massage and electrical treatment can be given to patients who are unable to pay the customary fees. One of the best examples of a successful Physical Treat-

z

337

ment Centre is the British Red Cross Clinic for Rheumatism which, with the encouragement of the Ministry of Health, was established at Peto Place, London, N.W.1. in 1926. Its success was so great and immediate that its accommodation was taxed to the utmost. Evening sessions are held on four days in the week, and, in addition, there are three morning and five afternoon sessions. All the treatments are given by appointment only, and thus the patient knows exactly how much time he will require. This enables him to undergo a course of treatment with the minimum disturbance to his work, or other appointments.

Many patients are sent by Approved Societies under a scheme which provides for special terms of payment; the Society guarantees treatment for each patient for a limited period only. A course usually consists of about nine treatments; and when this is completed a further guarantee is given if the patient shows definite improvement, or is considered to be a suitable case for palliative treatment. Eighty Approved Societies, in connection with National Health Insurance, and fifteen Benefit Societies sent patients to the Clinic during 1935—the last year for which figures are available—and the total number of attendances was 89,810. A year after the establishment of this Clinic an International League against Rheumatism was formed, with National Committees in various countries. This was not, however, primarily a Red Cross activity, but was designed to stimulate professional interest and encourage research into the causes of chronic rheumatic diseases, and to establish treatment centres.

There are now Red Cross Clinics, supported and administered by individual branches, for tropical diseases, massage, and orthopædic work; there are Camp Dispensaries for Hop-pickers arranged during the season, and there are Day Nurseries. In some localities there are Medical and Surgical Homes for people of limited means. There are nearly two hundred local Nursing Associations throughout the country, and free grants are made to each of them, every six months, of all the dressings and ordinary equipment they require. In addition, the local Red Cross Branches organise hospital libraries for patients of all hospitals, not only those under the auspices of their own Society.

The Red Cross Blood Transfusion Service.

One of the most remarkable services to mankind that have been organised in recent years is the Blood Transfusion Service. Men and women who are willing to give their blood, when required in the treatment of patients with certain diseases, or injuries which have resulted in severe depletion of blood, undergo a preliminary blood test with a view to ascertaining the 'group' to which they belong. They then have their names placed on the Society's Roll of voluntary 'Donors'; and such is the organisation and public spirited response to this need that any hospital, or private practitioner, merely by putting a telephone call through to Forest Hill 2264, London, and stating his requirements, can obtain the blood needed by his patient as quickly as the nearest donor can make the journey, at any time of the night or day.

The Aeroplane Hospital Service.

This is the youngest branch of the work of the Red Cross Societies. The first British Flying Hospital was named *Florence Nightingale*—by the orthodox method of breaking a bottle of champagne—at Hanwell Air Park on Sunday, 10th May, 1936. The ceremony was performed by Mrs Amy Mollison.

The machine is a low-wing, twin-engine monoplane, painted white with large red crosses. It represents a complete field dressing station, and it contains full medical and nursing equipment, including blood-transfusion apparatus, an oxygen tent and aluminium stretcher frames, whilst the cabin is designed and fitted solely for the carrying out of First Aid work.

The *Florence Nightingale* has recently been fitted with an antigas stretcher which incorporates the tent method of administering oxygen, and facilities for removing the parts contaminated by gas and replacing them by spares.

First Aid in Chemical Warfare.

During the past two years the Red Cross Society has carried out a great campaign for the teaching of First Aid in Chemical Warfare. Courses of lectures and practical instruction have been held all over the country, followed by examinations and the awarding of certificates to successful candidates. The main object of this teaching is to familiarise the general public, as well as doctors and nurses, with the types of gas likely to be used, the symptoms they would produce and their First Aid treatment; so that, in the event of such a catastrophe as a gas attack from the air, there will be no panic among the people, and casualty treatment stations could be improvised with as little delay as possible.

340

CHAPTER VI

THE ORGANISATION OF NURSING INTO A STATE-RECOGNISED PROFESSION

*The first organisation of trained nurses—The view of the Opposition—
The limitations of the Charter—The fight for State Registration—State
Registration in other countries—The International Council of Nurses*

IN England, the relation of the nursing profession to the general
public is now governed by the 'Nurses' Registration Act' of 1919;
but for more than thirty years before the passing of that Act the
nursing world was shaken by struggles and controversies regarding the desirability of such a standardising of training and theoretical attainments as must inevitably be required for State
Registration.

During the first twenty years after the inauguration, at the
Nightingale School, of training for nurses, the energies and interests of the newly qualified nurses were directed towards extending the reform into all the hospitals throughout the country;
but by 1880 the majority of hospital wards were controlled by
women who had undergone special training, and they were
training the probationers working under them. Medical science
had developed in many directions, and the general educational
and professional standards of nurses had needed, perforce, to
keep pace with the advances in surgery and in medical treatment. The period of training considered necessary had extended
to two years, and in some hospitals to three. The scope of
trained nursing had been greatly enlarged by the development of
district nursing, by private nursing in the homes of better class
patients, and by the organisation of midwifery training and certification.

341

It was now felt by many of the leaders of nurses and nursing organisations that State recognition was desirable in order to promote the efficiency of nurses by approving suitable schools, prescribing a minimum course of training and establishing qualifying examinations. Moreover, the interests of the public would be safeguarded by ensuring that a woman might not claim to be a professional nurse unless she were duly qualified.

The First Organisation of Trained Nurses.

In 1886, the Hospitals Association, which had been formed by Sir Henry Burdett, appointed a Committee to enquire into the possibility of establishing a General Register of Nurses. This Committee violently disagreed, a number of its members resigned and the remainder, under the leadership of Mrs Bedford Fenwick, formed the British Nurses' Association, in 1887, with a view to carrying forward a scheme for registration. Miss Nightingale was never in favour of this, and she expressed herself as 'in terror lest the "B.N.A.'s" and the "anti-B.N.A.'s" should form two hostile camps'.

As events turned out, the controversy was both hot and prolonged, and throughout the struggle each side continued to have very eminent supporters. Among the opposition were many of those who had had the longest and closest knowledge of nursing training, including Miss Nightingale and Mr Rathbone. The Association had Princess Christian as its President and Mrs Bedford Fenwick to direct its activities.[1] On 6th June, 1892, it was granted a Royal Charter by Queen Victoria as a result of her daughter's petition. It has always had a Royal President, for Princess Christian was succeeded by Princess Arthur of Connaught, who is still its President and is herself a State-Registered nurse who has also undergone a period of midwifery training.

[1]As Miss Ethel Gordon Manson, Mrs Bedford Fenwick had been Matron of St Bartholomew's Hospital, and she has remained, until the present day, a very powerful influence in every branch of nursing affairs.

The objects of the Royal British Nurses' Association—as it was designated after the granting of the Charter—were 'to unite all qualified British nurses in membership of a recognised profession, and to provide for their registration on terms satisfactory to physicians and surgeons as evidence of their having received systematic training'. It was felt that a Register of Nurses, duly certified as competent, would be a protection against impostors. The certification would be by a Board which would insist upon a *minimum* standard of professional proficiency. The suggested training was for three years in a hospital recognised by the Board as a training school.

The View of the Opposition.

Miss Nightingale held strongly to the view that:

'You cannot select the good from the inferior by any test or system of examination. But most of all, and first of all, must their moral qualifications be made to stand pre-eminent in estimation. All this can only be secured by the current supervision, tests, or examination which they receive in their training school or hospital, not by any examination from a foreign body like that of the proposed British Nurses' Association. Indeed, those who come off best in such examination would probably be the ready and the forward, not the best nurses.'

To her, this was a parting of ways, a possible sacrificing of high calling to professional advancement; and she thought that it might cause intending nurses to flock to the hospitals that gave the easiest certificate with the least possible trouble of training. On 26th February, 1891, she wrote to Mr Rathbone:

'Forty years hence such a scheme might not be preposterous, *providing* that the intermediate time be diligently and successfully employed in levelling up, that is, in making all nurses at least equal to the best trained nurses of this day; and in levelling up training schools in like manner.'

343

In view of the fact that it was thirty-four years after Miss Nightingale wrote that letter when the first State Final Examination for Nurses was held, one cannot but be, once again, impressed by her sound and well-balanced judgment, as shown in that paragraph. It was about that time that she made the acquaintance of Miss Lückes, the Matron of the London Hospital, who also strongly opposed the idea of registration; and throughout the struggle the most strenuous opposition to the passing of a State Registration Act continued to come from the London Hospital. There was a very sound reason for this. The proposed conditions for the registration insisted upon the whole of the training being consecutive, and the London Hospital nurses attended private patients in their own homes and were away from hospital for varying periods during their training. This rendered them ineligible for registration on the proposed lines, and therefore, the hospital had no choice but to oppose a scheme which would exclude its own nurses from recognition as qualified women in their profession.

The Limitations of the Charter.

The Charter, when obtained, was claimed as a victory by both sides. The truth was that the Lords of the Privy Council had steered a middle course by deleting the words 'the maintenance of a list, or register, of nurses showing as to each nurse registered', etc., and had substituted the words 'the maintenance of a list of persons who may have applied to have their names entered thereon as nurses', etc. There was nothing in the Charter which gave any nurse the right to call herself 'chartered' or 'registered'.

However, as far as the 'Woman's Movement' was concerned, the granting of this Charter was a great landmark, for it was the first time that an English Parliament had given a Charter to a body of professional women.

The Fight for State Registration.

From the time of its inception the Royal British Nurses' Association was very progressive in its outlook, it aimed at improving education and training, and it worked indefatigably for State Registration. In 1894, Mrs Bedford Fenwick founded the 'Matrons' Council', with Miss Isla Stewart, Matron of St Bartholomew's Hospital, as its first President, and having as its avowed object the hastening of some form of State recognition for fully trained nurses. In the following year the British Medical Association, on the motion of Dr Bedford Fenwick, passed a resolution that 'an Act of Parliament should, as soon as possible, be passed providing for the registration of nurses, and the Council of the Association are requested to consider the matter, and to take such measures as seem to them advisable to obtain such legislation'. This was not productive of any advance however, for doctors have never been unanimous with regard to ensuring the status of nurses, and a year later a Conference between the Parliamentary Bills Committee of the British Medical Association and representatives of nursing organisations passed a resolution, by a very small majority, against the registration of nurses.

The next important move occurred in 1902, when a 'Society for the State Registration of Trained Nurses' was formed; and from this time onward many unsuccessful Bills were introduced into Parliament. The first of these was drafted, in 1903, by the Royal British Nurses' Association. This was followed, in 1904, by one from the Society for the State Registration of Nurses. A Select Committee of the House of Commons was appointed to consider the question, and although it was in sympathy with the project, nothing tangible resulted from its findings. Then, in 1910, a Central Committee was formed, with representatives from each of the other bodies who were working for State Registration; and this Committee carried on the campaign until the beginning of the Great War, which did more than anything else could have done to focus public attention upon the nursing profession.

In 1916 the College of Nursing was founded, and it played a very active part in the contest. Finally, in 1918, a Bill drafted by the College of Nursing was before the House of Lords at the same time as a Bill drafted by the Central Committee was before the House of Commons; but both were withdrawn upon an assurance given by the newly constituted Ministry of Health that it would bring its own Bill for State Registration of Nurses before Parliament during the next session. The College Bill, however, proved to be the basis of the Bill which the Ministry of Health successfully piloted through its various stages until it became law in December, 1919; and thus ended a struggle which had lasted for over thirty years. This Government Bill is the Nurses' Registration Act which controls the profession to-day. Actually, three separate Acts were passed for the British Isles, one for England and Wales, one for Scotland and one for Ireland. This was rendered necessary because there was a different administrative head in each—the Minister of Health for England, the Scottish Board of Health, and the Chief Secretary for Ireland. Each country was empowered to set up a General Nursing Council for the purpose of carrying out the provisions of the Act. These involved the compilation of a recommended 'Syllabus of Instruction' and a compulsory 'Syllabus of Subjects for Examination'—the former naturally being more comprehensive than the latter—and the organising of qualifying examinations to be held at the same time throughout the country. The Council was also authorised to compile and maintain a Register of duly qualified nurses, and conditions were laid down for the inclusion in this Register of *bona-fide* nurses already in practice, and also for 'intermediate' nurses. The latter were those who were due to complete their hospital training within a stated period from the passing of the Act; after which time no nurse could be registered unless she had undergone the prescribed training and had succeeded in passing the examinations of the General Nursing Council.

The main Register is for General trained nurses, but there are

346

Supplementary Registers for Male Nurses, Infectious Diseases Nurses, Sick Children's Nurses, Mental Nurses and Nurses for Mental Defectives. For inclusion in any of these, all candidates take the same Preliminary Examination, but the Final is adapted to the demands that the specialised work will make upon the knowledge and efficiency of the nurse. The Preliminary examination is in two parts, Part I including anatomy, physiology and hygiene and Part II including theory and practice of nursing and first aid. Part I *may* be taken before entry into the hospital provided that the candidate has reached the age of $17\frac{1}{2}$ years and has taken a pre-nursing course approved by the General Nursing Council. Such courses have been established in many secondary schools and polytechnics. Part II may not be taken until the candidate has completed one year of her hospital training.

The Nurses' Act, 1943.

This Act provides for the training and enrolment of assistant nurses, giving them a recognised status in law. The training is shorter and the syllabus is less comprehensive than for State Registered nurses, but the assistant nurse fills a very necessary place both in hospital and in the patient's home.

State Registration in Other Countries.

The introduction of State Registration for nurses in this country did not establish a precedent in the recognition of nursing as a profession, for in many other countries such State Registration Acts had been passed quite early in the twentieth century, and the Cape Colony of South Africa had registered its nurses under the Medical and Pharmacy Act of 1891. The first Act entirely concerned with the Registration of Nurses was passed in New Zealand in 1901, and in 1903 the United States of America began to pass Registration Acts, those for North Carolina, New Jersey and New York being passed during that year. By the beginning of the Great War twenty-four of the

347

States had arranged for the registration of their nurses, and so also had Canada, Australia, Austria, Belgium and Germany. Since the Great War many other countries have introduced nursing legislation, until, at the present time, nursing is a registered profession practically throughout the civilised world.

The International Council of Nurses.

A proposal put forward by Mrs Bedford Fenwick, at the Annual Conference of the Matrons' Council held in London in July, 1899, 'That steps be taken to organise an International Council of Nurses,' was discussed at the Congress of the International Council of Women held in London in that year. The idea met with great approval, and the resolution was enthusiastically carried. A meeting was held on the following day at St Bartholomew's Hospital and a provisional committee was formed which included representatives from Great Britain, the United States, Cape Colony, New South Wales, Victoria, New Zealand, Denmark and Holland. Mrs Bedford Fenwick became, and remained, its President.

This Committee drew up a draft constitution which, with some slight amendments, was adopted in the following year. Its essential aim, as expressed in its own words, is 'the self-government of nurses in their Associations, with the aim of ever raising higher the standards of education and professional ethics, public usefulness, and civic spirit of their members'.

The International Council of Nurses has arranged Conferences and Congresses in many countries since its inception. The first was in Buffalo, N.Y. in 1901 at which thirteen countries were represented. Subsequently, Conferences were held every three or four years, except during the World War. The meeting places were as follows: Berlin (1904), Paris (1907), London (1909), Cologne (1912), San Francisco (1915)—this had the smallest attendance of any meeting, owing to the War. The first Conference held after the War was at Copenhagen in 1922, and then, in 1925, another was held at Helsingfors, Finland, at which there

348

were representatives from thirty-three countries and an attendance of one thousand. This number was considerably exceeded at the Congress held in 1929, whilst at that of Paris and Brussels in 1933 the attendance reached 2,284. In addition to these Congresses there have been interim conferences held at Geneva in 1927, 1931 and 1935.

The Quadrennial Congress of 1937 took place at the Central Hall, Westminster, London, from 19th July to 24th July. Four halls were available, and therefore meetings could be held simultaneously, under the following sections: (1) Nursing Education. (2) The Nursing Profession—Organisation and Administration. (3) Public Health. (4) Some Nursing Problems. It was opened by H.R.H. The Princess Royal, who said, whilst performing the ceremony:

'I fully appreciate how important it is that the International Council of Nurses should meet for discussions of mutual interest, and I desire to extend a warm welcome to that large representative body. In these days, when far-reaching medical and surgical researches are being made, it is more than ever necessary that nursing should maintain a very high standard. In the words of Florence Nightingale, "Nursing is something in which progress must be made every year".'

Her Royal Highness then declared the Congress open, and it was attended by 3,362 nurses. At the General Session on the evening of 21st July three countries were received as new members—Australia, Switzerland and Roumania—making a total of thirty-two, whilst seven other countries are associate members.

The next Congress is arranged to take place in the United States in 1941, and the newly-elected President of the Council is Miss Effie Taylor, M.A., R.N., Dean of the Yale University School of Nursing, Connecticut, U.S.A., where she succeeded Dean Annie Goodrich.

Such a world-wide organisation of professional women as the International Council of Nurses has, inevitably, resulted in associating the interests, aims and ideals of nurses of all nation-

349

alities; and because of the mutual helpfulness of its meetings and publications it has contributed to progress in many directions. It can undoubtedly claim to be the most progressive and far-reaching organisation of women in the world. Its headquarters have recently been moved from Geneva, and are now at 51 Palace Street, London, S.W.1.

Its members, in order of their affiliation, are: Great Britain, United States, Germany, Canada, Denmark, Finland, Holland, India, New Zealand, Belgium, China, Norway, South Africa, Bulgaria, Cuba, France, Irish Free State, Poland, Brazil, Greece, Yugoslavia, Philippines, Sweden, Austria, Czechoslovakia, Estonia, Hungary, Iceland, Japan (including Korea), Australia, Switzerland and Roumania.

Associate members are: Chile, Egypt, Latvia, Lithuania, Luxemburg, Siam, Syria and Turkey.

The National Council of Nurses of Great Britain.

This is an entirely self-governing organisation of nurses which was founded in 1904 with the objects of promoting mutual understanding and unity between Associations of Nurses of Great Britain, of acquiring a knowledge, through its affiliation with the International Council of Nurses, of nursing conditions in every country, of encouraging a spirit of sympathy with nurses of other nations and of affording facilities for National hospitality. It also seeks to increase the usefulness of the trained nurses as a social factor and to promote the educational, economic, and other interests of the nursing profession. Any Association of qualified nurses with a membership of not less than 50 is eligible for affiliation with the National Council of Nurses of Great Britain, for example, the Nurses' Leagues of approved training schools figure largely in its membership, and through it are in touch with the International Council of Nurses. Its official organ is *The British Journal of Nursing*, which is published each month.

350

CHAPTER VII

THE REFORM OF NURSING IN AMERICA

New York—Connecticut—Massachusetts—Philadelphia—Visiting Nursing—The Victorian Order—Organisation and University affiliation—Affiliation with Columbia University—The Minnesota Scheme—The School of Nursing at Yale University, Connecticut—Affiliation with other universities—Later developments—The American Red Cross—First organisation for War service—Reorganisation of the American Red Cross—Jane Arminda Delano and the work of the American Red Cross—The Delano Red Cross Nursing Service—Other activities of the American Red Cross—Red Cross 'Town and District Nursing Service'

New York.

THE first of the American hospitals to be reorganised on the Nightingale plan was Bellevue Hospital in New York. This hospital was inspected in 1872 by a representative of the New York State Charities Aid Society, who reported that the nursing was chiefly in the hands of women who were ex-convicts and who possessed all the undesirable characteristics of the worst nurses of that period. In the notorious 'Five Points Police Courts' of that time drunken prostitutes were often given the option of going to prison or into hospital service.

There were 800 patients in Bellevue Hospital when the inspection took place, each nurse had 30 or 40 patients under her care, and there were no night nurses—three night watchmen being employed who visited the wards in turn, and gave any essential attention.

A member of the Medical Staff, Dr Gill Wylie, visited Europe in order to study the nursing reforms that were then developing. He made Miss Nightingale's acquaintance and obtained much

351

valuable advice from her. Meanwhile, the Committee of Bellevue Hospital were exploring the possibilities and collecting funds for the establishment of a training school and a nurses' home. In May, 1873, the school was started with twenty-nine applicants for training. Many proved unsuitable, and some found the work uncongenial. Only six completed the full training, and the first among this number to receive a diploma as a graduate nurse was Miss Linda Richards.

The training school was commenced under the superintendency of an Englishwoman known as Sister Helen,[1] who was a member of the All Saints' Sisterhood. She had undergone a period of training at University College Hospital, London, and thoroughly understood the principles and ideals of the Nightingale Scheme. She had had subsequent experience of many kinds of nursing, including that carried out in hospitals, workhouse infirmaries, the poor homes of patients, and in connection with the Franco-Prussian War. She went over to America to work with a mission, and was at Baltimore at the time when she offered her services to the Bellevue Hospital. She accomplished a marvellous pioneer work, but she returned to England broken in health in 1876. However, she recovered, and afterwards nursed in African wars. She died at All Saints' House; and to her is accorded the honour, as the result of her reorganisation of Bellevue, of having founded the first secular training school for nurses in America.

Connecticut.

Six months after the commencement of nurse training at Bellevue, the New Haven Hospital at Connecticut started a school with three pupils. Very soon the number was extended to eight, and after two years' training and experience the nurses were employed for private work. In 1879 the doctors and nurses at this hospital compiled and published a textbook for the guidance and instruction of its probationers.

[1]Miss Helen Bowden.

352

This school was organised by medical men, and in that respect it differs from other early schools of nursing, which were the results of the work of women's committees.

Massachusetts.

The Massachusetts General Hospital (the Boston Hospital) started its training school a month later than the Connecticut hospital, on 1st November, 1873. This was opened under the direction of a woman named Mrs Billings, who had had charge of a hospital during the Civil War. She was not a nurse, so she went to Bellevue to work under Sister Helen for two months before taking charge of the new training school; but even after that special training, her stay at the Boston Hospital was very short, for she left three months after commencing her duties. Her successor remained for ten months. Naturally, with these somewhat rapid changes, the school was not proving an unqualified success; but the next Superintendent was Miss Linda Richards from Bellevue, who, on the completion of her first year had been appointed night sister at her training hospital. She reorganised the Boston Training School, and during the two and a half years that she was in control it reached a very high standard for the times.

Miss Linda Richards is said to be America's 'first trained nurse' for, although five other women completed the course with her at Bellevue, she was the first to receive a diploma and to hold a professional appointment as a qualified American nurse. After leaving Boston she studied nursing conditions and training in England. Later, she accomplished a remarkable work in regard to the adaptation of training school methods to the hospitals for the insane in America.

Philadelphia.

Nine years after the establishment of the training school at Bellevue, two nurses trained at St Thomas's Hospital under the Nightingale Scheme—Miss Alice Fisher and Miss Horner—

undertook the reorganisation of the old 'Blockley' Hospital, now the Philadelphia General Hospital. The reformation of these two important and well-known hospitals, together with changes that were developing as the result of the introduction of anæsthesia and antiseptics into surgical work, set the stage for a new era of professional nursing in America, and during the next twenty years more than two hundred Nurse Training Schools were established in the United States. In this reformation Bellevue Hospital was to the States what St Thomas's Hospital was to England—a centre from which radiating influences, through the persons of its trainees, spread into numerous other hospitals and institutions, introducing a new standard of theoretical and practical nursing.

Visiting Nursing. The Victorian Order.

In 1877 a movement started at Bellevue which resulted in an extensive organisation of visiting nurses. It spread into Boston, Philadelphia and Chicago, until, in 1897, it gave rise in Canada to the Victorian Order of Nurses. It was inaugurated by Lady Aberdeen, the wife of the Governor-General at that time, and it was the Canadian memorial of the Diamond Jubilee of Queen Victoria. The whole scheme was on the plan of the Jubilee Institute, but with a few necessary alterations which rendered it better fitted for Canada. The one outstanding difference was that, whereas in England no fees were asked, in Canada a small charge was made wherever this could be met by the patients. A characteristic of the Order was that it was founded on a national basis, having local centres which were connected with a central authority at Ottawa. As with Mrs Fry's Nursing Sisters in England it provided private nurses for people of moderate means, as well as visiting nurses for the poorer people.

The wife of each succeeding Governor-General is recognised as the head of the Order, and each nurse must be a graduate of a hospital training school approved by the executive council. After her graduation she must undergo a special course of training in district nursing. Upon the recommendation of the Chief Superintendent of the Order she is given a diploma, and also a medal which she is expected to wear during her service. The standard of nursing has always been high, and since 1921 the Order has granted scholarships to nurses enrolled for public health courses in the provincial universities. A considerable expansion of its activities took place as a result of the establishment of Lady Grey's 'Country District Nursing Scheme' in 1909. This supplied trained nurses to the homesteads, ranches and farms lying many miles from the towns, where distances were too great to permit of daily visits being paid. In 1919 the Department of Indian Affairs asked the Order to undertake district nursing for the Indians of three provinces. They numbered about sixty thousand, and the staff of nurses needed to be considerably increased to meet this extended demand for their services.

The Order is now, primarily, a Public Health Nursing organisation. Its activities include pre-natal and maternity work, post-natal care up to school age, school nursing, work in First Aid stations, and industrial nursing. Its members give classes in home nursing, assist in travelling clinics for dental care, ophthalmic conditions, and treatments for enlarged tonsils and adenoids. They also work in tuberculosis dispensaries; and they help in the Juvenile Courts and in relief work in all kinds of calamities and disasters.

Organisation, and University Affiliation.

A new standard of nursing education was introduced by the opening of the Training School in connection with the Johns Hopkins Hospital at Baltimore in 1890. In this school great emphasis was laid upon the intellectual aspect of nursing training and of hospital work. The President of the Trustees, Mr King, came over to England to discuss its organisation with Miss Nightingale. The first Superintendent of the Johns Hopkins Training School was Miss Isabel Hampton, afterwards Mrs Hampton Robb. Nine years previously she had undergone the

355

prescribed training at Bellevue Hospital, after which she had gained experience in the States and in Rome. Under her leadership the Johns Hopkins Training School formed an Alumnæ Society that was destined to set a standard of 'team organisation' to the American nursing world. Bellevue and the Illinois Training Schools had formed similar societies several years previously; but the Johns Hopkins Alumnæ Society was organised on less rigid lines, which allowed for its growth and expansion. Each successive class of graduates entered as a group. It was similar to the Nurses Leagues of the English hospitals in that it was entirely self-governing and made for unity amongst all the post-graduates of the same school. Such societies became a very definite characteristic of American Training Schools, and laid the foundation of national organisation long before such development had actually been planned. They helped the nurse to work for her school and her fellow nurses, but, as they did not bring her into the broader field by association with alumnæ societies of other hospitals, their danger lay in tending to make nurses self-centred with regard to their own training school. Many leaders saw this danger, and in 1896 the young alumnæ societies were united into a national body under the title of 'The Nurses' Associated Alumnæ of the United States and Canada', with Mrs Hampton Robb as its first President.

Although, since 1901, the American and Canadian nurses have been separately organised, the development of nursing into a State-recognised profession in America and Canada was largely due to the work of this Association. Since 1911 it has been known as the American Nurses' Association.

Affiliation with the Columbia University.

Mrs Hampton Robb was succeeded at the Johns Hopkins Hospital by Miss Adelaide Nutting, and when, in 1898, it was proposed to take steps to bring about some affiliation of nurse training schools with universities, for the purpose of arranging an advanced course in teaching and hospital administration for

356

which a recognised degree or diploma might be conferred, these two ladies were the leaders in the movement.

In conjunction with Dean Russell and Miss Kinne, of Teachers' College connected with the Columbia University of New York City, they founded the 'Department of Nursing and Health' and worked out a plan for a suitable post-graduate course. In this course, the first series of lectures on 'History of Hospitals and Nursing' was given by Miss Nutting herself in 1901.

Three years after its inception an endowment fund of 100,000 dollars was raised, in order that the cost of the scheme together with the salaries of the lecturers and instructors might be guaranteed. The course was then extended to two years. In 1907 Miss Nutting left the Johns Hopkins Hospital to take charge of Nursing Education at Teachers' College, and two years later she was elected to the newly instituted chair of 'Institutional Management' in connection with the Columbia University. In the same year the University of Texas gave a professorial chair of Nursing.

One marked result of University affiliation was the raising of the required standard of theoretical knowledge and the extension of hospital training in America to three years. This intellectual development did not proceed entirely unopposed. In particular, medical men seemed alarmed at such progress of nursing along an unexpected channel, and at a meeting at the New York Academy of Medicine in 1906 there was a discussion on 'The Overtrained Nurse'. Following this, a number of protests were made against the higher education of nurses; but the progress continued nevertheless.

The Minnesota Scheme.

In some medical quarters this development was welcomed. An article by Dr Richard Beard of the Minnesota Hospital University, on 'The University Education of the Nurse', was read, in 1909, in the States and in London. In the following year his scheme, with slight modifications, was put into practice. It involved a pre-nursing course of two years at the Minnesota University, followed by two years' experience in practical work in different hospitals combined with a certain amount of academic work. In the fifth year, general and specialised instruction was given; and on the satisfactory completion of the five years' course, and the attainment of the required standard of knowledge and skill, a Bachelor's Degree in Nursing was conferred.

The School of Nursing at Yale University, Connecticut.

The Rockefeller Foundation gave a fund to establish an independent school of nursing at the Yale University in 1924, and when this had proved its worth by the results of its first five years' work it received an endowment of a million dollars from the Foundation, which has done, and is still doing, a world-wide work in Public Health. This school is probably the best known of all the University Schools of Nursing in the world. Dean Annie W. Goodrich was its founder and head, and under her administration and direction it reached its present eminence. She has now retired, and, as Dean Emeritus, she still plays a very influential part in all developments in nursing education not only in America, but, through the medium of the International Council of Nurses, throughout the nursing world.

Affiliation with Other Universities.

Other American universities which have established courses in teaching and hospital administration are the Temple University of Philadelphia and the Marquette University; and there are about forty-five universities in the United States which give full courses in nursing. These schools are an integral part of the university itself.

In Canada a five years' course similar to that of the Minnesota University was introduced at the University of British Columbia, Vancouver, in 1919. The student may enter at the age of seventeen, and having successfully completed the course she is awarded the degree of B.A. in Applied Science

(Nursing), and also the certificate of the hospital school in which she obtained her practical experience.

Later Developments.

In 1925 Miss Nutting was succeeded as Professor of Nursing of Columbia University by Miss Isabel Stewart, who is a Canadian woman trained at Winnipeg General Hospital. She graduated from Teachers' College and became assistant to Miss Nutting. In 1923 she was elected Associate Professor, and she is a prominent member of the Educational Committee of the International Council of Nurses. It has often been stated that, although England leads the world in practical nursing matters, America has the higher academic standing. There is now, however, in America, a sharp distinction between 'nursing training' and 'education in nursing'; the latter including a wide scientific background for the nursing technique.

Another nursing development in the United States is the initiation of training schools for American-Indian nurses, and also for American-Negro nurses. These are under the superintendency and general administrative control of white nurses. The coloured women often make excellent nurses and they have met with great success, particularly in nursing the members of their own races. They have formed their own National Associations.

The American Red Cross.

In the Civil War of 1861–1865 the conditions under which the wounded were tended were much the same as those existing at the Crimea during the previous decade when Miss Nightingale set out from England. Women nurses went to the army hospitals to give what help they could, and Miss Dix made a gallant effort to organise them into a regular service. She was appointed Superintendent of Female Nurses in the first year of the war, but such an appointment was entirely without precedent in the United States and therefore her authority and her duties were not clearly defined. During the peaceful years that followed no

359

organisation of nurses for war service was undertaken, and the United States did not, at first, join the Red Cross Societies, refusing to sign the Convention of Geneva in 1866, and again in 1867.

The first move towards inaugurating Red Cross work took place in 1881, when Miss Clara Barton, who had nursed through the whole of the Civil War and had seen the work of the Red Cross in other armies during the war of 1870, organised a Red Cross Committee in the United States and incorporated the district of Columbia in it. She was its President, and it was designed to give help in all kinds of disasters and calamities—floods, earthquakes, fires, famines, massacres and epidemics—as well as in wars.

In March, 1882, the United States at last signed the Convention of Geneva, being the thirty-second power to join the Red Cross Societies. The work of the Red Cross Committee was then given official recognition. Miss Barton remained its President, and it found abundant scope for its energies in the forest fires, floods, droughts and yellow fever epidemics which occurred during the years following its organisation.

First Organisation for War Service.

The Spanish-American War was declared in April, 1898. At the beginning of this war the nursing was done by men orderlies of the Hospital Corps that had been inaugurated about 1887. These men were given a certain amount of instruction and training by the officers, but on the outbreak of hostilities their number had to be tremendously increased, and the new men were given no nursing training at all. Women helpers were introduced by Dr Anita Newcomb McGee, but, in the absence of efficient organisation and the hurry and confusion of unexpected happenings, volunteer nurses who chanced to be at hand were sent into camps with very little investigation of their credentials or their state of health. Moreover, many women who knew little or nothing of nursing were given posts of responsibility in military hospitals. Some, because of their natural gifts and their common sense, filled these posts excellently; but there were many who were quite unsuited to such responsibility, and, naturally, there were numerous regrettable occurrences. In order to meet this difficulty, Dr McGee suggested that a committee be formed from the National Society of the Daughters of the American Revolution (D.A.R.), of which she was a Vice-President, for the purpose of scrutinising all applications received, and selecting from them suitable nurses for both the army and the navy. Thereafter, only nurses who had graduated from a recognised training school, and could supply evidence of good health and character, were accepted. Nearly 1,600 nurses were appointed by this Committee, with consequent general improvement in the care of the sick and wounded both in the camps and the military hospitals.

After the conclusion of the war Dr McGee formed an unofficial organisation from these nurses. She was herself their President, and in 1901 they were given a recognised status as the 'Nurse Corps of the Army', the name being changed in 1918 into the 'Army Nurse Corps'. The Navy Nurse Corps was started in 1908, with Miss Esther Hasson as its first Superintendent.

Reorganisation of the American Red Cross.

The experiences during the Spanish-American War stressed the need for much better preparation and considerable extension of the work of the American Red Cross if it were to be in a position to cope efficiently with the hospital administration and nursing that might be required in a future war. The existing organisation was, therefore, dissolved by Act of Congress in 1905, and a new Red Cross Society was formed which was incorporated under Government supervision.

In 1909 representatives of the nursing organisations, including the Army Corps, met the Red Cross officials for the purpose of discussing plans for organising Red Cross nursing on a sound basis; and in December of that year the Red Cross War Relief

Board appointed a Central Committee on Nursing Service under the chairmanship of Miss Jane Arminda Delano. Ten nurses were appointed to serve on this committee, and its purpose was well expressed in the *Red Cross Bulletin* for October of that year, in the following words:

'The whole system of the Regular Army Nursing Corps and the Red Cross Nursing Corps will be placed under one head, so that in case of war the plans for Red Cross nursing assistance will fall into complete accord with the demands of the Army Medical Service. Miss Delano will, therefore, be not only fully advised as to the regular strength of the army corps, but will know exactly the status of the Volunteer aid of the Red Cross Nursing Corps.'

The general plan, as worked out by Miss Delano and her Committee, involved the formation of a branch of the Red Cross in each State, which included the leading nurses of that State, and was charged with the enrolment of its own nurses.

Under the conditions of the reorganised Society the American Red Cross *Nursing Service* is composed of fully trained graduate nurses only; whilst the American Red Cross *Society* is an organisation of lay persons—chiefly men—who help in times of disaster or national need. Before the World War its members numbered 500,000. During the War their number rose to 20 million, and it was the greatest army of relief workers ever mobilised; but since then the membership has decreased with the lessened need for their services. When America entered the Great War the Navy Nurse Corps had 165 members. Before the Armistice this had risen to 1285. The Army Nurse Corps reached ten thousand in number, and one-third of its members served overseas.

Jane Arminda Delano and the Work of the American Red Cross.

Jane Arminda Delano accomplished such a marvellous work in connection with Red Cross Nursing Service of America that the inclusion of some account of her life and activities would seem to be justified. She was born in New York in 1862, and whilst she was still in her infancy her father, a soldier in the Civil War, died whilst on a march to New Orleans. After her own school days she taught in a district school for a year or two, and then she entered Bellevue Hospital Training School, graduating in 1886. Two years later she volunteered for emergency nursing in Florida during a severe epidemic of yellow fever, and in the next year she worked in a mining camp in Arizona, organising a hospital and nursing the women and children during an epidemic of scarlet fever. Then for six years she was the Superintendent of Nurses at the University of Pennsylvania Hospital in Philadelphia. She afterwards studied medicine for a short time at the University of Buffalo, took a course in Civics and Philanthropy at the New York School and became Superintendent of the Girls' Department on Randall's Island—a house of refuge. After two years amongst these girls she returned to Bellevue Hospital as Superintendent of Nurses. So that, by the time she undertook the enrolment of nurses from every part of the United States under the newly constructed Red Cross scheme, she was a woman of wide experience.

She died at the Base Hospital, No. 69, Savenay, France, whilst on a tour of inspection: after having been operated upon several times for mastoiditis. Her death occurred on 15th March, 1919, and she was buried in the War cemetery for American soldiers at Savenay. Later, her body was taken to America and entered its last resting place among the ever-increasing army of the nations' illustrious dead in the beautiful Arlington.

The Delano Red Cross Nursing Service.

This was established by the will of Miss Delano, which provided a fund of 25,000 dollars to supply nurses to districts which were unable to afford Public Health work. It sends nurses to the mountains of North Carolina, to Alaska, to islands off the coast of Maine, to the Virginia mountains and to Idaho.

Other Activities of the American Red Cross.

As in England, the work of the American Red Cross extends far beyond the provision of proper care for the sick or wounded soldier in time of war. It includes the teaching of home nursing and hygiene, the organisation of Public Health services and the relief of distress from any cause.

Red Cross Town and Country Nursing Service.

This really commenced in 1912 when the Red Cross undertook to establish a nursing service for rural districts. Its purpose was not only to provide nurses for the sick, but to teach sanitation and hygiene in the homes of the people, and to endeavour to improve living conditions in the small villages and on the lonely farms of the country. It was under the direction of Miss Fanny F. Clement. It met a very great need and it has developed into an important work for which there is a rapidly increasing demand. It is now known as the Public Health Nursing Service of the Red Cross.

364

CHAPTER VIII

REFORMS IN MIDWIFERY AND MATERNITY NURSING

Short summary of history of midwifery—Development of midwifery training in England—The Midwives' Institute—The Midwives Act of 1936, and the establishment of a State Midwifery Service

IN Christian countries before the Reformation midwives were licensed by the bishops and worked under the control of the Church; but they were not given training or education for this work. It is generally conceded that most of the continental countries of Europe made much further progress in obstetrics during the sixteenth century than did England. As evidence of this we find that an ordnance for the direction of midwives was issued in Ratisbon,[1] Germany, as early as 1555; and a few years later, in 1580, a law was passed in Germany forbidding shepherds and herdsmen from attending midwifery cases. In Belgium and Russia a training extending over two or three years was considered necessary long before either training or qualifications were required in England. Austria also demanded that midwives should undergo some instruction and practical training before being allowed to practice.

In the first part of the nineteenth century midwifery shared in the very low standard of other branches of nursing in all countries, and the maternal mortality was very great. In 1846 it was estimated that 25 per cent of the mothers died who were admitted into the wards of the General Lying-in Hospital in London. The figure was just as high in other European hos-

[1]Now known as Regensburg.

365

pitals, and maternity wards were considered to be veritable death traps. The majority of the deaths were from puerperal sepsis, and the precise nature of this condition was quite unknown until 1843, when Oliver Wendell Holmes read a paper before the Boston 'Society for Medical Improvement', in which he stressed the infectious character of the malady.

Three years later, Ignaz Philip Semmelweiss, who was Assistant Physician at the Maternity Hospital at Vienna, observed that the death rate in the wards where students delivered was rarely under 12 per cent and often much higher, whereas in the wards where only midwives worked the mortality was barely 3 per cent. He found that the students were coming directly from the postmortem room and attending to the mothers without even washing their hands. He, therefore, insisted that not only should they thoroughly scrub their hands but should soak them in a solution of chlorinated lime. In a month the death rate had fallen to 3 per cent, and later it was reduced to 1 per cent. However, both these men encountered great opposition from their colleagues when they published their findings that the disease was conveyed from without, and made the suggestion that doctors were themselves carrying fatal infection to their midwifery patients.

Development of Midwifery Training in England.

After the establishment of the Training School for Nurses at St Thomas's Hospital in 1860, Miss Nightingale's next experiment was in connection with the training of midwives; and again she worked through an existing hospital—King's College Hospital. This training was started in October, 1861, and apparently, it worked successfully for a period of six years, but owing to a very serious epidemic of puerperal sepsis in 1868, it had to be adandoned. It must be remembered that, at this time, the principles of antisepsis had not been generally accepted, and the theories of Holmes and Semmelweiss had not definitely influenced obstetrical work in England.

Statistics of mortality from childbirth were then collected

from foreign countries as well as England, and it was found that the death rate was much greater in lying-in wards than in home deliveries.

In 1870 the London Obstetrical Society passed a resolution requiring the examination of midwives. In the following year Miss Nightingale published a small book entitled *Introductory Notes on Lying-in Hospitals* (Longmans, Green & Co., 1871, Octavo, p. 110). In this she included the collected statistics, and also a proposed scheme for organising an institution for the training of midwives and maternity nurses.

The first examination of midwives arranged by the London Obstetrical Society took place in 1872, and a certificate was given to those who had taken the prescribed training and had attended twenty-five labours.

The Midwives' Institute.

This Institute was founded in 1881 with the object of raising the standard of midwifery and the general status of midwives, but it was not until 1902 that the first Midwives Act was passed. The Central Midwives Board was then created in order to administer this Act. One of its important conditions was the prohibition, after a few years' interval, of the practice of midwifery by unregistered women. The Central Midwives Board was required to keep a Roll of certified midwives, and to regulate the conditions of their certification and practice. It entrusted the local supervision of midwives to Councils of Counties and County Boroughs, who became known as the Local Supervising Authorities. The Central Midwives Board worked, nominally, under the Privy Council and not under the Local Government Board. The Act of 1902 came into full operation on 1st April, 1910; and from that date it became an offence against the law for any woman not qualified, in accordance with the rules and regulations laid down under the Act, to attend women in confinement 'habitually and for gain'. When, in 1918, the second Midwives Act was passed it became the duty of the midwife to call a doctor herself when, in accordance with the rules of the Central Midwives Board, this was necessary. Hitherto, she was merely required to advise the patient's relatives to send for medical aid. In the following year, when the Ministry of Health was formed, the Central Midwives Board passed from the control of the Privy Council to that of the new Ministry.

Although the Act of 1918 was designed to secure the better training of midwives and to regulate their practice, much yet remained to be done in order that the hazard and uncertainty of childbirth should be decreased, and also the burden of disability and invalidism due to lack of knowledge, absence of preparation and facilities for the birth, and insufficient or unskilled medical or midwifery attention. It was realised that the maintenance of an efficient midwifery service was not only a medical and nursing duty, it was of paramount biological importance, and constituted a social, economic and administrative problem which it behoved the State itself to solve. But the solution could never be achieved merely by improved management of actual deliveries, for competent ante-natal and post-natal care was also necessary.

The Midwives' Act of 1936, and the Establishment of a State Midwifery Service.

To meet the great modern need, a new and much more comprehensive Midwives' Act was passed in 1936. A very important and far-reaching provision of this Act was that the State should organise a service of salaried midwives who should be available to give ante-natal advice and instruction to all pregnant women, attend the actual deliveries whether a doctor had been engaged or not, and undertake the management and nursing for 14 days after the birth. Hitherto, the lying-in period had been considered as 10 days, and there was no definite rule that the nursing must be done by a qualified midwife. The new provision, therefore, eliminated the 'handy woman' who, although most useful for the domestic management during the housewife's lying-in, should not be allowed to take part in the nursing.

This Act is not yet in full operation, but, according to its conditions, the institution and control of such a service in each district will be carried out by the Local Supervising Authorities.

Other Provisions of the New Act.

As with all other reorganisations of existing services, the new conditions may involve some hardship for nurses who have been working for many years under the old scheme. In order to minimise such effects from the transition, the Act has provided for 'compensation', either in one sum, or in the form of an annuity, to be paid to midwives who are practising independently, or who do not wish to enter the salaried service, providing that they surrender their certificates before July, 1939. This will also apply to those who are ineligible, owing to age or infirmity, for appointment under the new scheme, or who, having accepted an appointment, wish to retire before July, 1939.

The Act also provides for a scheme of superannuation on a contributory basis, as in all other Government services.

One of the greatest advances in connection with the new midwifery service is the institution of compulsory post-graduate courses. The Act empowers the Central Midwives Board to embody in its Rules a clause that all practising midwives should attend such courses of instruction. It also requires that every Local Supervising Authority should provide, or arrange for the provision of, courses of instruction which will enable the midwives to comply with the Rules that may be laid down by the Central Midwives Board. These courses have been made obligatory in order that it shall be possible for all practising midwives to attend them; at least in the salaried service, the Local Supervising Authorities must arrange that the necessary time is available. The frequency and duration of the post-graduate courses have not yet been settled. A suggestion that they should be for one month in every five years, and be supplemented by local lectures and demonstrations is under consideration.

In this direction the midwifery profession is giving the world a very valuable lead, for no other profession has, as yet, instituted a compulsory refresher course. Great advances are taking place in midwifery; and this provision ensures the continued interest of the midwife and makes it possible for her to keep pace with the march of her particular science, and thus to be in a position to give the best possible service to the mothers of the country.

370

CHAPTER IX

PUBLIC HEALTH NURSING

Development of the Public Health idea—The growth of some of the special branches of Public Health Nursing: Ante-natal care—Child Welfare Work—The movement in America—The movement in England —The influence of Milk Depots on the Infant Welfare movement—Influence of further legislative measures—The work of a modern Child Welfare centre—Toddlers' clinics—Day nurseries—Nursery schools— School nursing—The National Insurance Act of 1911—Industrial nursing—Tuberculosis care—Conclusion

ALL the nursing developments in England which are described in the foregoing chapters aimed at providing proper care and attention for the sick person, but directed no consistent efforts towards the prevention of illness, either by teaching the principles of hygiene and sanitation in relation to the homes of the people and the avoidance of disease, or by legislative control of the conditions under which the majority of the poorer people worked in order to earn their living.

Various Commissions had been appointed during the first half of the nineteenth century for the purpose of investigating the administration of the Poor Law, the state of prisons and asylums, and the conditions under which the poor worked in factories, mines and brickfields. The Reports of these Commissions brought vividly before the public the terrible hardships and filthy conditions under which the greater number of the labouring classes lived. The investigations into the causes of local epidemics received a flood of light from the developing knowledge of the relation between the unhygienic conditions and the spread

371

of infectious diseases, and this made it quite apparent that epidemics were, for the most part, preventable.

Slowly it dawned upon the minds of legislators, social reformers and all the intelligent section of the community that the problems had, hitherto, been attacked from the wrong standpoint. A social organisation which allowed the development of ill-health and then attempted to cope with disease by the building of large hospitals, the training of doctors and nurses, and the inauguration of medical and nursing services for the sick was certainly not an ideal state of affairs. It was a confession of the country's failure to promote and maintain the health of its people.

When once this idea had been firmly grasped the movement for the development of public health made rapid strides. The first epoch-making event was the passing of the Public Health Act of 1848, which resulted in the establishment of a General Board of Health with the power to form Local Boards throughout the kingdom and to enforce various measures for the protection of the health of the public.

Most of the activities of the Boards were, for many years, chiefly concerned with improving living conditions by the removal of refuse and excreta, the provision of pure water supplies and the improvement of housing conditions generally. In industry, measures were enforced to ensure proper ventilation of factories and workshops, and to mitigate the evil effects of dust and poisonous gases produced by certain manufacturing and trade processes. A limit was placed upon the number of hours a person might be employed each week, and also upon the age of employees. But none of these measures could be really effective in the prevention of disease unless the people themselves did their part in following the laws pertaining to hygiene and sanitation. Their greatest danger lay in their ignorance, and in order to combat this the Public Health nurse was evolved. Her mission is to care for the people before illness makes its appearance, and to carry such a message of health into homes and schools and work-

372

shops as will result in the building up of strong and effective bodies having the power to resist the onslaught of disease. This is an infinitely greater ideal than to attempt to render life endurable after health is lost, although it is accompanied by much less limelight and none of the dramatic thrill attendant upon helping a patient back from the very jaws of death, or assisting at an operation which constitutes one of the marvels of present day surgery.

It is not the purpose of this book to follow, in detail, all the steps in the development of Public Health Nursing from its inception to its present all-pervading sphere of activity. It can but give a brief outline of the manner in which the Public Health services are striving to promote and conserve the health of the individual from the time of conception to the extreme limits of old age; for there are branches of these services to meet the needs of human life in all its stages. These include ante-natal care and maternity services, infant welfare work, health visiting, school nursing, industrial nursing, and special clinics for such diseases as tuberculosis, rheumatism and venereal diseases. There is scope for still further extension of this work, for example, in the introduction of more nursery schools, or the inclusion of 'toddlers' clinics' at infant welfare centres. These would assist in the supervision of the healthy development of the child between two and five years of age.

The Growth of Some of the Special Branches of Public Health Nursing. Ante-Natal Care.

Although not the first of the Public Health Services to be initiated, ante-natal care takes precedence in regard to ensuring the health of the individual. This work was first started, in Great Britain, by Dr Ballantyne of Edinburgh in 1906; and at a National Congress on infant mortality held during that year in Caxton Hall, Westminster, a paper was read that had been prepared by him on 'Ante-natal Causes of Infant Mortality, including Parental Alcoholism'. He urged that many of these causes

373

were preventable, but that prevention must begin with the protection of the unborn infant. He claimed that this resolved itself, almost completely, into the hygiene of the pregnant woman and the treatment of her diseases. He laid stress on the need for more knowledge of the physiology of pregnancy, and the importance of detecting errors in diet, exercise, clothing, personal hygiene and surroundings, in order that these might be corrected sufficiently early to prevent their ill-effects. This was essentially work for which the nurse, as well as the doctor, was indispensable.

The care of the mother during labour had long been recognised as of great importance, and the establishment of a Board to regulate the training and certification of nurses in midwifery did much to improve the maternity nursing services, but it was realised that this was not, in itself, sufficient to ensure the maximum diminution of maternal mortality, the disabilities following childbirth, the number of neo-natal deaths and the proportion of weak and ill-developed babies among the poorer classes. The importance of ante-natal care can hardly be exaggerated if healthy nfants are to be born to mothers who will not suffer from any after effects of pregnancy and parturition, and an energetic educational campaign was initiated in order to convince prospective mothers of the necessity for watchful care and thorough examination during the months preceding birth. At first, this campaign was carried out from Child Welfare Centres; thus the ante-natal care was available for the second, although not the first, child; which was rather an unsatisfactory service to the community. Now, however, as a result of the teaching of mothercraft in schools, the wider and saner education in sex processes and the knowledge disseminated by health talks and literature, all intelligent young people have a better understanding, at the time of their marriage, of the facts relating to the production of a family, and they are anxious to do their best for the promotion of their own health and that of their children. Some localities have established 'Fathers' Clinics', and these are often very well attended by enthusiastic young men anxious to understand and to co-operate with their wives in the important duties of parenthood.

At the ante-natal clinic the prospective mother is taught how to regulate her diet in order to supply all the essential constituents both for herself and for her developing child, and at the same time avoid an undue strain upon her own excretory organs. She is instructed in the general hygiene of pregnancy, the adaptation of her clothing to her changing figure, and the importance of fresh air and sunlight. She is encouraged to take walks until the last month, when walking will be uncomfortable, and she is taught simple physical exercises designed to develop her abdominal muscles; for these are valuable factors in promoting a comfortable pregnancy and a safe delivery. She undergoes a routine physical examination in order that any abnormal condition shall be recognised, and corrected wherever possible.

However, even with the introduction of such ante-natal services, it soon became evident that there was still more to be done before a satisfactory stage was reached, for although the intelligent and careful woman would attend these clinics regularly, her more ignorant and feckless sister was still running many avoidable risks. It was obvious that a system of home visiting was required, and that this must be carried out by women who had not only undergone specialised training for the work of Health Visiting or District Midwifery, but who were possessed of sympathy and tact, a love of children and definite teaching ability.

Neither the District Midwife nor the Health Visitor has a right of entry into the homes of the people, and although, in order to be really useful, she must gain some knowledge of environmental conditions, she must avoid giving the impression that she is 'inspecting' the home. She must approach the prospective mother in a friendly spirit, and gain her invitation into the home because she is recognised as a friend and a helper. It is not usually difficult for a nurse to gain the confidence of a young wife, and even when attendance at an ante-natal clinic is not possible—owing

375

to distance, for example, for not all localities have initiated such a service—the District Midwife can give all the necessary advice both with regard to the pregnancy and the preparation for the confinement.

When the new State Midwifery Service, to be developed under the provisions of the Midwives Act of 1936, the ante-natal advice and instruction will be given by the midwife who will attend the confinement and also be responsible for the nursing for fourteen days following the birth. She will, as under the provisions of the Act of 1915, notify the birth to the Medical Officer of Health, and from his department a notice will be sent to the Health Visitor for the district who is responsible for the Child Welfare work. Before leaving her patient, the midwife will endeavour to arouse the mother's interest in the work that is being done in the Child Welfare Clinics in her neighbourhood, and encourage her to attend them with her baby.

Child Welfare Work.

The honour of inaugurating the modern Child Welfare Service really belongs to France. The movement was especially directed towards the reduction of the devastating mortality amongst infants from summer, or epidemic, diarrhœa, and the subsequent heavy loss of potential citizens.

The first crèche had been established in 1844, by Firman Marbœuf. It was a result of the industrial development in France which led to the employment of married women in factories and workshops. French crèches soon became very numerous, but they were frequently in the charge of ignorant and incompetent women and many of them proved to be hot-beds of infection for summer diarrhœa.

A dispensary for infants was opened at Havre by Dr Gebert in 1875. Its object was to provide medical treatment for sick babies without removing them from their homes to a residential institution. The little patients remained under the care of their

376

parents, so that the bond between parent and child could continue unbroken by a sojourn in hospital.

The originator of the modern infant welfare movement was Professor Pierre Budin. He became the chief of staff at the Maternitè Hôpital, Paris, in 1895, where he established a 'Consultation de Nourrissons'. The mothers of the babies born in the hospital were encouraged to bring their infants back at the end of a month from their confinement. The baby was weighed and examined, and the mother received a sum of money which varied with the progress made by her baby. About the same time Dr Dufour founded an institution called the 'Goutte de Lait', at Fécamp. It was not attached either to a hospital or a dispensary, and it was supported by voluntary contributions. Any mother might bring her baby, and according to her circumstances she was ranged in one of three sections—Gratuitous, Half-paying, Paying. Each infant had, for his sole use, two numbered baskets containing a set of bottles corresponding to the number of feeds he was to have in the twenty-four hours, and each bottle contained just sufficient for one meal, the quantity varying, of course, with the age of the child. Once a week the mother brought her baby to be weighed and medically examined.

The establishment of Consultations des Nourrissons and Gouttes de Lait rapidly extended through France during the last few years of the nineteenth century. Their objects were to keep all children under two years of age under regular supervision with weekly weighing and examination, to encourage breast feeding, and, where this was not possible, to provide specially prepared cows' milk for the infants.

The fundamental principle of Child Welfare work is that in order to help the baby the mother must be educated in childcare; and almost simultaneously with the development in France a 'School for Mothers' was established in Belgium. But, as with ante-natal care, the necessity for home visiting very soon became apparent. This was required for two reasons—to keep in touch with children who had been brought to the clinic and give advice with regard to improvements in home conditions where necessary, and also to find out what was happening in the homes from which the children did not attend the clinics. Thus, another very wide field of activity opened up for the Public Health Nurse.

The Movement in America.

The improvement in methods of artificial feeding was an essential element in the prevention of infant mortality, and the success of the work in France attracted the attention of milk reformers in America, who were at that time investigating the contention that milk was a dangerous carrier of all the kinds of infection that proved the most fatal to infants. There were two schools of thought in America with regard to the best way of dealing with this problem. The leader of one was Dr Henry Leber Coit, the founder of the 'certified milk' movement. He and his followers held that if steps were taken to ensure that milk was obtained from healthy animals, and that it was effectively protected from contamination at all points between the cow and the consumer, 'raw' cows' milk was the best and most suitable article of diet for infants who had to be artificially fed. This movement aimed at placing on the market a supply of milk so pure that it could with confidence be given to infants and sick persons, for whom it was primarily intended; and to Dr Coit, as the originator and guiding influence in this movement, must be largely attributed the advances in clean milk production that have been made during the past thirty to forty years.

The other school, led by Mr Nathan Straus, contended that the possibility of infection was so great that pasteurisation of all milk intended as food for children was the only safe procedure, and therefore it should be made compulsory that all milk should be pasteurised. From this faction arose the Straus Milk Depots which started in New York and spread during the next few years to Chicago, Philadelphia, Rochester and other parts of the United States. Mr Straus claimed that the fall in infant mortality in New York during the next ten years was largely the result of the work at his depots, which not only had a direct effect upon the infants themselves but had an educational influence that led to improved methods in the feeding of children in the city generally.

The Movement in England.

The first milk depot in England was opened at St Helens in August, 1899, and at the end of the first year 140 babies were being fed on milk from this depot, at a charge of 2d. per day. Very soon Liverpool followed St Helens' example and the movement spread to many other towns throughout the British Isles. In London, the most active and progressive milk depot was at Battersea. As in France, the infants were fed directly from the bottle in which the milk was supplied, and that obviated the necessity for a feeding bottle, thus avoiding one fertile source of contamination.

Influence of Milk Depots on the Infant Welfare Movement.

The object of the milk depots was to instruct the mothers in the art of rearing healthy babies, but in the British milk depots the babies were not weighed or medically examined as in France. Instead, the mothers were supplied with printed instructions and they were visited by women sanitary inspectors, who worked on the same lines as the health visitors do now in endeavouring to ensure that the instructions were carried out.

The first International Congress devoted exclusively to Child Welfare was held in Paris in October, 1905. It was attended by all sixteen of the important European countries, the Argentine, Cuba, Brazil, Egypt and the United States; and this Congress proved to be a very important step in the development of child welfare work. One result was that in June of the following year the National Conference on Infant Mortality already mentioned in connection with ante-natal care, was held in the Caxton Hall, Westminster. One of the many important papers was read by Dr

Niven, of Manchester, on 'The Teaching in Schools of Elementary Hygiene in Reference to the Rearing of Infants'. He gave particulars of the work done by a trained nurse specially appointed for that purpose. Six lectures, with practical demonstrations, were given to the older girls in the elementary schools. Two were on washing and dressing a baby, two on infant feeding and two on the general managements of babies. The results were tested by examination.

Influence of Further Legislative Measures.

The development of Child Welfare work was considerably helped about this time by the passing of two Acts of Parliament, the Notification of Births Act of 1907 and the Children's Act of 1909. The latter enabled legal action to be taken when children were neglected; and neglect and cruelty were interpreted as occurring when necessary medical treatment had been omitted, or when hygiene conditions were bad enough to be definitely detrimental to health. Local authorities and the inspectors of voluntary societies, such as the National Society for the Prevention of Cruelty to Children, were enabled to warn neglectful parents, and in extreme cases to take legal action for their punishment and for the removal of the children to a more satisfactory environment. The Notification of Births Act did not apply to the whole country, but only to those districts in which it had been adopted by the local authorities. It provided that the parent, in addition to registering the birth of his child within six weeks of its occurrence, should send a notification to the Medical Officer of Health within 36 hours of the birth.

This made early and systematic home visiting of infants practicable; and then, in 1915 another Act was passed which made the notification of a birth within 36 hours of its occurrence compulsory throughout the country, and also conferred upon Local Authorities statutory powers to make arrangements for the care of expectant mothers, nursing mothers, and young children. The visits of advice made after the birth of an infant gradually be-

380

came more general, and practical help was given wherever it was obviously needed. This might include a regular supply of milk or free meals for an expectant or nursing mother. All mothers were encouraged to bring their babies to an infant welfare centre, where medical advice was also available when required.

A good deal of health visiting was done by voluntary workers in the early part of this century, especially in Salford, Manchester and Huddersfield, but gradually it has been taken over by qualified women who have undergone specialised training in Public Health Nursing and who understand the management of healthy as well as sick children. A further impetus was given to the work by the passing of the Maternity and Child Welfare Act of 1918. This authorised Treasury grants for the extension of these public health services; and then in the following year the Local Government Board was merged into the newly established Ministry of Health. All forms of public health work have progressed continuously since that date.

The Work in a Modern Child Welfare Centre.

The Centre is under the control of a doctor, usually a woman, assisted by one or more Public Health nurses. Following the reception of the notification of a birth, the department of the Medical Officer of Health sends a notice to the Public Health nurse, and she visits the home as soon after the conclusion of the midwife's visits as possible. She gives what advice appears necessary and invites the mother to bring her baby to the clinic. Here, the doctor sees the baby on the first visit, and at regular intervals subsequently. The nurse weighs the babies, gives individual advice to the mothers and group-teaching by means of short 'health talks' on how to keep well, on the best kinds of food and clothing for children of all ages, or on making the best use of housekeeping money. Classes are held in such subjects as sewing, cooking and home nursing, and there are special clinics for dental care, artificial sunlight treatment, remedial exercises, and other examinations and treatments that are found to be necessary.

Toddlers' Clinics.

The weakest point in health supervision at the present time is that in relation to the child between the age of two and five years. After the introduction of school nursing services it was found that at least 16 per cent of the children admitted to elementary schools were suffering from defects or diseases which had developed since babyhood. These included carious teeth, enlarged tonsils and adenoids, various manifestations of rickets and tuberculosis, ophthalmic conditions, diseases of the ear, nose and throat, and skin conditions. Many of these defects could have been detected and corrected much earlier if there had been adequate supervision during the pre-school years. This was emphasised in a circular issued in December, 1929, by the Ministry of Health in conjunction with the Board of Education (circular 1054). It commenced with the bold statement that 'the State made itself responsible for the health and education of all children from the age of five onwards', and then proceeded to point out that, for three or four years before going to school, hundreds of thousands of children 'have no help, direction or succour from public sources, however much they may need it'. It stressed the conclusion that 'it is grossly uneconomic to allow the health and stamina of infants to deteriorate until five years old, and then to spend large sums of money in trying to cure them between the ages of five and fifteen'.

Systematic health visitation can be invaluable in detecting abnormal conditions in these children and in arranging for treatment at a clinic or hospital. It was suggested that it might be possible to utilise school clinics for this purpose; but where special 'Toddlers' Clinics' could be introduced these would, quite obviously, be far more likely to meet the need of both the healthy and the physically defective child. Such clinics are now being developed throughout the country, and so also are nursery schools and toddlers' playgrounds. These are usually under the supervision of a health visitor, and they secure an open-air life for the child of the poor and over-worked mother.

A circular issued by the Minister of Health in May, 1936 (circular 1550) again draws attention to this need in the following words: 'The Minister is concerned to find that in many areas insufficient attention is being given to the health of young children between the ages of 18 months and 5 years'; and that many diseases and defects discovered when the child enters school 'could have been prevented from developing, or could have been quickly cured, if adequate supervision of the health of the children had been exercised during the pre-school years. . . .' 'It should be the duty of the Health Visitor to see these children at regular intervals, to make enquiries as to their state of health, and to be on the look-out for any signs or symptoms that suggest a departure from normal health. In all cases where there is ground for suspecting disease or defect, the mother should be advised to consult the family doctor, or to take the child to the appropriate clinic for medical examination, without delay.' It lays stress on the importance of continuity of supervision, concluding that 'the adequate supervision of the health of the pre-school child will be best secured if the responsibility for attending to the health of children, from birth up to school-leaving age, is concentrated in the hands of one and the same authority'. An alternative to this might be the linking up of Maternity and Child Welfare services with that of the Education Authorities by the passing on of records concerning each individual child, and the maintenance of the continuity of these records.

Day Nurseries.

The modern Day Nursery receives children from the age of three months to five years, and often from 7 a.m. till 5 p.m. Each child is carefully examined upon admission and no ailing child is allowed to stay. Especially does this rule apply to a child with a heavy cold, for the spread of infection must always be guarded against as far as possible. The children are bathed and fed, and the nursery provides a very happy routine of play, meals and sleep which is often followed by considerable improvement in health and spirits. Usually the mother pays for the cost of food, but the rest of the expense of these nurseries is borne by the rates.

The Nursery School.

In a Nursery School the children usually come after breakfast, and the school may be for mornings only, or for the whole day; the children being provided with a mid-day meal. The age for admission may be two or three years, and these schools often accept children from a different social class; fees being paid according to the type of school and the ability of the parents to meet the financial demands.

Gradually, in England, the partial gap between the infant welfare centre and the school medical inspection and nursing is being filled up, and when this is finally effected it is felt that the hygienic or preventive side of the school medical work can be more fully developed because its clinical activities will be greatly lessened.

The Polish Factory Crèches.

In Poland there is an interesting co-operation between the Child Welfare and the Industrial Nursing Service. In every factory which employs a hundred women it is compulsory, by Law, to establish a crèche where a mother may leave her young children during her working hours. These crèches are staffed by trained nurses, and the mothers are, therefore, quite relieved from anxiety with regard to the welfare of their infants; and it is claimed that the standard of their work has consequently improved.

School Nursing.

Elementary education became national in 1870, but school attendance was not compulsory until 1880; and then it was gradually realised that sickness was the chief cause of absence from school and of subsequent inefficiency in adult life. In 1892 an enquiry was instituted into the feeding of London school children, and during the investigations it was discovered that many of the children attending elementary schools were suffering from the neglect of minor ailments or injuries. Also, quite a number were present who were obviously unfit to attend because of some infectious or verminous condition. It was suggested that a nurse should be appointed to visit schools and attend to minor ailments before they became serious. This work started at a Board School in Wild Street, Drury Lane, London, and Miss Amy Hughes, who was at that time Superintendent of Queen's Nurses in Bloomsbury Square, undertook to carry out daily visiting at the school followed up by home visiting. The children attending this school were among the poorest and most neglected in London.

Five years later the London School Nurses' Society was formed as a private charity; for, as with all the developments of public health work in this country, school nursing started as a voluntary effort as the outcome of local, not central, initiative. But the forthcoming subscriptions to the Society were entirely inadequate to cope with school nursing in such a vast city as London, which had nearly five hundred elementary schools; for it could afford to employ only five nurses. Each nurse was able to visit about four schools in one day and to examine or give nursing treatments to about one hundred children. This constituted a very heavy day's work, for only children who were obviously in need of the nurse's attentions were sent in by the teachers. Among the conditions treated were suppurating ears, infected cuts or abrasions, inflamed eyes, skin diseases, and verminous heads and clothing. In spite of financial difficulties the efforts met with great success and the nurses had so thoroughly demonstrated their usefulness that the work was taken over by the London County Council in 1904; and the School Nurses' Society was then dissolved.

During the industrial depression of 1906 an Education Act was passed that authorised the giving of food to insufficiently nourished children. This was followed in 1909 by the Education (Administrative Provisions) Act which imposed upon education committees the duty of providing for systematic medical inspection of all children, whether sick or well, as soon as possible after admission to an elementary school, and of providing treatment for those in need of it. This treatment was given in a school clinic when it could not be secured by the parents in any other way; for example, by attending at hospital out-patient clinics.

The Education Act of 1918 extended this duty of medical inspection, but without the provision of treatment, to all pupils in secondary or continuation schools. Subsequent Acts have amplified the provisions of those already mentioned, and the work of the School Nurse now affords steadily increasing employment to women who are genuinely interested in health problems among children of school age; for at the present time there are between 5,000 and 6,000 nurses working under the Education Authorities in this country. Some give their whole time to the school medical service whilst others include health visiting, following up the work of the school clinics in the homes of the children. In many rural districts school nursing is a part-time service of the District Nurse. In addition to the actual physical examination of the children and the giving of treatments, the teaching of practical hygiene is an important duty of the school nurse although the theoretical part of this subject is usually included in the general educational curriculum of the school.

The time is not far distant when the work done for infants, toddlers and school children will be a unified organisation, and then its scope will be greatly increased; but at the moment there is yet another hiatus in the health services. This affects the child between the age of leaving the elementary school—which has hitherto been fourteen but is now raised to fifteen—and the age of sixteen, when he or she comes under the health insurance scheme. During this time defects may develop which could have been checked by medical supervision, and by the time he comes under the medical care as an insured person his health and efficiency may be seriously impaired. If he enters a large industrial concern he will probably come under a medical service initiated by the firm for which he is working, but there is no guarantee that this will happen, and this still leaves a large section of the community unsupervised by a Public Health Service during an important period of life.

The National Insurance Act of 1911.

Although the provisions of this Act are essentially concerned with medical care and monetary benefits rather than with nursing developments, the establishment of a National Health Insurance has indirectly affected the scope of nursing work in many directions. The Act applies to all persons over the age of sixteen[1] who are employed in manual labour, and to all other employed persons whose income does not exceed £250 a year. Both the insured persons and their employers pay weekly contributions. At the age of 65 the insured person ceases to contribute. He, or she, is then entitled to an 'old age' pension, but not to sickness or disablement benefit; although the employer must still continue to pay his part of the contribution.

Under the National Scheme the insured person is entitled to medical attention and treatment, and also to sickness allowance and disablement benefit, and the wife of an insured person to maternity benefit. Therefore, not only is efficient medical care assured, but sickness of the worker no longer entails destitution, and this in itself is a great factor in promoting a better general standard of health throughout the country.

In 1928, another Act was passed which, in addition to modifications in other directions, extended the sickness insurance to some classes of workers who had not been included under the provisions of the Act of 1911.

[1]A recent amendment, which came into operation on January 1, 1938, has decreased this age to fourteen.

387

Industrial Nursing.

America claims to have led the way in Industrial Nursing, for as early as 1895 the Vermont Marble Company employed a nurse to visit the families of its employees; but by the end of the nineteenth century only two other firms in the United States had followed this example.

However, England appears to have an equal claim to have been first in the field. About the year 1875, a trained nurse named Philippa Flowerday was employed by Colman's Mustard Factory in Norwich, to supervise the health of its workers, and this precedent was followed by Cadbury's Chocolate Factory in 1897. But the development of industrial nursing is essentially a twentieth-century achievement. The Great War gave a tremendous impetus to the work, for it considerably increased the need for such a service; especially in munition factories where workers were prone to develop diseases as a result of chemical irritation, and where minor casualties were of frequent occurrence. Welfare departments were established in these, and in other factories which came under Government control, not only in Great Britain but in all belligerent countries. At first the efforts were directed, mainly, towards the reduction of the time lost by workers as a result of sickness or minor injuries, and the consequent waste of industrial energy involved by the absence of even one 'cog' in the human machinery.

Then it began to be realised that there was a very close relationship between the contentment and the health of the worker; and also that the success of a business enterprise depended, ultimately, upon the willing co-operation of individuals, which was the outcome of health, and of happiness in the human relationships, of all grades of employees.

Long hours, hasty and inappropriate meals, insufficient exercise, low wages, large families and unhygienic home conditions, are all factors which threaten the health of the individual. The

388

more progressive modern firms are fully alive to these considerations, and they have carried their health propaganda and service much further than actual statutory rules and orders demanded. Working conditions are rendered as healthy as possible, buffets and rest rooms are introduced, and facilities are provided for recreation and athletic training. Many firms arrange for an initial and a periodic medical examination of their workers. This does not, necessarily, mean that an applicant is rejected, or a worker discharged, because of some physical disability; but that he, or she, is given work in a suitable department. For example, a sedentary occupation may be found for an applicant when continued standing or running about would be too strenuous, or work in the open air when the confined space of a packing room would be injurious. In addition to this, some advice or treatment may be given which would result in a general improvement in the worker's physical or mental condition. In all these health organisations of modern industry, especially where there is a liability to develop certain industrial illnesses or diseases, the nurse has a very definite place. She is a Public Health nurse specialising in an industrial organisation; and she must be fully competent to render First Aid, and also to recognise early signs of a breakdown in health. In connection with the latter, she must be familiar with the manufacturing or chemical processes in the factory in which she works, especially when these are conducive to 'occupational disabilities'. She not only attends to casualties in her surgery but she carries out routine nursing, makes sanitary inspections, supervises health educational activities, and she may even be required to do some home visiting. She must be capable of keeping accurate and systematic records, particularly when the provisions of the Workmen's Compensation Act might operate; and she must be conversant with the aims and scope of organised social services, of unemployment and sickness insurance, and of Trade Unions. Another important science of which she needs some knowledge is Industrial Psychology, for it is now realised how great a part fatigue, boredom, monotony, or an uncongenial occupation play in the undermining of mental health.

At the present time over a thousand nurses are employed by British industrial firms, and, to meet the special needs of those who intend to take up this work, there has recently been established by the College of Nursing a full-time course of study covering a period of not less than nine calendar months. The subjects of study are: Health of the Industrial Worker; The Nursing Service in Industry; Psychology (general and applied); Principles and Administration of the Social Services; The Modern Industrial System; and First Aid in Chemical Warfare. Practical experience is gained at centres in London and in the provinces, and a certificate is awarded on the results of an examination together with satisfactory reports on practical work.

A part-time course, extending over a period of six months, has been arranged for nurses already employed in industry. This includes lectures on two evenings a week throughout the whole period, an interchange of practical work being arranged where possible.

Industrial nursing is the youngest branch of the Public Health Nursing Service, but it is an extremely important development, for the promotion and conservation of the health of the worker not only makes for the comfort and economic independence of the individual and the family, but also for national prosperity.

Tuberculosis Care.

Tuberculosis is a condition which brings, perhaps, more privation in its train than does any other disease. This privation affects not only the patient, but also his dependants; and therefore the disease is of grave economic, as well as of medical and nursing, importance.

Under the provisions of the Health Insurance Act of 1911, a great impetus was given to work in connection with the control of tuberculosis, a special 'benefit' being included in order that tuberculous insured persons might be enabled to undergo sanatorium treatment. The Tuberculosis Care Organisation does not now work under the provisions of this Act, for subsequent legislation—of 1912, 1921, 1924 and 1930—has been directed towards establishing a very efficient service associated with the County and County Borough Councils; and many Voluntary Societies assist in this organisation. In the present scheme the nurse plays an important part, and her success or failure depends, more than in any other branch of preventive work, upon her enthusiasm, her personality and her experience in social welfare.

Her duties are to assist in the prevention of the spread of the infection, to encourage the patient to take advantage of sanatorium or hospital treatment, and to help during the long period of after-care that is required in these cases.

She needs a wide knowledge of the workings of Insurance Societies, and of the avenues by which assistance can be secured from various charities or public bodies. She must be able to give tactful and helpful advice with regard to improving conditions in the home. One of the functions of the Tuberculosis Care Organisation is to help in making home conditions suitable, for instance, by the loan of beds and bedding so that the patient is not compelled to sleep with another member of the family; and, in some cases, by transferring the family to a larger house. Sometimes, children need to be 'boarded-out' in order to allow a mother to undergo treatment in a sanatorium, and whilst she is away it is often necessary to take steps to ensure that the home is being maintained in a reasonably satisfactory condition, so that when she returns her progress is not retarded by worry or anxiety which might have been avoided.

In the new concept of the fight against tuberculosis it is an essential point that the patient must remain under medical observation for a number of years, and it may be necessary that he, or she, should find a more suitable occupation than that followed before the sanatorium treatment. To help in this way, in addition to tuberculosis dispensaries and treatment centres, small workshops and handicrafts classes are being developed in the sanatoria themselves and also by the Local Authorities and the Voluntary Societies.

One great aim of the campaign against tuberculosis is to educate the general public to a realisation of the fact that a tuberculous patient has the best prospect of recovery from the disease if treatment is begun in the earliest stage. The vital importance of seeking skilled medical advice at the first possible moment, if there is any suspicion that the lungs are affected, will then be appreciated; and with the present increasing facilities for diagnosis and treatment, and for the examination of contacts, it is hoped that the mortality from this insidious scourge may be lessened. In this campaign, not only health visitors but all nurses may take some part.

Conclusion.

Although this review of the Public Health activities of the present age has been confined, almost entirely, to developments in England, all these forms of nursing work have now become embodied in the public hygienic practice of almost every civilised country of the world. The organisation in each country follows the same broad lines, having the same fundamental aims and objects, but it differs in detail in accordance with the constitution of the country, the special needs of its people, and the degree of the development of these services; and since public health nursing has been so organised that services are available to all members of the community, including those who can, and wish, to pay the cost of them, it has grown out of the class of private charity or philanthropic activity.

These health services are now linked up by national and international contacts, through the medium of Congresses, Leagues and Literature, so that all are enabled to advance along the lines developed by the more progressive countries.

CHAPTER X

SOME MODERN DEVELOPMENTS IN NURSING EDUCATION IN EUROPE

Two Hungarian systems of nursing education—The State School of Budapest—Nursing education in Finland—Central preliminary training schools and State schools of nursing—The University School of Nursing in Brussels—The 'Block' System

Two Hungarian Systems of Nursing Education.

As in most Catholic countries, the nursing in Hungary was carried out almost entirely under the auspices of religious Sisterhoods until quite late in the nineteenth century. The first steps towards professional training were taken by the Hungarian Red Cross Society in 1879, and between that date and the beginning of the Great War the foundations of scientific nursing training were successfully laid, courses for Red Cross nursing being organised in ten different cities, and always in connection with large general hospitals. More than 1,300 nurses were trained during this period, and they were in charge of the nursing work in thirty-seven institutions.

During the War the Red Cross continued to train professional nurses, over 8,000 qualifying during the War period. But, as with all other countries, the number of nurses available for service were quite insufficient to meet the demand, and, therefore, on the initiative of the Ministry of War, the Red Cross organised a body of 'voluntary aids', with at least one year of practical experience.

After the War the 'voluntary aids' were dispersed, many Red Cross nurses had to retire on account of age or illness, and seven out of the ten Red Cross training schools were lost under the terms of the Peace Treaty. Moreover, the Hungarian Red Cross was bankrupt and there was no possibility of re-establishing their

393

training of nurses. Between 1918 and 1921 no training school for nurses existed in Hungary; and then, in November, 1921, the University Hospital of Debreczen, acting upon the initiative of the Red Cross, organised a new training school which proved to be a milestone in the history of Hungarian nursing. Here, for the first time, both theoretical and practical training were given in the hospital itself and the superintendent of the hospital also acted as the supervisor of the training school. Later, when the State School of Nursing was established at Budapest, the Debreczen Training School was taken over by the University. Its present teaching programme is considerably more extensive than that of the majority of English hospitals. It includes, in the first year, a total of 275 lectures, and the practical training during this period involves a preliminary course of two months in the demonstration room and diet kitchen, and then three months each in the medical, surgical and pediatric wards. The twelfth month is vacation. During the second year the students are divided into two groups, those who are working for a diploma in bedside nursing, and those who wish to specialise in public health nursing; but both groups attend the same lectures, which total 189. The practical work is much more varied than in the first year, but is different for the two groups. Since September, 1932, the practical work in public health has been arranged in a five-month course that has followed the two years' bedside training.

The State School of Nursing at Budapest.

This school was erected in connection with the State Institute of Hygiene under the auspices of the Ministry of Public Welfare. It is not attached to a hospital but the students obtain their practical experience in the General Hospital of the city, which is staffed by a religious Order assisted by partly trained lay nurses. Some of the Sisters have themselves had training in the State School, and in time all those who are in charge of wards or departments will be graduate nurses.

The School is built on four floors and each floor is divided into two parts, one part being devoted to classrooms, demonstration rooms, dining rooms and common rooms, and the other part to dormitories. It has accommodation for eighty students.

The course of training includes a preliminary period of sixteen weeks, during which 225 lectures are attended and 214 hours of practical work is done. The whole course covers two and a half years. The School has two organised teaching wards, in the medical and surgical services respectively, and each is under the charge of a teaching supervisor of the school who has been accepted by the hospital as a head nurse. The regular hospital nursing staff has been retained. This consists of three nurses to each teaching ward; but their appointment is proposed by the School and they work under the direction of the School authorities. The linen and equipment necessary to make the nursing care and teaching as adequate as possible has been supplied by the School from a special fund. Under these conditions it is possible to teach the students in the wards on exactly the same principles as those used in the demonstration room.

The preliminary course covers sixteen weeks, and the curriculum is as follows:

	Theory	Practice
Anatomy	17 lectures	17 hours
Physiology	20 ,,	15 ,,
Bacteriology	15 ,,	12 ,,
Chemistry	15 ,,	10 ,,
Materia Medica	30 ,,	
Personal Hygiene	10 ,,	
Immunology	15 ,,	
Pathology	13 ,,	
Theory of Nursing	30 ,,	120 ,,
Hospital Administration	6 ,,	
History of Nursing	20 ,,	
Professional Ethics	4 ,,	
Psychology	20 ,,	
Nutrition	10 ,,	40 ,,
Total	225 lectures	214 hours

This involves 28 hours each week. The rest of the time is available for study. During the remainder of the first year three courses of 30 lectures are given—in surgical diseases, medical diseases and pediatrics respectively.

The second year curriculum includes:

Child psychology	10 lectures
Diseases of the eye	10 ,,
Ear, nose, and throat diseases	12 ,,
Obstetrics	10 ,,
Gynæcology	10 ,,
Infectious diseases	20 ,,
Clinical tuberculosis	10 ,,
Venereal disease	10 ,,
Mental diseases	20 ,,
First aid	10 ,,

and during the third year:

Hygiene and Public Health	30 lectures
Preventive hygiene: mother and child welfare, school hygiene, prevention of venereal diseases, tuberculosis, etc.	60 ,,
Social problems and social administration ..	30 ,,
Statistics	10 ,,
Elements of economy	15 ,,
Special problems of the rural field ..	10 ,,
Public Health legislation and administration ..	10 ,,
Eugenics, health propaganda, and technique of organisation	20 ,,
Work of the Public Health nurse	20 ,,

The practical training includes:

Teaching ward in the medical service	16 weeks
Teaching ward in the surgical service	16 ,,
Babies' and children's ward	10 ,,
Obstetrical ward	4 ,,
Nervous and mental ward	2 ,,

396

Eye diseases: ward and out-patients' dept. .. .. 4 weeks
Ear, nose and throat diseases: ward and out-
  patients' department .. .. .. 2 ,,
Public Health nursing theory .. .. .. 22 ,,
Field work:
  Maternity and infant welfare, including nursery
    schools and social service .. .. .. 12 ,,
  Tuberculosis .. .. 4 ,,
  Teaching districts and generalised public health
    programmes .. .. 12 ,,
  Vacations .. .. 10 ,,

The 'field experience' in public health nursing includes, besides the work with specialised organisations, general work in teaching districts where the students are under the direction of specially trained teaching field supervisors. All nurses in training spend a certain amount of time in the public health field because it is considered essential that the bedside nurse should know the type of home from which her ward patients come, and should be able to give them definite and extensive health teaching whilst they are under her care in the hospital.

Nursing Education in Finland.

A new type of development in nursing education has taken place in Finland during the past decade. It has involved the establishment of Central Preliminary Training Schools and State Schools of Nursing under the control of the State Board of Health.

Until the end of the nineteenth century there was very little professional nursing in Finland apart from the work of the Deaconesses, but some of the leaders in nursing affairs were feeling that there was an urgent need for reform both in the standard of work and the conditions under which nursing was done. Therefore, in 1898, they founded the Nurses' Association of Finland with the avowed objects of raising the standard of nursing by scientific training, and improving the working conditions, the

397

education, and the economic and social status of nurses. It established a Nurses' Home for probationers in connection with the General Hospital of Helsingfors, the Red Cross giving a small yearly allowance towards its upkeep until 1904. In that year the late Baroness Mannerheim, who had received her nursing training at St Thomas's Hospital in England, was appointed Superintendent of the Hospital and President of the Nurses' Association of Finland. In 1906 the Association founded a preparatory school for intending probationers of the General Hospital, with Miss Ellen Nylander as its first director—a position she held for fifteen years, during which time many advances took place. These included the raising of the standard of admission to that of high school education, the organising of courses of study, the lengthening of the training period and the shortening of the hours of hospital duty. In 1909 a similar school was established at the City Hospital, Helsingfors (the Maria), and the graduates of these two schools were registered by the State Board of Health as 'older trained nurses', as distinct from the 'younger trained nurses' who had taken courses of training in State hospitals which required only elementary education for admission, and who worked either under fully trained nurses in institutions or independently in rural visiting nursing services.

In 1929, mainly as a result of repeated appeals from the Nurses' Association to the Government, the Diet passed a law on nursing education and reserved a sum of money in the Budget for the initial expense of the necessary reorganisation.

Under the provisions of the law, the supervision of nursing education is now vested in the State Board of Health which appointed a Director of nursing education. All the training schools of Finland are under State control, with the exception of the municipal school of Helsingfors. Each State school has its own Board, and the medical director of the school, the superintendent of nurses of the hospital, and the nurse-director of the preliminary training school associated with it, are *ex officio* members of this Board, the other members being appointed by the State Board of Health for a term of three years. The financial proposals drawn up by each individual school has to pass the State Board of Health, and the Government, before they are voted upon by the Diet; but since the organisation of State Schools of Nursing in 1930 practically all the Budgets of the State Board of Health for nursing education have been supported by the Government and by the Diet. The Budget of the municipal school in Helsingfors is provided by the city funds.

The Central Preliminary Training Schools.

Preparatory to training in any of the State schools of nursing in Finland, a candidate must undergo a four-months' course in one of the central preliminary schools connected with the schools of nursing. The Board of each training school selects its candidates, who then apply for admission to the preliminary school with which the training school is connected. The curriculum of the four-months course is practically the same in all accredited schools and is as follows:

Anatomy and physiology	35 hours
Elementary bacteriology	15 ,,
Elementary chemistry	30 ,,
Elements of pathology	10 ,,
Hygiene	15 ,,
Nutrition and dietetics	80 ,,
Principles and practice of nursing	84 ,,
Care of infants	12 ,,
Bandaging	34 ,,
Elements of massage	20 ,,
Occupational therapy	20 ,,
Psychology	20 ,,
Ethics of nursing	15 ,,
History of nursing	15 ,,
Total	400 hours

In addition, the students have classes in physical education and practical work for not more than 112 hours during the course.

399

The schools which are situated within the grounds of a hospital have initiated practice in the wards of those procedures taught in the practical classroom.

During the four-months' preliminary period the student is required to live in a students' home, and the fee for tuition and board is 1,700 marks in the municipal school and 2,000 in the State schools. Having completed the preparatory course, the student nurse's training is divided into a basic course of 26 months, which is the same for all students, and an additional 6 months of specialisation in some branch of hospital nursing or in public health work, according to the wishes of the student.

Training in the State Schools of Nursing.

The theoretical part of the basic training includes:

	Lectures by doctors	Classes by nurse instructors
Medical nursing	15 hours	12 hours
Materia medica	10 ,,	8 ,,
Surgical nursing and theatre technique	15 ,,	12 ,,
Obstetrical and gynæcological nursing	11 ,,	8 ,,
Ophthalmological nursing	5 ,,	3 ,,
Nursing in diseases of the ear, nose and throat	5 ,,	3 ,,
Pediatric nursing	13 ,,	10 ,,
Nursing of communicable diseases ..	5 ,,	4 ,,
Nursing of venereal and skin diseases	4 ,,	3 ,,
Tuberculosis nursing	5 ,,	4 ,,
Psychiatric nursing	12 ,,	10 ,,
First aid	5 ,,	3 ,,
Public health nursing	5 ,,	5 ,,
Survey of the nursing field	—	5 ,,
Total	110 hours	90 hours

The practical experience in the basic course includes work in the following fields of nursing:

Medicine	4 months
Surgery (including 2 months in the operating room)	6 ,,
Gynæcology	2 ,,
Ear, nose and throat diseases	1 ,,
Eye diseases	1 ,,
Pediatrics	3 ,,
Psychiatry	2 ,,
Tuberculosis, venereal and skin diseases, epidemic diseases, obstetrics, and Public Health nursing —1 month of each	5 ,,
Total	24 months

The student works not only in the wards on the various services but also in the out-patients' departments or health centres. Many of the schools of nursing in the more sparsely populated districts are unable to give their students the experience desired in each department. In some instances the students are in residence for one year only, and then go to different towns for experience in the various services. The distances are often rather great, but free transportation on railways is provided for the students. During the last six months of training those who elect to specialise in hospital work go to the particular department they desire, such as the surgical, medical or mental wards, the theatre, the X-ray department or the laboratories. They may also specialise in midwifery.

The students who wish to take the course in public health nursing are transferred to the School of Public Health Nursing in Helsingfors, where a total of 165 lectures is given in the following subjects:

Physiology	8 lectures
Personal hygiene and Public Health	36 ,,
Child welfare and pre-natal work	18 ,,
Tuberculosis	16 ,,

Venereal diseases	..	..	..	..	6 lectures
Care of crippled children	..	..	..	2	,,
Eugenics	..	..	..	..	2 ,,
Mental hygiene	..	..	..	..	4 ,,
Nutrition	..	..	..	..	5 ,,
Public Health nursing	..	..	..	22	,,
Social administration	..	..	..	10	,,
Industrial welfare	..	..	..	..	4 ,,
Poor Law administration	..	..	..	4	,,
Psychology	..	..	..	..	20 ,,
Child psychology	..	..	..	..	6 ,,
Book-keeping	..	..	..	..	2 ,,

The theory is concentrated in lectures given on two days a week, the practical work occupying the other four. Field work is provided by various municipalities and private organisations, and includes:

Care of the infant and pre-school child	..	1 month
Child welfare, including pre-natal work	..	1 ,,
School nursing	.. ..	..	2 weeks
Preventive tuberculosis work	.. ..	..	2 ,,
Generalised Public Health nursing in rural areas	.. ..	..	$1\frac{1}{2}$ months
Home nursing or district nursing	..	..	2 weeks

The last month is devoted exclusively to study and examinations.

Throughout the training course the students live in Nurses' Homes. No fees are charged, and board, lodging and laundry are provided. In addition, the students in the State schools receive 50 marks a month during the last twenty months of the three-years' course. In the municipal school at Helsingfors the allowance is 35 marks a month during the second year and 350 marks a month during the third year.

The University School of Nursing in Brussels.

The inauguration of yet another new system of nursing education has occurred in Brussels, with the opening of the University School of Nursing in connection with the St Pierre Hospital in 1936.

This hospital has a very long history. It was first founded as a leper hospital in the twelfth century, and was organised into a general hospital under the Emperor Joseph in the eighteenth century. By a decree of Napoleon, dated 2nd July, 1806, it was recognised as a centre for the teaching of medicine and surgery, and it became a School of Medicine in connection with the University of Brussels in 1823. It underwent reconstruction in 1849 and again in 1878; but it was completely modernised in 1923. It is now a city hospital of 700 beds, with a separate block for patients suffering from infectious diseases, and very well organised out-patient departments and emergency services. In its grounds has been built the School of Nursing dedicated to the memory of the two famous War heroines of Belgium—Edith Cavell and Marie Depage.

The school was equipped and endowed by a grant of 262,000 dollars from the Rockefeller Foundation, and it has accommodation for 200 student nurses. Its official designation is 'École Universitaire D'Infirmières—Fondation Edith Cavell—Marie Depage'. It is controlled from the University, and Mlle Mechelynck, the Directrice, holds her appointment from the University; but she is also the Matron of the hospital. Under her, in the School, are two assistant directrices appointed by the University, as are all the lecturers in special subjects.

The full course in the school is three years, including the preliminary period. If desired a post-graduate course can be taken during the fourth year for the Health Visitors' Certificate.

Each year is arranged into four terms; but all the lectures are concentrated in the first and second terms; the third is devoted to study and revision combined with practical work; a month's holiday is taken during the fourth term, and the student completes her preparation for, and takes, her examinations.

The preliminary course commences always in September, and it includes:

Anatomy and Physiology .. .. 24 lectures
Bacteriology .. .. 12 ,,
General hygiene .. .. 24 ,,
Hospital hygiene .. .. 12 ,,
Hygiene of the nurse .. .. 12 ,,
Ethical standards and their application .. .. 12 ,,
History of nursing .. .. 12 ,,
Domestic economy—Theory .. .. .. 24 ,,
  ,, ,, —Practical work .. .. 88 hours
Practical demonstrations in nursing technique .. 48 ,,
Practical nursing work by the students .. .. 144 ,,
Study and revision .. .. 180 ,,

An examination is held in both theory and practical work at the conclusion of this term, and successful candidates then proceed to the second term's work, during which the following are given:

Anatomy and physiology .. .. 8 lectures
General biology and cytology .. .. .. 20 ,,
Pharmacology .. .. 12 ,,
Preventive medicine .. .. 20 ,,
Practical demonstrations in nursing technique .. 24 hours
Criticism and correction of students' work .. 24 ,,
Study and revision .. .. 72 ,,
Practical work in the wards, each week .. .. 30 ,,

During the third term no lectures are given, nine hours each week are devoted to study and revision, with correction and criticism of the work done by the students, and each student works for 39 hours in the wards and departments of the hospital, making the usual total of 48 working hours a week.

In the fourth term each student has one month's holiday; during the rest of the time she works for 44 hours in the wards and spends 4 hours each week in classroom work preparatory to the examinations. During the second year the general arrangement of theoretical and practical work is the same, but the ward work is much more specialised; and more advanced and specialised subjects are included in the lectures. In the first six weeks 72 lectures are given, and the student works for 38 hours in the wards each week. For the rest of the term she works in the wards for 44 hours and spends 4 hours in the school each week. The heaviest lecture syllabus is arranged for the second term, commencing 1st January. This includes:

Obstetrics	16 lectures
Pathology of infectious diseases	16 ,,
Diseases of the ear, nose and throat	3 ,,
Ophthalmology	3 ,,
Diseases of the skin	3 ,,
Massage	8 ,,
Child care	16 ,,
Preventive medicine	16 ,,
Orthopædics	8 ,,
Criticism and correction of work	50 hours

Practical work in the wards and departments occupies only 28 hours a week during the two months in which these lectures are given; but 44 hours a week during the remaining month.

The arrangements of the third and fourth terms are the same in each year of the training.

The third-year lectures include:

Hospital administration	8 lectures
Surgery and theatre technique	12 ,,
Mental hygiene	10 ,,
Preventive medicine	10 ,,
Professional problems	12 ,,
Dietetics, theory—10, practical—16 ..	26 hours

These are given during the first term. For the rest of the year the student concentrates upon practical work and the preparation for her final examination. No student nurses are engaged in night duty during the first year, nor whilst they are attending the courses of lectures.

405

Post-graduate Course for Health Visitors.

During the first two weeks the student attends a preparatory course which includes:

Social conditions	6 lectures
Ethics, history and work of the visiting nurse	10 ,,
Demonstrations of work in the home ..	10 lessons
Demonstrations of first aid in street accidents	3 ,,

In the Public Health course, as with the general training, all the lectures are given in the first and second terms. They include, in a comprehensive curriculum, all the special subjects required. The examinations are held in September.

Concluding Note—The 'Block' System.

The developments in Hungary, Finland and Belgium typify the trend of modern nursing education; each has contributed something new in the history of European nursing, and for that reason they are selected as examples. Many other countries have made great strides in recent years; but for the most part they have progressed along paths already indicated by former developments.

The modern tendency in nursing training is to regard the undergraduate nurse as a scientific student whose education and instruction must not be allowed to conflict with the practical nursing work in the wards. It is recognised that each may so encroach upon the other that neither is truly efficient, and in order to allow for concentration upon practical nursing duties without the distraction of attendance at lectures and classes the 'block' system has been introduced. This has been tried with success in Warsaw and in some Scandinavian hospitals, and also—as has already been shown—in a modified form at the University School of Nursing in Brussels. It has recently been adopted at University College Hospital, London. At various stages in their training the probationers return to the 'school' for a few weeks, during which they devote their whole time to lectures, classes and private study. It is felt that this alternation between periods of theoretical instruction and periods of physical activity will preserve a fresh and vigorous mental outlook and will prevent fatigue in the student nurse, and it will also obviate the constant depletion of staff in the wards for the purpose of attendance at lectures.

CHAPTER XI

POST-GRADUATE EDUCATION OF NURSES IN ENGLAND

The Founding of the Royal College of Nursing.

THE Great War which started in 1914 raised problems which had not hitherto faced the nursing profession. The care of the wounded called for a very high standard of knowledge and nursing skill. The civil hospitals were endeavouring to carry on their work with very depleted staffs. Overworked nurses were breaking down in health both at home and abroad, and this in itself threatened to constitute a very serious problem after the ending of the War. It was obvious that some kind of central organisation was needed, and its establishment could not wait until peace should be declared.

Early in 1916, some of the leaders of the nursing profession, under the guidance of Dame Sarah Swift and Sir Arthur Stanley (the Matron-in-Chief and the Chairman of the British Red Cross Society), together with Sir Cooper Perry, the Medical Superintendent of Guy's Hospital, met at the Royal Automobile Club to discuss the possibilities of forming an organisation which should be self-governing and which should assist and direct nurses in all stages of their professional life. They drafted the Constitution of the College of Nursing on simple and democratic lines, and it was registered, in March, 1916, under the Companies Act of 1908–1913, as a company limited by guarantee and not having a share capital. The late Miss Mary S. Rundle was appointed its Secretary and its headquarters were one small room in Vere Street, furnished as an office, and lent by the late Sir James Boyton. A wide appeal for membership was launched,

407

which met with an overwhelming response from nurses both at home and abroad, and thousands of applications poured into that little room.

The first object of the College was to set a definite uniform standard for membership; and also of nursing training, to be adopted by English hospitals, for this was before the advent of State Registration.

By 1919 the work had so developed that it was impossible to carry on without larger premises. The financial position of the College was now much more stable, and so No. 7, Henrietta Street was rented and the College occupied the whole house.

The Great War had now ended, and the British Women's Hospital Committee, of which the late Viscountess Cowdray was the Honorary Treasurer, felt that it would like to do something for nurses whose health had broken down under the strain of the War, and also to assist the College. This Committee therefore inaugurated 'The Nation's Fund for Nurses', which is now administered from offices in the new College building. The objects of this fund were two-fold, to assist nurses broken in the War, or in distress through no fault of their own, and to help to endow the College. The former was the more urgent of these objects, and so, naturally, it received the primary consideration. The endowment was accomplished later, mainly by the activities of the members themselves.

The next great development came in 1922, when the College became established in its permanent home at 1a, Henrietta Street, which had been most generously built and furnished by the late Lord and Lady Cowdray. On 31st May, 1926, Her Majesty, Queen Mary, the Royal Patron of the College, opened the new headquarters; and in 1928 the College was incorporated by Royal Charter, and thus ceased to be a limited liability company. In 1939, authority was granted for the use of the prefix 'Royal'.

It is now 26 years since the inauguration of the Royal College of Nursing. Its headquarters stand in the heart of the West End of London, at the foot of Harley Street and Wimpole Street, and next door to the Royal Society of Medicine. The quiet dignity of the grey stone building, the entrance hall, staircases, Council and Committee Rooms and Lecture Hall, is in keeping with the standard it has always striven to maintain; the department devoted to educational work, with its library, classrooms, demonstration rooms and laboratories, exemplify its purposeful efficiency, and its social activities find an excellent setting, both in the College premises and in the adjoining Cowdray Club. It has 106 branches in the British Isles, and also many clubs and social centres throughout the country.

Among its principal achievements are improvements in the conditions under which nurses work, the drawing up of a minimum scale of salaries—which has been adopted in the majority of hospitals in this country—the initiation of a Federated Superannuation Scheme for Nurses and Hospital Officers (contributory), which gives provision for later years, and the safeguarding of the public against unskilled nursing by assisting to promote the State Registration of Nurses Act, 1919, the Nursing Homes Registration Act, 1927, and the Nurses' Act, 1943.

The College is recognised by the Ministry of Health as a training centre for Health Visitors, it co-operates with the Midwives Institute by giving courses of instruction in preparation for the Midwife-Teachers' Certificate of the Central Midwives Board, and it arranges courses of study in preparation for the Diploma of Nursing of the University of London. It has co-operated with the University in the establishment of post-graduate courses for International students at Bedford College for Women although these are in abeyance during the present war. It established a course for Sister Tutors at King's College of Household and Social Science and, in 1940, it initiated a similar course at the College headquarters under the designation of Nurse-teachers' Course. Special courses of lectures and visits are arranged for industrial nurses and for those in charge of war nurseries. An eighteen months' course in dietetics was introduced in 1942. In addition, it has furthered post-graduate education both in London and the provinces by its branches, where throughout the year special courses of lectures are arranged and 'Study Weeks' are held. Its departments include a Public Health Section, a Sister Tutor Section, a Private Nurses' Section, a Ward Sisters' Section and a Student Nurses' Association.

In connection with the College a number of scholarships and bursaries are awarded for special study in this or other countries. It has for many years been interested in, and encouraged, international developments, arranging special tours to other countries and giving facilities for nurses from abroad to see some of the nursing work that is done in this country. By its affiliation with the National Council of Nurses of Great Britain, which took place in 1927, it is linked with the International Council of Nurses.

One of its most cherished aims for the future is the endowment of a Chair of Nursing at a University, and the nucleus of a Fund for this purpose has already been formed.

The official organ of the Royal College of Nursing is *The Nursing Times*, which is published each week.

The Sister Tutors' Certificate.

When the syllabus of the General Nursing Council was accepted as the standard of training for student nurses it became imperative that some qualified nurses should specialise as teachers in preliminary training schools and as tutors in hospitals; and thus a new field of professional activity was opened up, and a new qualification came into being—the Sister Tutors', or Nurse-Teachers', Certificates.

Several educational bodies have arranged courses of instruction and examinations for this qualification. The first of these was initiated by the Royal College of Nursing and held at King's College of Household and Social Science (University of London) in the Session 1919-1920, and it opened with 14 students. Since then the number of students has remained fairly constant, fluctuating between 8 and 20 each session.

The Course consists of an academic year of three terms. The curriculum includes all the scientific subjects which the Sister Tutor is required to teach, and, in addition, a course of 20 lectures on Institutional Administration, 12 lectures on the Principles of Education and Methods of Teaching and 25 lectures on Business Affairs. Students who are preparing for Part A of the examination for the Diploma in Nursing of the University of London can attend a course of 15 lectures in General Psychology.

Another course is arranged by the Battersea Polytechnic. It can be taken either as a full-time course of three terms from September to June or as a more intensive course which covers a period of six months, commencing in January.

For nurses who are engaged in other work during the day a part-time evening course was arranged, extending over a period of two years and involving attendance at lectures on two evenings a week. The course has now been spread over three years. The Battersea course also covers the syllabus for Part A of the examination for the Diploma in Nursing of the University of London.

The Nurse-Teachers' Course which opened at the Royal College of Nursing, in 1940, is intended for trained nurses who wish to qualify as teachers of nursing and allied subjects. It is a whole-time course extending over the academic year and the students spend a fortnight during both the Christmas and the Easter vacation in observation work in schools of nursing.

The syllabus includes lectures, and practical work where required, in the following subjects:

Anatomy	..	..	..	..	..	24 hours
Physiology	..	..	..	..	..	70 ,,
Bacteriology	..	..	..	..	..	24 ,,
Hygiene and Public Health		..	..	..	17 ,,

Physics and Chemistry in relation to the Theory and Practice of Nursing	60 hours.
Psychology	20 ,,
Biology	24 ,,
History of Nursing	12 ,,
Infant and Child Hygiene	10 ,,
Nutrition	8 ,,
Communicable Diseases	6 ,,
Educational Psychology and Methods of Teaching	15 ,,
Teaching in Schools of Nursing	7 ,,
Training School Administration	10 ,,

In addition, visits are arranged in connection with the Public Health lectures, each student gives two practice classes or lectures in connection with Methods of Teaching, and tutorials are given in all subjects. A number of scholarships are awarded each year for this course and some of these cover fees, books and maintenance. 31 students are enrolled for the 1943-1944 session. Like other courses, it covers the syllabus for Part A of the examination for the Diploma of Nursing of the University of London.

University Affiliation in England: The University of Leeds.

The University of Leeds was the first to initiate a Diploma of Nursing in this country. Its medical school is the General Infirmary at Leeds, and lectures given in this hospital are deemed, for the purpose of qualifying as a candidate for examination, to have been delivered in the University itself.

Before presenting herself for examination for this Diploma a candidate must have completed four years' training in a general hospital recognised by the University for this purpose, or must have completed three years' training in an approved general hospital and, after having obtained her State Registration certificate, have gained two years' experience of a character approved by the University. She must furnish certificates of attendance at prescribed lectures, including a course on Social Economics or other approved subject, and at least three months must be spent in attendance on courses in the University of Leeds, or the Hospital.

The examination is held twice a year; it is arranged in two parts, and includes written papers, practical work, and *viva voce* examinations. The first awards of the Diploma of Nursing of the University of Leeds were made in 1921.

The University of London.

The question of introducing a Diploma in Nursing, and the conditions under which it should be awarded, had been under consideration by the Senate of the University of London for some time, and an Advisory Committee consisting of persons with a special knowledge of the subjects involved had been appointed to enquire into the matter and make a considered report. Draft regulations and syllabuses were sent to the principal hospitals and training schools of this country for their observations and comments; and then the Senate, at their meeting in July, 1926, resolved that a Diploma in Nursing be instituted by the University, and that the Regulations and Syllabuses be adopted; the latter being designed to be covered by a course of one year of serious study after the qualification of State Registration had been obtained. The Diploma is thus of post-graduate type, and the examination may not be taken until the candidate has had a further two years of experience after the completion of her general training; this experience being of a type to comply with the regulations of the University governing the award of the Diploma in Nursing. The examination is arranged in two parts. Part A includes the 'Scientific Basis and General Principles of Nursing, including Elementary Psychology', and all candidates must pass in this before proceeding to Part B, which includes 'History of Nursing and Nursing Ethics' and one of the following: (1) General Nursing, (2) Obstetrics and Gynæcological

Nursing, (3) Nursing of Children, (4) Mental Nursing, including Psychology (more advanced), (5) Fever Nursing and Epidemiology, (6) Elementary Economics, Sociology and Hygiene, in relation to the duties of Public Health Nurses, (7) Hospital Administration.

The syllabuses of subjects for examination for the Diploma in Nursing of the University of London are wider and more comprehensive than for any other post-graduate qualification in nursing in this country. The examinations are held once a year, for Part A in October and for Part B in November. They were first held in the autumn of 1927.

414

CONCLUSION

ALTHOUGH the seeds of the modern profession of nursing were undoubtedly sown in the remote past, its full growth has been shown only during the last century. Its roots have now penetrated into every part of the earth, and by national and international association the whole profession shares in every movement or development that occurs in any of its branches.

In its modern guise, nursing offers a very wide sphere of useful and interesting activity to the women of our land, and of every other civilised country in the world. It is no longer the expression of a mystic art possessed only by the favoured of the gods—or demons. Nor is it a work of self-abnegation or religious fervour undertaken as a penance, or for spiritual solace and uplift; nor even is it, entirely, a selfless answer to the call of human suffering. Much less is it a shunned and rather repulsive activity of the ignorant woman to whom no other calling is open. And yet, in its long history, it has been all of these things. But Florence Nightingale made of it a dignified secular profession for which a thorough and arduous training is necessary.

Since the days of her activity it has been granted a legalised status. It demands of its members a good general education followed by a specialised course of study, and experience in practical work, in addition to suitability of character and personality.

It provides a means of earning a salary which will give a woman independence and a reasonable degree of comfort, and ensures, through its various contributory schemes, that when her working days are over she shall receive an annuity which will, at least, protect her from want in her old age.

It has not, however, even yet found a solution for all the

415

problems attendant upon the safeguarding of health and the adequate care of the sick, nor even of the training of the student nurse; for each era brings its own difficulties which must be faced and solved by the leaders of the profession in that age.

But something of the art, and much of the vocation, must still remain, to illumine with its mystic light some inevitable tasks which would otherwise be wearisome and unlovely, perhaps even sordid, and to irradiate the paths which lead into the unknown future.

416

BIBLIOGRAPHY

PART I

Jacques de Morgan. *Prehistoric Man.* Routledge, 1924.

J. G. Frazer. *The Golden Bough.* Macmillan, 1906-30.

Gustave Glotz. *The Aegean Civilisation.* Routledge, 1925.

L. Delaporte. *Mesopotamia.* Routledge, 1925.

A. Lods. *Israel & Judaism.* Routledge, 1932.

S. Bhagavat. *A Short History of Aryan Medicine and Science.* Macmillan, 1896.

Susruta Ayur-Vedas. Translated by K. L. Bhishnagratna. Calcutta, 1907.

Charaka-Samhita. Translated by K. A. C. Kaviratna. Calcutta, 1904-16.

Susruta-Samhita. Translated by K. K. Bhishnagratna. Calcutta, 1907.

D. Muthu. *Antiquity of Hindu Medicine.* Bailliére, Tindall & Cox, 3rd ed., 1930.

Edward Upham. *The Sacred Books of Ceylon.* Parbury & Allen, 1833.

K. C. Wong & Wu-Lien-Teh. *History of Chinese Medicine.* The Tientsen Press, China, 1932.

G. Eliot Smith. *The Ancient Egyptians and the Origins of Civilisation.* Harper.

A. Moret. *The Nile and Egyptian Civilisation.* Routledge, 1927.

F. H. Brooksbank. *Legends of Ancient Egypt.* Harrap, 1923.

A. Jardé. *The Formation of the Greek People.* Routledge, 1926.

L. Robin. *Greek Thought and the Scientific Spirit.* Routledge.

Sir Clifford Allbutt. *Greek Medicine in Rome.* Macmillan, 1921.

Charles Singer. *Greek Biology and Greek Medicine.* Oxford University Press.

Hippocrates. Selected works translated into English by W. H. S. Jones & E. T. Withington (4 vols.). Loeb Classical Library.

Genuine Works of Hippocrates. Translated by Francis Adams. 1849.

PART II

Cardinal Gasquet. *English Monastic Life.* Methuen, 1924.

J. C. Hannah. *Christian Monasticism.* Allen & Unwin, 1924.

J. M. Ludlow. *Woman's Work in the Church.* Strahan, 1865.

Lina Eckenstein. *Woman Under Monasticism.* Cambridge University Press, 1896.

A. Chevalier. *L'Hôtel Dieu de Paris et les Sœurs Augustines.* Champion, Paris, 1911.

P. Helyot. *Les Orders Monastiques.* (8 vols.). Paris, 1714, reprinted 1838.

Montalembert. *Life of St. Elisabeth of Hungary.* Translated into English by F. D. Hoyt. Longmans, Green, 1904.

D. Campbell. *Arabian Medicine.* 1906.

H. W. Fincham & W. R. Edwards. *The Order of the Hospital of St. John of Jerusalem.* Collingridge, 1915.

E. W. Schermerhorn. *Malta of the Knights.* Heinemann, 1929.

E. J. King. *Knights of St. John in the British Empire.* St. John's Gate, 1924.

Johannes Jörgensen. *Life of St. Francis of Assisi.* Longmans, Green, 1912.

C. Creighton. *History of Epidemics in Britain, from 664 to the extinction of the Plague.* Camb. Univ. Press, 1914.

R. Crawfurd. *Plague and Pestilence in Literature and Art.* Oxford University Press.

Eileen Power. *Mediaeval English Nunneries.* Methuen, 1922.

R. M. Clay. *Mediaeval Hospitals of England.* Methuen, 1909.

F. G. Parsons. *History of St. Thomas's Hospital.* Methuen, 1932-6.

G. O'Donoghue. *The Story of Bethlehem Hospital.* Fisher Unwin, 1914.

E. K. Sanders. *Vincent de Paul, Priest and Philanthropist.* Heath, Cranton & Ouseley, 1913.

Sister M. J. Gately. *The Sisters of Mercy.* Macmillan, 1931.

A. M. Lovat. *Life of the Venerable Louise de Marillac.* Simpson, 1916.

M. Goodman. *Experiences of an English Sister of Mercy.* Smith, Elder, 1862.

A. Jameson. *Sisters of Charity, Catholic and Protestant.* Longmans, 1855.

Memoirs of the Life of Elizabeth Fry, edited by two of her daughters—K. Fry and R. E. Cresswell. Charles Gilpin, 1847.

S. Corder. *Life of Elizabeth Fry.* Cash, 1853.

C. F. Montague. *Sixty Years of Waifdom.* Lippincott, 1928.

F. Tiffany. *Life of Dorothea Lynde Dix.* Houghton Mifflin, Boston, 1891.

418

PART III

Life of Pastor Fliedner. Translated from the German by C. Winkworth. London, 1867.

M. R. S. Andrews. *A Lost Commander*. Doubleday, New York, 1929.

Sir Edward Cook. *Life of Florence Nightingale*. Macmillan, 1913.

T. B. O'Malley. *Florence Nightingale, 1820-1856*. Thornton, Butterworth, 1931.

J. C. Willis. *Florence Nightingale*. Unwin, 1931.

Agnes Jones, Memorial by her Sister. Strahan, 1871.

E. F. Rathbone. *William Rathbone*, a Memoir. Macmillan, 1905.

W. Rathbone. *The History and Progress of District Nursing*. Macmillan, 1890.

J. Conolly. *The Construction and Government of Lunatic Asylums*. Gilpin. 1847.

D. H. Tuke. *The Insane in U.S.A. and Canada*. Kegan Paul, 1885.

C. W. M. Jacobi, *On the Construction and Management of Hospitals for the Insane*. Translated into English by J. Kitching, London, 1891,

R. G. Hill. *Lunacy, its Past and Present*. Longmans, Green, 1857.

J. H. Dunant. *Un Souvenir de Solférino*. Translated into English by Mrs. D. M. Wright as *The Origin of the Red Cross*, 1918.

Col. Sir James Magill. *The Red Cross, its Idea and its Development*. Cassell, 1926.

M. T. Boardman. *Under the Red Cross Flag at Home and Abroad*. Lippincott, 1915.

P. M. Ashburn. *A History of the Medical Department of the U.S.A. Army*. New York, 1929.

W. E. Barton. *Life of Clara Barton*. Houghton Mifflin, Boston, 1922.

L. P. Brockett & M. C. Vaughan. *Women's Work in the Civil War*. Philadelphia, 1867.

Various Authors. *History of American Red Cross Nursing*. New York, 1922.

Annie M. Brainard. *Evolution of Public Health Nursing*. W. B. Saunders, 1922.

G. F. McCleary. *The Maternity and Child Welfare Movement*. P. S. King, 1925.

G. F. McCleary. *The Early History of the Infant Welfare Movement*. Lewis, 1923.

J. E. Lane Claypon. *The Child Welfare Movement*. Ball, 1920.

M. S. Gardner. *Public Health Nursing*. Macmillan, 1924.

M. E. Chayer. *School Nursing*. Putnam, 1931.

Harley Williams. *A Century of Public Health in Britain*. A. & C. Black, 1932.

On the State of the Public Health. Annual Report of the Chief Medical Officer.

Nursing Education and Schools of Nursing. The Rockefeller Foundation, 1932.

GENERAL

HISTORY OF MEDICINE

F. H. Garrison. *Introduction to the History of Medicine*. Saunders, 1929.

Dr. Charles Singer. *A Short History of Medicine*. Clarendon Press, 1928.

S. G. B. Stubbs & E. W. Bligh. *Sixty Centuries of Health and Physick*. Sampson Low, 1931.

J. J. Walsh. *Mediaeval Medicine*. A. & C. Black, 1920.

D. McKenzie. *The Infancy of Medicine*. Macmillan, 1927.

W. R. Dawson. *Magician and Leech*. Methuen, 1929.

R. Crawfurd. *Pestilence and Plague in Literature and Art*. Oxford University Press, 1914.

Cambridge Mediaeval History. *Cambridge Medical History*. Cambridge University Press, 1911.

HISTORY OF NURSING

N. & D. Nutting & L. L. Dock. *A History of Nursing*. Putnam, New York, 3rd edn., 1931.

L. L. Dock & I. M. Stewart. *A Short History of Nursing*. Putnam, New York, 3rd ed., 1932.

Sarah Tooley. *A History of Nursing in the British Empire*. Bousfield, 1906.

L. R. Seymer. *A General History of Nursing*. Faber & Faber, 1932.

J. J. Walsh. *Those Splendid Sisters*. J. H. Sears, New York, 1927.

H. McLean. *Nursing in New Zealand*. Tolan Printing Co., New Zealand, 1932.

V. McCormick. *Historical Sketch of the American Nurses' Association*. Published by American Nurses' Association, 1929.

H. W. Munson. *The Story of the National League of Nursing Education*. Saunders, Philadelphia, 1924.

M. Breay & E. G. Fenwick. *History of the International Council of Nurses*. Published by the I.C.N., 1921.

INDEX

421

422